The HEALTHY HEART Program

Cardiac transplant patient, Brian Price (centre), accompanied by Dr. Terry Kavanagh (left) and Robin Campbell (right), finishing the 1985 Boston Marathon. Another world's first! (see page 203)

The HEALTHY HEART Program

Terence Kavanagh, M.D.

 Rodale Press, Emmaus, Pennsylvania

For my mother
and
for Jo and "the guys"
who made it happen

This edition published by arrangement with Key Porter Books Limited

Copyright © 1985 by Key Porter Books Limited

Library of Congress Cataloging-in-Publication Data

Kavanagh, Terence.
    The healthy heart program.

    Rev. ed. of: Heart attack? counterattack. c1976.
    Includes index.
    1. Cardiacs—Rehabilitation.   2. Exercise therapy.
I. Kavanagh, Terence. Heart attack? counterattack.
II. Title. [DNLM: 1. Exertion—popular works.
2. Heart Diseases—prevention & control—popular
works. WG 113 K21ha]
RC684.E9K38   1985   616.1'206   86-3238
ISBN 0-87857-632-0   paperback

Editorial consultant: Diane Mew
Graphs by Julian Cleva
Printed in the United States of America on recycled paper containing a high percentage of de-inked fiber.
First Rodale edition July 1986

2 4 6 8 10 9 7 5 3 1   paperback

Photograph Credits

The Publisher is grateful for the assistance of those who have provided the photographs used in this book. Every care has been taken to acknowledge below the correct sources. The Publisher would welcome information that will permit the correction of any errors or omissions.

Page ii: Mary Ellen Carlyle
Page 4: David Lee
Page 100: Steven Behal
Page 195: Robin Campbell, Toronto Rehabilitation Centre
Page 201: Dr. A. W. Chisholm and Dr. S. J. Witchell, Department of Cardiovascular Services, Sunnybrook Medical Centre
Page 218: Greg Merhar, American Running and Fitness Association
ALL OTHER PHOTOGRAPHS PROVIDED BY THE AUTHOR

Contents

Preface

This book describes the approach used in the Toronto Rehabilitation Centre's Cardiac Exercise Program. This program was instituted in 1968, with a view to improving the physical and mental well-being of sufferers from coronary heart disease, particularly survivors of a heart attack. Over the ensuing years, the program has grown until today it is probably one of the largest of its type in the world, with an ongoing caseload at any given time of about one thousand patients.

The book is aimed not only at those attending the Toronto program, but also those individuals who have heart disease living in an area where a formal physician-supervised exercise rehabilitation program is not available. Intelligent use of the information and training tables contained here should make it possible to set up a personal rehabilitation regime that is both safe and effective.

It has always been my contention that patients should be taught as much as possible about their disease. Admittedly, this is not always easy. Medicine is a complex and fast-changing subject, requiring the undivided attention of even the most erudite specialist if he or she is not to fall behind. And yet it seems to me totally unrealistic to expect a patient to cooperate with a treatment strategy, particularly one involving lifestyle changes such as stopping smoking or exercising regularly, without explaining the rationale behind your approach. Frank discussion of disease does not, as some think, create neuroses. Only ignorance and fear can do that.

I have therefore included as much elementary physiology as is needed to explain the changes which occur with physical fitness, and enough medicine to help the layman understand the nature of heart disease. The approach is essentially pragmatic, and the goal quite clear-cut — to reduce the risk of heart attack by encouraging the development of a healthy, active lifestyle. To that extent, I am sure that, given the extremely high prevalence of heart disease in our society, this book can be of value to all those apparently healthy males who are at or are fast approaching middle age, one out of three of whom will die from a heart attack.

This is as good a time as any to record my indebtedness to all who have played such an important part in this book and in the program upon which it is based.

Johanna Kennedy, R.N. and Professor Robin Campbell, both of whom started the program with me back in 1968, have contributed so much in enthusiasm, loyalty, clinical and administrative skills over the years that it would be truly impossible to over-estimate their worth. They, together with their hand-picked staff (which grew from three part-timers in 1968 to fifty full- and part-time therapists, nurses, exercise physiologists, technicians and physicians by 1980) are without doubt the reason for the Toronto program's phenomenal success.

No one person, and no group, operates in a vacuum. The Toronto Rehabilitation Centre is a public hospital. To its Board of Directors, and in particular its late President, John Farmery, who died this year, goes the credit for encouraging me, as Medical Director, and my staff in our efforts to institute an exercise program for heart patients.

It is, I know, customary from time to time for health workers to rail against government-controlled medicine. Be that as it may, we at the Centre are entirely funded by the Ontario Ministry of Health, and I would not have it any other way. Need I say more?

There are two essential ingredients to any successful medical rehabilitation program: the patients, and the physicians who refer them. I always look upon any referral as both a compliment and an act of faith. My heartfelt thanks for both.

There is one other group to which I feel a deep sense of obligation. Over the years, our patients' spouses and families have been our most ardent supporters. As is inevitable in any long-term follow-up program for heart attack patients such as ours, we must experience the reality of fatal recurrence, sometimes in those we have known for many years. In these circumstances, the relatives have gone out of their way to thank the program for helping to ensure that those final years were savoured with zeal and enthusiasm. If nothing else, it is that attitude which makes our task one of the most satisfying in all of medicine.

Working physicians probably should never undertake the task of writing a book. We really don't have the time. Delays are unavoidable, deadlines are broken, and frustration abounds. Manuscript typists and editors have to have the patience of Job— and really enjoy their work! Anna Ceci, who cheerfully typed the whole thing, and Diane Mew, who edited with great tact and supreme skill — all at odd hours, when they should have been relaxing and going about their own business — deserve medals. Will they accept instead my respect and gratitude?

In the long run, to coin a phrase, I accept full responsibility for errors of omission and commission, medical and otherwise.

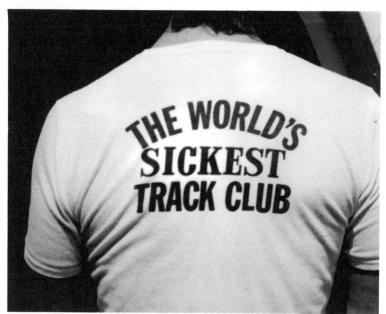

The T.R.C. Joggers logo.

Prologue

On April 15, 1973, a group of seven men, ages ranging from 30 to 56, made rehabilitation medicine history. They had all suffered one, two or three heart attacks, and on that date in 1973 they successfully took part in the seventy-seventh running of the Boston Marathon. As far as I know, they were the first such patients to attempt this feat. The purpose? To demonstrate the effectiveness of an exercise program for heart attack survivors which had been instituted by the author five years previously. They, as it were, "put the show on the road," a feat which not only gained world-wide publicity, but also went a long way towards justifying a program which was ultimately to become the largest of its type in the world. I feel, then, that this story is important enough to be told as a prologue to the pages which follow.

THE T.R.C. JOGGERS

The kernel of the Toronto Rehabilitation Centre's post-coronary program is exercise, the major activity being long distance jogging (that is, slow, relaxed running). In my experience, this is the best way to attain endurance fitness, which is the only form of fitness of benefit to the heart. But, as you will learn later, endurance fitness cannot be stored. This means, for our cardiacs, staying on a jogging program for the rest of their lives — which we anticipate will be lengthy.

Man is by nature gregarious, and long distance running is a lonely sport. Running in groups helps to alleviate the boredom and tends to prevent back-sliding from the regular training routine. Thus it was that our most enthusiastic post-coronary joggers began to meet regularly on weekends for long, easy runs through the pleasant park system which surrounds the Centre. Our first five-mile jog was a great achievement, only to recede into mediocrity as we managed seven miles, and then ten. As we ran, we discussed the pros and cons of different routes through the park, the advantages and disadvantages of various brands of running shoes, the physiology of "continuous" as opposed to "interval" training, and so on. Heart disease was forgotten, and gradually over the weeks my title changed from "doctor" to "doc" to "coach." We were no longer a doctor/patient group. We were a running club.

The driving force of any track club is competition, the desire to run faster, at your chosen distance, than any member of your own or any other club. Obviously, I could not allow such an approach in our group; the men were running for their health. For us to indulge in racing one another would have been (and still is) not only imprudent, but pointless. Yet how to maintain club interest and motivation without the stimulus of competition? The answer was, of course, simple. Each man would compete against himself. There was no reason why each could not attain fifteen or even twenty miles. Distance, not speed, would be the goal. The only limitations would be those imposed medically.

But, said the men, if distance was to be our aim, why not pick a distance which had the stamp of official recognition? Ever since the birth of the modern Olympic Games in 1896, the 26¼ mile marathon run has been the pièce de résistance, the longest foot race in any official track and field contest.

Our aim, then, would be to complete an official marathon run. To come unscathed through such an ordeal without excessive strain or damage to the heart would not only be an achievement in itself, but it would have the added advantage of focusing attention on the value of exercise therapy in cardiac rehabilitation. Furthermore, it would restore confidence to other heart attack victims who felt their active lives were over, and that all they had to look forward to was a life of semi-invalidism.

As for the specific race, what better than the famous Boston Marathon. Held annually every Patriots' Day, and dating back to 1897, this event attracts runners from all over the world. Just four hundred miles or so down the highway from Toronto, we could drive there in a day.

If you want to run twenty-six miles non-stop, you have to attain an average weekly training mileage of nearly twice that. The men were running twenty miles or so weekly at this stage, so they had a long way to go. The progression had to be slow and careful, otherwise their middle-aged muscles and tendons would injure, and they would miss valuable training sessions. Progress was checked by regular laboratory tests on the bicycle ergometer and treadmill. From time to time, they were telemetered while running (a small radio-transmitter is attached to the runner's chest, and this transmits his electrocardiogram back to a receiver in the Centre as he runs around the track). It was agreed that at any time, the "coach" could revert to the role of "doc" and imperiously forbid a man to take part in the run, even right up to the time of the starting gun.

By Christmas, everyone was fitter than I would have believed possible, but the days were getting shorter and colder. Running in the dark became a necessity as the mileage increased. Luminous strips on the shoes and sweat suits were adopted after Harry B. narrowly missed injury from an overtaking truck which had decided to share the soft shoulder with him. We learned to run in temperatures as low as 10°F above zero (-12°C), by the use of suitable layers of clothing, and much of the knowledge we acquired that winter was later applied to the entire post-coronary class.

We left Toronto to drive to Boston two days before the race. Accompanying the men were a medical team of three: myself, Johanna Kennedy, the nurse coordinator of the program, and Salah Qureshi, our chief medical technician. In addition to our running gear, we carried instruments to sample blood, measure body weight, take blood pressures, and record electrocardiograms. We intended to learn as much as we could about the effect of such physical and mental stress on the post-coronary patient.

If you've never witnessed the start of a large marathon, you may find it hard to understand what an emotional experience it can be. The tension mounts as the minutes tick off to the start. The officials bustle and shout instructions. The runners dance restlessly or stand morosely, as their personalities decree, some talking incessantly and laughing loudly, others tight-lipped and tense. The motorcycle police who are to cover the whole route race their

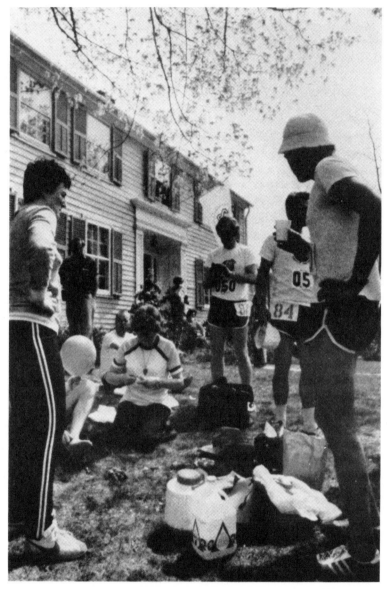

T.R.C. marathoners: above, preparing to begin the 1976 Boston Marathon (in 100 degree heat); opposite: blood pressure check, Boston Marathon, 1973; pride of achievement after Honolulu Marathon, 1974; trophy presented to "Supercoach," Dr. Terry Kavanagh, by his patients, the world's "sickest" track club.

engines in an increasing crescendo of noise, as if anxious to be on their way. Finally, just as you think it will never come, there is the hoarse familiar command, ''On your marks,'' the starting gun fires, the noise of the motorcycle engines increases to a deafening roar, and the whole pack is on its way, the top runners already fighting to get clear of the ruck and establish a strategic position.

On this occasion, I had little time to dwell on the scene. As our men left, Jo Kennedy and Salah Qureshi quickly gathered the discarded sweat suits, and the three of us ran to the waiting cars ready to drive to our first rendezvous a few miles down the course. We made the meeting place with minutes to spare. As each man passed, he seemed relaxed and running easily.

Throughout the remainder of the race, the medical team must have driven the course three times over. We knew that after the 13½ mile mark, provided all was going well, our runners would be strung out considerably. This meant that we could not accompany them as a group, but would have to ''leapfrog'' the cars, trying to check each man's condition every mile or so, while at the same time briefly meeting with each other to compare notes and decide who needed the most attention.

As the miles wore on, Herman R., 32 years old, gradually pulled ahead of his clubmates. He went on to cross the finish line, the first of our group to do so. Don C., age 40, was close behind and came in running strongly. Then one by one and so fast that I barely had time to get my measurements, each appeared at the finish line. Dino V., followed by Harry B., then John N., John R. and finally Ken S. They were all tired, but happy and in excellent physical condition. Not only that but, wonder of wonders, they had actually overtaken hundreds of competitors on their way to the finish line, and watched countless others, exhausted, being picked up by emergency trucks and ambulances.

That night, back in the motel, after all the post-race examinations and tests were completed, we celebrated. The hard training had paid off, and we had proved our point. The program worked.

The story of the T.R.C. Joggers did not end in 1973. The club has expanded to accept any ''post-graduate'' from the regular cardiac exercise program who aspires to finish a marathon or, indeed, who enjoys runs of six miles and upwards. We still meet regularly on weekends for long runs, and to date can boast of finishing 196 official marathons in places as far afield as Honolulu, New York, Ottawa, Detroit, Reno and Dublin. We have entered the Boston Marathon a total of six times and, in 1983, we marked the tenth anniversary of our first attempt by having twenty-six entrants (including on this occasion Jo Kennedy and myself) and twenty-six finishers. You can imagine how the champagne flowed that night!

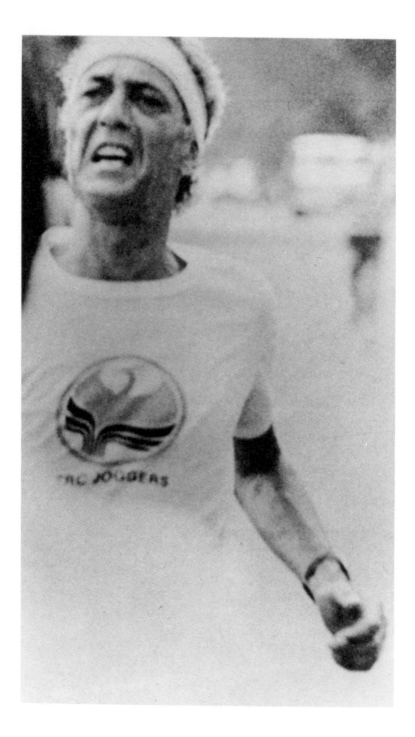

Part One

THE ANATOMY OF
A DISEASE

Courage was mine, and I had mystery
Wisdom was mine, and I had mastery.

Wilfred Owen

CHAPTER ONE

Atherosclerosis: The Modern Plague

The ancient Greeks believed in gods who could be both spiteful and capricious, from time to time playing cruel tricks not only on one another but also upon that vulnerable creature, man. Certainly the study of human history cannot help but leave one with the impression that whoever or whatever controls our fate possesses a malevolent sense of humour—with the joke inevitably being on us. If the current vogue in sick jokes is an updated version of this idea, then surely the sickest one-liner in history is that simple three-word title, ''coronary care unit.''

For those of you who have had a heart attack, a detailed description of a coronary care unit is likely both unnecessary and depressing. For those of you who have bought this book because you wish to avoid finding yourself in such a situation in the future, suffice to say that the CCU is one of the ultimate expressions of man's achievements in the field of medical electronics: a private observation ward where no privacy exists, where the patient's blood pressure, respiratory rate, heart action and other vital signs are constantly monitored, 24 hours a day, by automatic instruments which not only record every breath and every heart beat, but also alert the watching nurse by audio and visual signalling devices of any irregularity.

Until the 1960s, we possessed only two of the three essential ingredients for a CCU — the nurse and the patient. The third ingredient, the highly sophisticated electronic instrumentation, is the product of our technological age. And herein lies the joke, for it now seems likely that this same era of science and the computer which gave us mastery of the air, journeys to the moon, and machines which think, has also imposed upon the human being a lifestyle incompatible with survival. An exaggeration? The World Health Organization has recognized the increased incidence of heart disease in modern times to be "of the utmost urgency," and in a report published in 1982 commented that coronary heart disease "causes death or disability in many who are still in the active years of life and whose children are still young. Its personal and social costs are profound, both for the individuals and families involved and for the countries in which it is common." Dr. W. Kannel, medical director of a large-scale investigation of cardiovascular disease in the United States, goes further and refers to it as "the greatest sustained epidemic confronting mankind."

The plain facts are that heart attacks kill and disable more people in the western world today than any other single disease, and that includes cancer, chest disease, alcoholism and motor vehicle accidents. As the affluent life spreads to the non-western countries, so their incidence of heart disease begins to climb. Ironically, society seems to have developed the ability to furnish the CCU with both equipment and patients in the same era. Whether or not this curious relationship is coincidental or causal is a matter which we will explore later but, in the meantime, we will take a closer look at the villain of the piece, myocardial infarction, or the heart attack of popular parlance.

PROFILE OF A HEART ATTACK VICTIM

John S. was entitled to feel pleased with himself. A professional engineer, at 41 he possessed all the contemporary hallmarks of success: a happy marriage, two teenage boys who were doing well at school, a comfortable house (almost paid for) in a desirable neighbourhood, and the imminent prospect of promotion to company vice-president. Mind you, he hadn't had too much time of late to count his blessings; a year previously the company plant started moving to a new location and, as production manager, he had found himself involved in a hectic work schedule. Even Mary, his usually so-patient wife, began to express concern as six- and seven-day work weeks became routine. Still, the job had to be done and "goodness only knows what a mess things would get into if I wasn't there to keep tabs on everything." Besides, when the move was completed, he could ease off a bit, maybe "play a little golf, or take a week's vacation and get in a little fishing." Maybe he would cut back on his smoking too; with all his stress and strain he was up to a pack and a half a day now . . . wouldn't do any harm to lose a little weight also, but that was difficult when one's meals consisted of an endless succession of hurried sandwiches interspersed with "two-martini luncheon meetings" and expense-account dinners.

Yes, he probably was a little out of shape — which no doubt accounted for the heartburn and indigestion pain he had begun to experience in recent months whenever he got up-tight at work or tried to lift anything heavy. He was "probably developing a peptic ulcer," the almost prestigious occupational disease of all successful executives.

In due course, John's plant completed its move to the new location. But the transition phase brought with it teething problems which, naturally, only John could solve. Admittedly, weekends at the office were no longer routine (although they did occur from time to time), but the twelve- and thirteen-hour workday became commonplace. Always a hard driver, he was now hotly in pursuit of the presidency, and he dedicated himself to the task with all the energy and determination which had characterized his performance as one of the best linemen of his university football team. Unfortunately, he wasn't in his early twenties any more and while he still possessed the spirit and motivation of bygone years, his body was no longer fit enough to endure the tasks he placed upon it. His "indigestion" pain was bothering him more frequently now, and not only after eating. From time to time he experienced severe discomfort in his upper abdomen and chest when he ran up a flight of stairs, or walked quickly up an incline (not that he did too much walking nowadays). Usually, the pain would go away if he belched or rested for a minute or so.

He began to feel chronically tired. Never at any time, however, did he feel that he had any serious health problem. After all, he had always come through the annual company medical examination with flying colours; blood pressure, electrocardiogram, blood and urine checks always normal — which was, after all, only to be expected in a strong, 6'2" ex-college football player.

Then one day, while sitting dozing in front of the television set, he got a fright; the stomach pain came on quite suddenly. Only on this occasion, it was more severe, and seemed to have moved up into his chest. For a moment or two, he had difficulty breathing, as the pain radiated first into his neck and jaw, and then down both arms to his hands. He found he was sweating profusely. He didn't know what to do. When he tried to lie down, the pain seemed to get worse; moving around didn't do any good, and neither did belching gas. Mary, noticing his agitation and pale, sweating features, learned for the first time of his recurrent bouts of "indigestion." She wanted to call a doctor, but John persuaded her to wait and see if his condition improved. Fortunately (or unfortunately as it turned out), the pain subsided after about thirty minutes, although for the next day or two his chest felt very sore. In deference to Mary's wishes, he called in to see his family physician the following week, and told him that he had been getting the "occasional niggling stomach pain when I am over-tired or tense." A combination of John's natural tendency to downplay any evidence of physical weakness, together with what may have been a too-easy acceptance of his tale by the physician, led to a diagnosis of "nerves." An electrocardiogram was not carried out. Still, as John himself says, "hindsight is always 20/20."

During the following weeks, John continued his heavy work schedule, suffering only occasional and relatively mild "nerve" pains in his chest — until the week the plant workers went on strike. If the job was hectic before, it was frenetic now. Extra duties, extra hours, unpleasantness on the picket lines, all contributed to bring about a desperate situation. There seemed to be no solution. As a matter of fact, there was, and in John's case, it was almost the final one.

At four o'clock one morning, he was awakened by the most severe pain in his chest he had ever experienced. It was as if a terrible weight was pressing on his chest bone, squeezing and squeezing until he felt he could no longer breathe. He thought he was going to die. He put up no argument when Mary called the ambulance and, within half an hour, an electrocardiogram was carried out in the emergency department and the young, serious-looking doctor quietly gave him the news; he had sustained a severe heart attack and was to be admitted to the coronary care unit immediately.

John was six weeks in hospital, during which time he experienced a series of emotional reactions to his predicament. At first, he was stunned by the doctor's diagnosis. It was impossible for him to have had a heart attack; his heart wasn't weak, he had never had a day's illness in his life—there must be some mistake. This period of "denial" lasted about 48 hours. Some patients never lose it even after discharge from hospital, persisting in their belief that the doctors have "made a mistake." In John's case, it was replaced by a sullen anger. What right had fate to treat him in this unfair fashion? Hadn't he worked hard to make his mark in life, to provide for his wife and family, to get on? What reward was this for living according to the rules?

After he came out of intensive care, his cardiologist told him he would probably be able to go home "in a couple of weeks." Always a stickler for accuracy, John interpreted "a couple" as being exactly two. When these two weeks were up, he was told he might be in hospital for another "few weeks." He now became dreadfully depressed. He felt the doctors were keeping something from him: he was going to die, or at best be an invalid for the rest of his life. He would never see his children again.

At the end of six weeks, he went home still in a depressed mood. The first day back in familiar surroundings was almost too much for him. He felt so fatigued he had to go to bed after only a few hours. He had lost his old aggressive self-confidence and was fearful of responsibility. Even after his return to work, ostensibly fully recovered, Mary was at first surprised and then perturbed to find that he continued to lean on her, reluctant to take the initiative in financial or domestic matters requiring a decision.

This state of affairs continued until his doctor, sensing a deterioration in the family relationship, had a talk with him and asked him if he would like to attend a new exercise rehabilitation class which had recently been instituted at the Toronto Rehabilitation Centre. John agreed. Later, he commented that the rehabilitation program was "like a lifebelt to a drowning man. It's the best thing since sliced bread."

THE GENERAL PATTERN

Of course, there is no such thing as a typical heart attack victim, patients coming in all shapes, sizes and types. John's story is a composite case history, drawn from the files of patients referred to me for post-coronary rehabilitation. But interestingly enough, an analysis of a hundred of these patients carried out in conjunction with Professor Roy Shephard of the Department of Preventive Medicine and Biostatistics, University of Toronto, in 1973 and published in the *Canadian Medical Journal*, revealed a surprising similarity in the patterns of life prior to their heart attacks. Comparison with a matched group of healthy individuals showed that the patients who had sustained a heart attack also experienced a greater than average degree of business, financial and domestic stress in the year prior to their illness. In many cases, the stress factor was extreme.

In the last few weeks before the attack, a significant proportion had experienced vague pains in the chest, neck, jaw or arms, but had ignored these symptoms, ascribing them to "indigestion" or "nerves." Most described a feeling of incredible fatigue, one man actually falling asleep while dining with a business client, and another instinctively reacting to the news of his heart attack with the thought, "at least I'll be able to get a good sleep in hospital." Overweight, heavy smoking and lack of regular physical activity were all too common.

Often the attack itself occurred within 24 hours of a severe emotional experience or unaccustomed physical stress: for example, a violent row with the boss, or half an hour of trying to start a recalcitrant outboard motor. In at least one case, the emotional and physical were combined, when a patient undertook a long and exhausting journey to see a boyhood house full of bittersweet memories of early struggle.

Another study I carried out at the Centre, also published in the *Canadian Medical Journal*, showed that many of these patients go through a phase of denial after the infarction, but then all too frequently become depressed, lacking in confidence, and fearful for the future. They feel they have lost their masculinity, and they worry about their future ability to perform the role of husband and father with the same success as previously. They hide their depression very well, even from their wives, and it requires careful questioning by the physician and the psychologist to uncover it. Where depression exists, however, it is always profound. Oddly enough, the depressed post-coronary patient invariably feels that he is the only one in the whole group who feels this way. His fellow sufferers are as convincing in their show of false bonhomie and cheerfulness as he is.

By now, you should be getting a picture of the manner in which coronary artery disease can strike its victim, often nowadays an apparently healthy, busy man in his forties. Women are much less affected, and we will see the reason for this later. But what exactly is coronary artery disease, and what causes it? In order to answer these questions, we must take a brief look at the anatomy and physiology of the heart and blood vessels, and then make a short excursion into the field of epidemiology.

WHAT IS CORONARY ARTERY DISEASE?

The heart functions just like a mechanical pump. Its sole function is to supply the force by which blood is driven through the blood vessels to all parts of the body. Its walls consist of muscle tissue which possesses the unique property of contracting involuntarily; it works day and night, irrespective of whether its owner is awake or asleep. But, like all of the body's tissues, the heart muscle needs to be supplied with oxygen-rich blood. This it receives from two small arteries which branch off from the base of that major artery, the aorta, through which the rest of the body's blood supply needs are met (Figure 1). These small arteries are known as coronary arteries, and they are the heart's private blood supply system, operated by the heart and for the heart.

Each cycle of the heart's pumping action is divided into an active contracting stage when the various chambers are ejecting blood into the general circulation, and an inactive resting stage when blood is being sucked from the great veins into the non-contracting, almost empty heart. The active stage is referred to as *systole*, the inactive stage as *diastole*. If you place the palm of your hand over your left breast, you may be able to feel the impulse of your heart beating regularly against your chest wall (provided, of course, that you are not covered by a too generous layer of fat); this impulse is due to the heart contracting in its stage of systole. A unique feature of the coronary circulation is that blood flows through it most actively when *the heart is in the phase of diastole*. This is in direct contrast to the blood flow to the rest of the body which occurs, of course, in the stage of systole. It will be seen later when we come to consider the effect of exercise training on the heart, that this fact is of considerable significance.

What happens when someone has a heart attack? What causes the "attack"? The disease responsible is called atherosclerosis, a medical term for fatty thickening which occurs in the walls of blood vessels. The condition, when it develops, may affect any of the arteries in the body, but the consequences are most serious in the coronary vessels. These are often not much thicker than a drinking straw. The fatty infiltration of their walls leads to a gradual narrowing of their inner diameter, with the result that they are

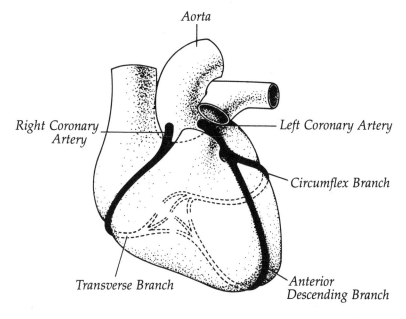

Aorta

Right Coronary Artery

Left Coronary Artery

Circumflex Branch

Transverse Branch

Anterior Descending Branch

Figure 1   The Coronary Arteries, Your Heart's Blood Supply

unable to supply sufficient blood to the heart during times of high demand. When a hard-working muscle is partially deprived of its blood supply, it develops a cramp-like pain; put a tourniquet around your upper arm so as to cut off the blood supply, and then clench and unclench your fist for a few minutes, and you will quickly see what I mean. The heart muscle is no exception. Thus a patient who is suffering from atherosclerosis of the coronary arteries may find that emotional tension or physical exercise induces a form of cramp in his heart which he feels as an acute pain in the chest or, to use the medical term, angina pectoris — which is Latin for the same thing.

Walking up stairs or uphill, hurrying on the level, or suffering a severe shock, are notorious examples of daily incidents which bring on angina pectoris. A common situation in which both emotional and physical factors occur together is the all-too-familiar struggle through one of our modern overcrowded airports carrying a heavy suitcase. As soon as our atheromatous victim slows down or stands still, the workload on his heart is reduced; the

narrowed coronary arteries can now cope with the blood requirements of the heart, and the cramp-like pain subsides.

Is angina pectoris, then, the same thing as a heart attack? Not
really. The heart attack represents a further stage in the progress
of the disease, and it should be noted that this may occur in a
patient who has never experienced anginal pain. The narrow bore
of the coronary artery may be plugged by the fatty substance which
is accumulating in the walls (referred to medically as "plaque");
or a piece of the fatty substance may break off and be carried down-
stream by the blood flow until it reaches a portion of the artery
which is too narrow to penetrate. Sometimes the cause of the blockage may be a blood clot (thrombus) which has formed on the surface of the fatty patch and then breaks loose.

Sometimes no blockage can be demonstrated at post-mortem
examination, and we then must assume that a sudden increase in
the workload of the heart has created a situation where the blood
supply simply could not keep pace with the demand. Whatever
the mechanism, the end result is the same. A portion of the heart
muscle is deprived of its blood supply and dies. Our patient classically complains of severe and continuous chest pain which,
unlike angina pectoris, refuses to go away despite resting, taking
indigestion pills, or belching gas. He shows all the signs of shock,
such as sweating, pallor, slow pulse rate, and falling blood pressure. Within a few hours, his electrocardiogram tracing will show
changes from the normal because the electrical potentials from
the heart muscle are being modified by the presence of dead tissue.
There is also an early rise in the blood level of various substances
released by the breakdown of heart muscle tissue. These substances are known as enzymes; their diagnostic importance lies in the
fact that they can often be detected by special laboratory tests prior
to the appearance of electrocardiogram changes.

If the area of damage to the heart is great, then death is likely.
There may be an immediate electrical failure to the entire heart
("cardiac arrest" or "ventricular fibrillation"), or it may occur up
to 48 hours after the attack. If it does, then we may be able to
restore the normal electrical activity of the heart quickly by applying an external "defibrillating" electrical current to the chest wall,
in which case the subject may live. This is one of the values of
having the patient in the coronary care unit, for here his heart can
be monitored continuously and if electrical failure develops, he
can be resuscitated within seconds.

Unfortunately, cardiac arrest is most likely in the first few hours of the attack when decisions are still being made to call a doctor or arrange admission to hospital.

Provided the patient survives the immediate emergency of the attack, his outlook rapidly improves. The dead heart muscle is replaced by fibrous scar tissue, and in about six weeks the process of repair is complete. Patients often ask if the repaired area is as strong as before. It depends on what you mean by "strong." If the damage is not too extensive, then the fibrous patch will stand the strain of the heart's pumping action without difficulty. Occasionally, when the area of damage is large, or if the patient remains too active during the acute stage of the attack, the patch may weaken, thin and bulge outwards; this bulge is known as an aneurysm, and its presence can be a contraindication to intensive exercise therapy. However, this is a rare occurrence, and the physician can easily detect it by electrocardiograms and specialized x-ray techniques.

Obviously, although fibrous repair tissue may be strong, it does not possess the specialized heart muscle cells' ability to contract rhythmically and regularly so as to produce the "heart beat." To this extent, therefore, the more replacement fibrous tissue present, the less flexible will be the heart wall and so the less efficiently will it stretch during the resting phase (diastole) or shorten during the pumping phase (systole). Essentially then, a heart attack is death of heart muscle due to blockage of blood supply; or, to put it medically, myocardial infarction (heart muscle death) due to coronary occlusion (blockage).

A LOOK AT THE EPIDEMIOLOGY OF CORONARY ARTERY DISEASE

Epidemiology is the study of diseases occurring in groups of people. One of its many uses is to help answer the questions related to the cause, incidence and prevention of a specific disease in the community. Because of the high incidence of coronary heart disease, a solution to the problem becomes urgent. It is no longer enough to study each case on an individual clinical basis; we must also examine large numbers of persons suffering from the disease, hoping to find some common denominator.

While we now have evidence that the death rate from heart attack is decreasing slightly in some countries, such as the United States and Canada, it shows no signs of abatement in others, for example England, Israel, and most of Europe; and it is on the increase in places as far afield as Scotland, Singapore, Switzerland, and Malaysia. However, lest we in North America become complacent, it should be noted that heart attack is still responsible for one-third of all deaths in the United States and Canada, results in more hospitalization costs and work loss than any other single disease, and is by far the leading cause of death in middle-aged men.

The alarming rise in coronary artery disease dates back only to the 1920s. Prior to that, physicians were familiar with the disease, but came across it infrequently in practice. Angina pectoris was first described by Heberden, an English physician, in a paper presented to the Royal College of Physicians in London in 1768. By that time, he had observed about twenty cases; eighteen years later he wrote, "I have seen nearly a hundred people with this disorder." Not a great number for a lifetime of practice. The famous physician, Sir William Osler, in 1892 described coronary heart disease as being "very rare." What was it, then, about the early decades of the twentieth century that spawned this modern plague? Since we don't know the cause of the disease, we can only attempt educated guesses in answer to the question.

To discover the causes of a disease is no small task. It may take years, even generations, of observation and research. The Black Death, a grimly accurate description of bubonic plague, ravaged the known world throughout recorded history, and still occurs sporadically to this day in certain parts of the globe. Yet it was only in 1894 that the causative agent, the deadly plague bacillus, was jointly discovered by a Japanese, Shibasbauro Kitasato, and a Frenchman, Alexandre Yersin. Even that knowledge was not as valuable as it might have appeared, as we still had no idea how the bacillus actually infected man. It was not until 1914 that the true culprit was discovered—the rat flea. Sucking blood from the stricken rat, it ingests hordes of the plague bacilli into its gut, and then transmits them into the blood stream of its healthy, human host. It took over two thousand years to find the answer, following a myriad of false clues, dead ends and spurious leads. Hopefully, we will be more speedy with coronary heart disease; but no matter how we telescope it, the process remains the same: observation, experimentation and more observation — together with that stroke of luck, or genius, that is the brilliant deduction.

But perhaps we don't need to actually know the cause of a disease in order to deal effectively with it. Let me draw another example of what I mean, again from the fascinating pages of medical history. John Snow, a nineteenth-century English physician, was concerned about the recurrent epidemics of Asiatic cholera which ravaged London in 1831 and again in 1848 and 1853. Considered by earlier healers to be a visitation from God upon the evil-doer, the condition was a deadly killer, with no known cure. Once contracted, it was invariably fatal in a matter of days. From his epidemiological observations, Snow inferred that the disease was caught by healthy individuals from persons who were already afflicted. He furthermore theorized that, whatever the actual causative agent, it was in some way eliminated in the patient's excreta, which was then accidentally swallowed by the next victim in whom it multiplied and reproduced cholera. Since all of the cases occurred in a district of London which obtained its drinking water from the River Thames, he blamed the spread upon the pollution of the river by infected human waste. Accordingly, he advised the then up-to-date measures of improved sewage disposal, as well as purification of the water supply by filtration through sand and gravel.

In 1854, Snow had the opportunity to test his theory. In a small area of central London a particularly virulent outbreak of cholera resulted in five hundred deaths in a two-week period. Following a painstaking house-to-house survey of each case, he established that all had a common source of drinking water, a pump in nearby Broad Street. He advised the removal of the pump handle, and immediately the number of new cases diminished to zero — a dramatic vindication of his theories, despite the fact that the cholera bacillus was not identified until many years after his death!

These cases illustrate why the epidemiological approach is sometimes the only one open to us, and how at times it can be of immense practical value in helping us to control or even eliminate a disease — even if it may sometimes lead us to do the right thing for the wrong reason.

RISK FACTORS

We have seen that atherosclerosis consists of an infiltration of the blood vessel wall by a fatty substance, which, in time, calcifies in the form of plaques, narrowing and possibly even blocking the artery channel. Its three clinical manifestations (angina pectoris, heart attack and sudden cardiac death) now seem almost inevitable accompaniments of our modern lifestyle. The development of atherosclerosis is a highly complex process which still largely defies precise scientific explanation. Broadly speaking, there are two main theories of causation. Both date back to the mid-nineteenth century and represent the views of rival German pathologists.

The first, attributed to Rudolf Virchow and later to another of his countrymen, Ludwig Aschoff, focuses attention on the high fatty content of the atherosclerotic plaques. Large particles, consisting of a mixture of fat and protein, are said to infiltrate the wall of the artery and accumulate in excessive amounts. These fatty bumps are known as atheroma (Greek for porridge). As they grow, they destroy the smooth inner lining of the artery, leaving a roughened surface upon which red cells accumulate and clot. Thus the plaque, consisting of fatty material, muscle cells from the artery wall, blood cells, clot and other accumulated debris, grows larger and larger until it effectively reduces normal blood flow through the vessel. Why does the fat particle become trapped in the vessel wall in the first place? At this point, we have to fall back on conjecture; the process has been variously traced to (1) inflammatory reaction in the artery; (2) wear and tear to the inner lining of the vessel (particularly where it bends and curves) due to the effect of prolonged and sustained high blood pressure; or (3) toxic damage to vessel wall cells from constant exposure to a chemical, such as the carbon monoxide in cigarette smoke. Finally, a closely associated factor in the Virchow hypothesis is the requirement that there be a high level of fat in the blood, particularly in the form of low-density lipoprotein (more on that later).

A knowledge of this theory explains why physicians wishing to prevent the development of atherosclerosis in their patients prohibit cigarette smoking, regularly check for high blood pressure, and advise against a high-fat diet.

An alternative theory on the causation of atheroma was proposed by a contemporary of Virchow, by name Rokitansky. Unfortunately for him, he did not have the same high reputation and influence with his peers as did Virchow, and there is no doubt that this is one reason why his views were given little credence at the time. According to Rokitansky, the prime villain in the piece was not the errant action of the lipoproteins, but rather a defect in the clotting mechanism of the blood whereby thrombi (blood clots) form in and on the inner wall (endothelium) of the affected artery. Once formed, the thrombi enlarge by enmeshing other constituents of blood, including the fat particles. A disciple of Rokitansky would therefore attempt to prevent atherosclerosis by prescribing substances which thinned the blood and reduced the likelihood of clotting.

While the Virchow theory reigned supreme for a century or more (and it is fair to say that subsequent evidence tends to support him), since the 1970s Rokitansky's views have begun to assume a degree of relevance in the enigma of heart disease. One of the present-day champions of the Rokitansky thesis, the Scottish physician Dr. Duguid, has consistently reminded us that there are not one, but two events necessary for a heart attack to occur: first, the gradual formation over years of the atherosclerotic plaque which narrows the artery; second, the sudden development of a blood clot on top of that plaque which within seconds or minutes blocks the artery. If the second event were rarely to occur, then the history of the disease would be totally different. Individuals might suffer from varying degrees of angina pectoris, but in the absence of the critical heart attack their life expectancy would be considerably prolonged. Looked at in another way, one might speculate that while atherosclerosis has been with us for generations, the current epidemic of cardiac deaths might well be due to some aspect or aspects of twentieth-century living which has increased the tendency of our blood to clot. Nowadays we tend to look at both these aspects of the heart attack.

Of late, interest has focused on the action of a group of tiny, round, disc-like cells, called platelets, which circulate in the blood and play an important part in the formation of blood clot. Their role is to seal off breaks or openings in the wall of a blood vessel by accumulating in clumps around the damaged area, and by releasing a substance called thromboxane, which constricts the vessel wall and reduces the flow of blood. Theory has it that in certain circumstances, platelet activity can become excessive, leading to the formation of a clot *inside* the intact vessel (an intravascular clot) rather than on the broken surface of the injured vessel wall. It is, of course, an intravascular clot within a coronary artery that leads to a heart attack. What would cause the platelets to misplay their role in this way? The answer could well be an atherosclerotic plaque, which disrupts the smooth inner lining (endothelium) of the blood vessel, simulating a full-thickness break in the wall. Why, then, doesn't intravascular clotting always occur in the presence of atherosclerosis? The answer lies in the endothelium itself.

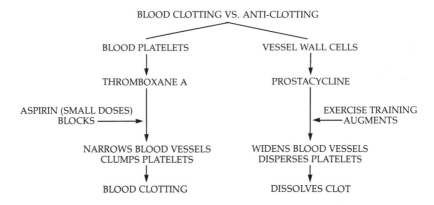

Figure 2   The Interaction Between Blood Platelets and Vessel Wall Cells in Blood Clot Formation

Specialized endothelial cells generate a powerful anti-thromboxane substance called prostacycline, which disperses the clumped platelets, dissolves the clot, and dilates the vessel. Thus we have, in the healthy state, a natural balance between two opposing systems (Figure 2).

Looked at in this way, we could explain coronary thrombosis on the basis of excessive platelet activity due to extensive destruction of endothelium by widespread atherosclerosis. Then again, it has been shown that the hormones, epinephrine and norepinephrine, increase platelet stickiness and clumping tendency. Both these hormones are secreted by the body during emotional stress. We know that prolonged periods of stress may trigger a heart attack. Nicotine also stimulates the production of epinephrine and norepinephrine, which could explain why cigarette smokers are prone to heart attack.

Interest in this aspect of coronary artery disease has also led to the trial use of various substances to inhibit the production of excessive quantities of thromboxane by the platelets. Aspirin is one such drug. Given in small quantities (300 milligrams once a day, or even every other day) it has been reported to reduce the incidence of heart attack and stroke. There is still some uncertainty as to the optimum dose for protection. Some scientists maintain that larger doses will not only inhibit thromboxane production but also that of prostacycline, thereby cancelling out any good effect and possibly even worsening the situation. Two other anti-platelet drugs which are used for the same purpose are sulfinpyrazone (Anturan) and dipyridamole (Persantin).

Before leaving this subject, I would also mention that regular physical activity has been shown to play a beneficial role in this mechanism, both directly by reducing platelet stickiness, and indirectly by causing a reduction in the secretion of stress-induced epinephrine and norepinephrine. Bit by bit the pieces of jigsaw seem to be fitting together.

Let us return to the practical aspects of atherosclerosis. The atherosclerotic plaques take years to form. This is the quiescent stage of the disease. The patient is not aware of any abnormality; in fact, he often feels in excellent health. Routine check-ups, including electrocardiograms, are often negative. Occasionally, a laboratory test may show a higher than normal amount of fat in the blood, but more frequently this reading will be normal. The newer and more sophisticated methods of measuring coronary blood flow such as exercise stress testing, coronary angiography (x-ray of the coronary arteries using a radio-opaque dye), radio-isotope studies, may be of value in early detection, but as yet are not available routinely. Eventually, with the passing years, the process of artery-narrowing matures until it leads to alteration in blood flow of sufficient magnitude to affect the function of the heart. When this occurs, the subject for the first time experiences symptoms, usually chest pain or breathlessness on minimal exertion. The overall process may occupy a span of forty years.

Nowadays, we are used to seeing the acute episode, myocardial infarction, at an earlier and earlier age. The youngest patient who came to my attention was a 27-year-old doctor who was training as a cardiologist. He first noticed chest pain when he ran up a flight of stairs to attend a cardiac arrest! Three days later, he sustained a heart attack. Herman R., the first post-coronary patient to finish the Boston Marathon in 1973, suffered his attack when he was 29. While atherosclerotic changes of one sort or another are present in practically all of us from infancy, there is individual variation in their degree of severity. Slight fatty infiltration of the coronary vessel wall may never progress to the stage where it causes symptoms. But heavy involvement at an early age will invariably lead to a full-blown clinical picture of coronary heart disease. Since we do not as yet understand the mechanism by which the fatty invasion of the vessel wall occurs, we are unable to say why some of us seem more susceptible than others. Our lack of conclusive and statistical proof as to the exact cause of atherosclerosis does not mean that measures cannot or should not be taken towards primary and secondary prevention. There is now a vast body of evidence from numerous epidemiological studies linking coronary artery disease to various risk factors. These are traits or common denominators shared by individuals or groups of individuals in whom the disease has a high incidence. If you possess a large number of these factors, you are "coronary-prone," and the likelihood of your developing the disease is high. Obviously, it is of great practical importance to know what these risk factors are since, as we will learn later, a significant number of them are subject to change or control.

One of the most famous epidemiological investigations is the Framingham Study. Sponsored by the United States Public Health Service and started in 1948, it studied the pattern of coronary heart disease developing over twenty years in a group of 5,000 residents (2,336 males and 2,873 females) in the small town of Framingham, Massachusetts. Each subject was medically examined every two years; body weight, blood pressure, chest x-ray, electrocardiogram, blood fat levels, smoking habits, and other details were carefully noted. The findings demonstrated that males who had elevated levels of fat in their blood, suffered from high blood pressure or diabetes, and smoked had ten times the standard risk of developing coronary heart disease; if those factors were absent, the likelihood was reduced to one-third the standard risk.

Other studies elsewhere emphasize additional risk factors, including race, family history, emotional stress, and physical inactivity. This book is mainly concerned with the effects of physical training but, for a complete understanding of the problem, each of the factors will be dealt with under a separate heading.

Sex, Race

Young women are relatively free from coronary heart disease, provided they do not suffer from diabetes, high blood pressure or very elevated blood fats. After they reach the menopause, however, their immunity is partly lost, and the incidence climbs until it is the same as males of comparable age. The reason for this is unknown, but it may be connected with the possible protective effect of female hormone. One study in the United States attempted to establish this by administering female hormone to coronary-prone males; unfortunately, the incidence of annoying and harmful side-effects caused the experiment to be abandoned.

One of the highest incidences of coronary heart disease is reported from Finland, particularly the eastern part of the country. There is no valid single explanation for this, although dietary habits and smoking have been variously incriminated, and it has been reported that blood cholesterol levels as well as blood pressures are higher than average.

Post-mortem examinations on young American soldiers killed in battle in Korea, average age 22, showed that a high proportion of these young men had atherosclerotic narrowing of one or more coronary arteries in excess of 50 per cent; similar evidence of advanced coronary atherosclerosis has been shown in young soldiers killed in Vietnam, and also in young accidental death victims in Great Britain and in Israel. Chinese soldiers, on the other hand, did not have these changes to anything like the same extent. Similarly, the death rate from heart disease in Japan is only one-sixth of that in the United States. One might be tempted to say that the Asiatic has a racial immunity to the disease, were there not now evidence to suggest that Japanese who emigrate to the United States and who adopt the western way of life lose their apparent immunity and succumb to the same extent as the Caucasian.

I am inclined to reject the influence of race in favour of environment and cultural factors. It seems to me that the low mortality rate from heart disease in the Scandinavian countries is less likely to be due to the inhabitants' Teutonic origin than it is to their lifestyle—just as the Finns must surely owe their coronary-proneness to some factor other than their supposed Mongolian antecedents. After all, the Inuit of Canada's far north are pure Mongolian, and yet have very little heart disease.

High Blood Pressure

The association of high blood pressure, or hypertension as the condition is referred to medically, and coronary heart disease has been known for some time. The Framingham Study showed that hypertensives have about four times the likelihood of developing severe coronary atherosclerosis as the normotensive subjects. Electrocardiogram changes indicative of diminished coronary blood flow are seen more frequently during exercise tests in subjects with high blood pressure. Unfortunately, we still don't know the cause of 90 per cent of cases of hypertension encountered in practice. Nevertheless, there are now a series of prescription medications which can be used to reduce high blood pressure and keep it within normal limits. This obviously is a risk factor which can be detected during the regular physical check-up and then controlled by medical treatment.

The Cholesterol Connection

If there is one word that has made the scene in North America in the past twenty years, it's cholesterol. The paradox is that while everyone has heard of cholesterol, few know precisely what it is. There seems to be a number of misconceptions. For instance, most people think that cholesterol is some kind of dangerous fat that is present in certain foods, that it causes heart attacks by ''furring'' the inside of the blood vessels, and consequently should be eliminated entirely from our diet. At best, this picture is too simplistic, at worst, it's just plain nonsense. Let us try to clarify the situation. What exactly is cholesterol and how did it gain its bad reputation? To answer that question and to understand the various terms used, we must take a brief look at the chemistry of fatty foods.

When we eat fat, it is broken down into what we call *fatty acids*. These are substances which are mostly made up of carbon atoms and hydrogen atoms. The carbon atoms are arranged in long chains, and the hydrogen atoms are attached to the carbon atoms at intervals along the chain (Figure 3a). Each carbon atom has four grappling hooks, or bonds as the chemist calls them, which allow it to link up with any four other atoms. As you can see from the illustration, one bond is attached to each of two hydrogen atoms, and the remaining two to two adjoining carbon atoms. When all four bonds of the carbon atoms are occupied in this way, we refer to the fatty acid as being *saturated*. Where the hydrogen atoms are sparsely scattered along the carbon chain, however, many of the carbon atoms have bonds to spare. The spare bond usually ''doubles up'' with another carbon-to-carbon bond where it is readily available for use if needed (Figure 3b). This type of fatty acid is known as a *polyunsaturated* fatty acid (*monounsaturated* if only one double bond).

The saturated fatty acid is almost invariably found in animal fat, has a relatively high melting point, and is solid in consistency at room temperature. Typical examples of saturated fats are meat

Figure 3a Saturated Fatty Acid

Figure 3b Unsaturated Fatty Acid

Figure 4 Fatty Acid Type and Content (%)

Figure 5   Triglyceride

fat, dripping, lard, butter. Polyunsaturated fatty acids have a low melting point, and constitute the vegetable and fish oils — for example, corn oil, safflower oil, sunflower oil and cod liver oil (Figure 4).

When not being used as fuel for the various metabolic processes of the body, fatty acids join up with an alcohol called *glycerol*, three fatty acid molecules to one glycerol molecule, and the resultant package is known as a *triglyceride* (Figure 5). This is the form in which fat is stored in your body.

Cholesterol, although it has some of the physical properties of a fat, is really not a fat at all. It resembles more closely an alcohol. It is in fact a sterol and is an essential constituent of all the cells in the body; in particular, those which go to make up the tissues of our brain, spinal cord and nerves. It is a major ingredient of bile juice and helps to manufacture our body's supply of natural cortisone and sex hormones. Its presence in the deeper layers of the skin prevents us from being poisoned every time we handle or touch potentially dangerous acids or solvents which would otherwise penetrate the skin barrier and enter the blood stream. It also saves us from dying from dehydration by helping to prevent excessive evaporation of body water from the skin. As you can see, without cholesterol, the human body could not survive. Thus it is widely distributed in nature and can be found in many of our foods, being particularly abundant in egg yolk and "organ" meats such as liver, kidney and brain. However, just in case we don't get enough cholesterol in our diet, our bodies have the ability to manufacture their own cholesterol. This process takes place principally in the liver, which is capable of synthesizing up to six times more cholesterol daily than is found in the average diet!

But if cholesterol is so vital to our continued health, how did it become the villain in the piece? To answer that, you have to go back to 1911 when a Russian, Dr. Nikolai Anitschkov, carried out an experiment in which he demonstrated that he could cause atherosclerosis in rabbits by feeding them on a diet of egg yolk. Since the atherosclerotic plaques which developed in the linings of the rabbits' blood vessels contained quantities of cholesterol, he concluded that the cholesterol in the egg yolk diet had been absorbed into the blood stream and then, because of its high concentration, had eventually clogged the arteries by forming a deposit along their inner walls. At that time it seemed reasonable to assume that atherosclerosis in humans as well as rabbits was due to a diet too rich in cholesterol-containing foods. Taking the argument one step further, it was thought possible to prevent the development of atherosclerosis by restricting our cholesterol intake. In practice, however, this didn't work too well. Only in a minority of cases was it possible to alter blood levels of cholesterol by varying only the amount of cholesterol eaten.

We now recognize that this was too simplistic an approach. Excessive caloric intake from any source, regardless of whether it is carbohydrate or fat, leads to overweight and obesity and can elevate blood cholesterol levels. It seems that the situation is aggravated if fat contributes more than one-third of one's daily calorie intake. Finally, the type of fat consumed is important. Only one-third should be from animal fat, the other two-thirds from vegetable or fish oil.

Why do we think that blood cholesterol levels might be important? Well, for some time scientists have noticed that in countries like Japan, where the population derives much of its source of dietary fat from vegetable fats rather than animal fats, the average blood cholesterol levels are lower than in, say, North America and the incidence of atherosclerosis is very low indeed. As a result of these observations, it was recommended that in countries where there was a high level of coronary atherosclerosis, the diet be changed so as to reduce the amount of animal fat and increase the amount of vegetable oil used.

This is pretty well the state of the art today. The majority of physicians would recommend that those of us who live in the more affluent countries reduce our intake of animal fats and dairy products and, where possible, substitute vegetable oils. The results of such an approach are, unfortunately, not as clear-cut as we would like. The all-important experiment of altering the dietary habits of infants and children in order to assess the effect on heart disease incidence in adult life has not yet been undertaken. We are still uncertain as to whether reducing blood levels of fat is synonymous with reducing the likelihood of having a heart attack.

Furthermore, while it is relatively straightforward to demon-strate the association between a low animal fat diet, low blood fat levels and low incidence of heart attack in a whole population such as the Japanese, it is much more difficult to explain discrepancies within a given population. For instance, why is it some North Americans have extremely high blood cholesterol levels and others have very low ones despite the fact that their overall dietary habits may be similar? To make the situation even more complex, a number of studies purporting to show the beneficial relationship between a low fat diet, low blood fat levels and protection from heart disease have given conflicting results.

To date, there have been five major studies which have attempted to show that reducing blood cholesterol levels lowers the incidence of coronary heart disease. The most recent, the United States Lipid Research Clinic trials, extended over ten years and involved 3,806 men in twelve medical centres in the United States and Canada. The results were published in 1984 and showed that the regular taking of a cholesterol-lowering medication (Cholestyramine) dropped average total cholesterol blood levels by 14 per cent, and that this was associated with a 19 per cent reduction in the incidence of fatal and non-fatal heart attacks. This is encouraging news. However, the following points should be borne in mind. First, although the subjects in the trial were in apparent good health, they all suffered from abnormally high blood cholesterol levels, particularly the ''bad'' or LDL cholesterol (see below). Whether the same benefits could be obtained in individuals with lower blood cholesterol readings is still unknown. Secondly, the medication used in the trial is expensive (approximately $200 a month), is tedious to take (a bulky powder-liquid mix taken with every meal), and is frequently associated with gastrointestinal side effects such as constipation, heartburn, abdominal discomfort, gas and nausea. Finally, it should be noted that the study did not test the value of a well-followed low animal fat diet alone.

The World Health Organization conducted a trial involving 15,745 men living in Edinburgh, Budapest and Belgium. This was published in 1978. It also dealt with men whose blood cholesterol levels were very high. The use of another cholesterol-lowering agent (Clofibrate) over a five-year period decreased cholesterol readings by 9 per cent, and while this was accompanied by a 25 per cent decrease in the incidence of *non-fatal* heart attacks, there was no reduction whatsoever in the development of *fatal* primary heart attacks. Furthermore, there was a disturbingly high incidence of gall-bladder problems and bowel cancer in those individuals taking the Clofibrate. Again, the effect of diet alone was not studied.

A trial which took place in Norway and the results of which were published in 1981 did involve intervention by diet alone, and here there was a 40 per cent reduction in death from coronary artery disease. Unfortunately, the number of subjects involved was small, and only included those with high initial blood cholesterol levels. Also, the reduction in heart attack deaths could hardly be solely attributed to diet since there was also a very significant reduction in cigarette smoking habits. A United States Veterans' Administration trial looked at the effects of a more stringent low-saturated high-polyunsaturated fat diet on elderly men and found it to be successful in reducing heart disease, but again only in those who had very high blood fat levels to begin with.

Lastly, the United States Coronary Drug Project, a study involving fifty-three centres and some eight thousand heart attack patients, failed to show with any degree of certainty that the reduction in blood cholesterol brought about by diet and/or medication had any effect on subsequent mortality from recurrent attacks.

Yet, despite some of the discrepancies in the above trials, few sensible physicians would deny that there is a strong association between excessive ingestion of fats and the development of atherosclerosis. There is strong evidence also that a high intake of animal fat stimulates the liver to produce more cholesterol, while a high intake of unsaturated fat has the opposite effect. It seems that while most pieces of the puzzle appear to be available to us, they just don't fit together to form a clear picture. A further compounding factor in the interpretation of all these data is that we continue to see a significant number of patients who have had a proven heart attack and yet do not have elevated total blood cholesterol readings.

What's new on the horizon? In recent years there has been less interest in cholesterol itself, and more attention paid to its travelling companion, the lipoprotein. When fat is required as fuel by a muscle remote from the fat storage site, it has to be transported to

Low Density Lipoprotein Particle

High Density Lipoprotein Particle

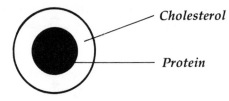

Figure 6   Lipoprotein

the scene of the action. As we have seen, the bloodstream is the body's main means of transportation, and herein lies the snag. Since blood is 80 per cent water, substances using it as a freeway must be water-soluble. As any schoolboy knows, fat and water do not mix. The problem is solved by the use of two blood proteins each of which, when attached to a particular portion of the fat molecule, renders it water-soluble and thus capable of being borne along the bloodstream to the working muscle. The fatty acids are detached from the triglyceride and transported in the blood on a protein called albumen. Cholesterol is attached to lipoprotein.

It turns out there are two forms of lipoprotein which can be associated with cholesterol. One is large and light, like a soccer ball; the other is smaller and heavy, like a billiard ball. The larger type is referred to as the low density lipoprotein (LDL), and the smaller type as the high density lipoprotein (HDL) (Figure 6).

It has been known for some time that individuals with abnormally high levels of LDL cholesterol are prone to heart attacks. Since the mid-1970s it has been observed that there is an equally striking but inverse relationship between the amount of HDL cho-

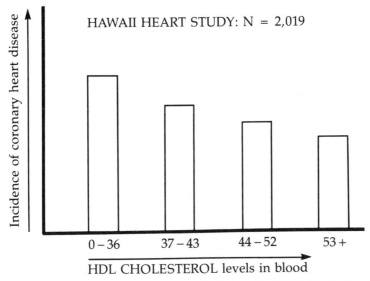

Figure 7 **Coronary Disease Inversely Related to HDL Cholesterol Level**

lesterol in the blood and the incidence of atherosclerosis. In other words, the higher the proportion of HDL cholesterol you possess, the lower your chances of a heart attack. This inverse relationship has been demonstrated in population studies carried out in Hawaii (Figure 7) and in Framingham, Massachusetts, which might explain why some individuals with high total (i.e., HDL and LDL cholesterol) blood cholesterols do not suffer heart attacks. Females, for reasons as yet unknown, tend to have higher average levels of HDL than males, and this may be the reason why they are less likely to suffer from coronary artery disease. It is possible that LDL cholesterol cannot pass through the blood vessel wall, becomes trapped, and over the years forms the familiar fatty plaques of atherosclerosis. On the other hand, HDL cholesterol apparently encounters no such difficulty.

Assuming that such a theory is found to be true, the next step would be to find a method of changing our LDL cholesterol into HDL cholesterol, at least in those individuals in whom LDL levels are high. So far, no drug has been found that will accomplish this. A very strict low-fat diet is useful, but it takes considerable time to work and is not successful in everyone. Exercise, on the other hand, has been consistently shown to be associated with high HDL levels.

In 1974 Dr. A. Lopez, Associate Professor of Medicine at the Louisiana State University Medical School, published a report describing the effects of a seven-week training program (30-minute sessions, four times weekly) on thirteen young medical students. There was a significant fall in LDL and a concomitant increase in HDL. Two years later, Dr. Peter Wood, an English biochemist now working in the Stanford University School of Medicine, reported his investigation of forty-one joggers, average age 47, who had been jogging in excess of 15 miles a week for a year. When compared with a group of sedentary men of similar age, all the joggers had considerably higher levels of HDL. He remarks in his article that "these very active men exhibited a plasma lipoprotein profile resembling that of younger women rather than of sedentary middle-aged men. This characteristic, and apparently advantageous, pattern could be only partially accounted for by differences in adiposity [amount of body fat] between runners and control subjects."

In this regard I have had the opportunity to look at the effect of a distance walking/jogging program on two groups of heart attack patients referred to the Centre and followed for one year. Group 1, thirty-five subjects in all, commencing the program three months after their heart attack, showed a 10 per cent gain in fitness in response to an average of 10 miles of walking weekly. A small but significant increase in HDL cholesterol occurred over that period.

Group 2, twenty-seven in all, trained an average of 30 to 48 miles a week. In this group HDL cholesterol correlated very well with weekly running distance, declining in those subjects who eased up on their program, and increasing in those who intensified their training. Interestingly, the threshold dose of exercise needed to surpass the normal sedentary HDL cholesterol values was about 12 miles per week. Greater training distances were accompanied by larger increases in HDL levels, but while the average training pace for the group was a 10½ minute per mile pace, distance covered was more critical than pace. It would seem certain that exercise exerts a beneficial effect on the amount and type of fats in the blood stream (Figure 8).

These findings might also explain the apparent paradoxes which have dogged the experimental work associated with blood cholesterol in the past. It could, for instance, explain why individuals

Figure 8   Effect of Training Distance on HDL-C; T.R.C. Patients

with blood cholesterols in the 400s and 500s still avoid heart attacks while others with blood cholesterols in the high 200s succumb. If those with the high cholesterol counts had most of their lipoprotein in the form of HDL, or alternatively, those with the low cholesterol counts had most of their lipoprotein in the form of LDL, this would explain the apparent discrepancy.

There is yet another area of controversy. I have already said that the present dietary trend is to substitute animal fats with vegetable oils—that is, to replace saturated with unsaturated fats. This, however, poses a problem for the food industry. One can use liquid corn oil as a substitute for cooking lard, but what about a liquid substitute for butter? How would you like to pour margarine onto your toast in the morning? The solution is something of a compromise. Food chemists have devised a method of partially saturating the unsaturated vegetable oils. They place the oil in a large tank and bubble hydrogen gas through it. This adds hydrogen atoms to the carbon chain. The process is known as hydrogenation or hardening, and the result is a vegetable oil which has a higher melting point and is closer in consistency to an animal fat. Consequently, it is easier to package and use. In the words of the ad, your margarine is now as "spreadable as butter."

Hydrogenation is also used for another purpose. The empty spaces in the unsaturated fatty acid chain are just a little bit too available to any passing molecule that happens to be homeless at the time. The most commonly available molecule is oxygen; so, over a period of time, the inclusion of oxygen in the carbon chain causes the fatty acid to change its properties. It develops a rather unpleasant odour and taste. In other words, it has become rancid. Obviously, if you attach hydrogen atoms to the spaces along the chain, you reduce the likelihood of rancidity. In short, if you want to prolong the shelf-life of any foodstuff which contains an unsaturated fat, you merely hydrogenate that fat.

Herein lies the controversy. Some experts say that hydrogenation defeats the whole purpose of eating unsaturated fats; since you have now turned the unsaturated fatty acid into a saturated fatty acid by hydrogenating it, you might as well have stuck with eating animal fat. Some scientists go even further, maintaining that you are actually worse off because instead of eating the natural fat, you are ingesting an artificial material which, for all we know, might be dangerous. How could that be so? Well, the molecules of the unsaturated fatty acid can present chemically in two forms, each a partial mirror image of the other. One form, known clinically as the *cis* form, looks like this:

The other, the *trans* form, looks like this:

It so happens that the cis configuration is the one most frequently found in naturally occurring unsaturated fatty acids. However, the process of hydrogenation converts the cis into the trans form and it is this type, therefore, that is found in certain brands of margarine, peanut butter, etc. When we eat these substances, the fatty acids are incorporated into the cells in our body and while the evidence to date suggests that they do not produce any ill effects, there are some food scientists and physicians, among them the eminent Dr. Mann of Vanderbilt University in Nashville, who feel that the ingestion of abnormal trans fatty acids is injurious to health. At the present time the whole matter remains unresolved.

There is one vegetable oil used extensively in the food industry which is probably more dangerous in terms of causing atherosclerotic heart disease than any animal fat. That is coconut oil which, despite the fact that it is an oil, contains a high proportion of saturated fatty acids. Why is it used? Largely because it is relatively cheap, and also because when added to a variety of food stuffs, it gives them a creamy consistency and a pleasant taste. In addition, because of its high saturated fatty acid content, it keeps well and is not subject to oxidization and rancidity. Today it is used widely, and is found in cookies, salad dressings, bread, margarine, coffee creamers, even certain infant formulas. The amounts used are probably small, but remember that the highest incidence of coronary artery disease in the world has been found in primitive tribes which, lacking both meat and dairy products, have relied on a combination of fish and coconuts as the two main staples in their diets.

Having read all this, you are bound to be perplexed. Accordingly, I have attempted to summarize in point form the dietary policies which are most generally accepted by the medical profession at this time. I have avoided the more extreme and bizarre recommendations — of which there is no shortage in this day and age — confining myself to suggestions which are founded on a legitimate body of data.

1. The most important rule is to maintain your ideal body weight (see page 310). If you can achieve this, it means that there is a perfect balance between food intake and energy expenditure. It really doesn't matter what you eat, it's all fuel to drive the body machine. I have often thought that if I were in a remote area, miles from any laboratory service and with no means of measuring blood fat levels, I could probably estimate fairly accurately those individuals with a low cholesterol count mere-

ly by putting them on a scale and pinching the skin folds of their abdomen, chest and waist. The light, lean, skinny individual with minimal subcutaneous fat is usually free from atherosclerosis. If you eat more than you need, then you will invariably store it in the form of fat. The 30-mile-a-week jogger can eat a great deal more than the sedentary office worker and still stay slim and trim.

2. Reduce your intake of fat so that it accounts for about 30 per cent of your daily caloric intake (see page 311). These days, the average Western diet contains far too much fat — about 50 to 60 percent of the calories eaten each day. The trouble is that not all of the fat you eat looks like fat. It's easy to see the fat on a piece of pork or a slice of bacon. But many hot dogs contain anywhere from 50 to 60 per cent fat, a hamburger is considered lean if it contains only 20 per cent fat, and there is often beef fat or lard in white bread, cookies, packaged pastries, prepared salad dressings, fried chicken and a whole host of packaged edibles.

    So if you want to reduce the amount of fat in your diet, you not only have to cut down on fatty meats, you must also read the contents label carefully before you buy. In general, you might try to eat more veal, poultry and fish. Approximately one-third of the fat you consume should be animal fat (saturated), and the remaining two-thirds vegetable fat (unsaturated). One way to achieve this is to cook in vegetable oil rather than lard or butter. When you buy packaged or canned foods, read the label to see whether the fat or ''shortening'' which has been included is saturated or unsaturated. But again a warning: the more hydrogenated the vegetable fat, the more it will resemble animal fat. Needless to say, it is almost impossible to avoid some degree of hydrogenation in modern foodstuffs, but settle for partial rather than full hydrogenation. Also, where the ingredients are listed something like this: vegetable oil and/or beef fat and/or lard — assume the worst. If you buy margarine, choose the soft type that comes in a plastic tub; if it's wrapped in parchment, you know that the vegetable oil in it has been heavily hydrogenated, in which case you might as well buy butter.

3. Butter, along with other dairy products such as whole milk and whole milk cheese, are classed as animal fats. Although I

would not advocate their complete exclusion from your diet (unless you have a major problem with high blood fat levels), they should be used in moderation.

4. We have seen that reduction of cholesterol in the diet usually results in only modest changes in blood cholesterol levels. We also know that the absorption of cholesterol is enhanced by your intake of animal fat. Nevertheless, most authorities agree that we should hedge our bets and cut back on those foodstuffs which contain cholesterol in particularly high concentrations. These are egg yolk (use the whites of the egg, or limit yourself to three whole eggs a week, and remember this includes whole eggs or egg powder used in cooking), organ meats (liver, kidney, brains), and certain shellfish (oysters, shrimp, lobster, crab).

5. Finally, don't forget the Golden Rule: All things in moderation. Only if you have grossly elevated blood fat levels and have been given strict instructions from your physician to follow a rigid diet should you become too meticulous. The above guidelines represent the middle-of-the-road thinking. But then, the middle of the road isn't a bad place to be — especially when the traffic starts to reverse! In the present state of our knowledge, you can't afford to pin all your hopes on diet. Regular exercise, stopping smoking, regular check-ups to detect the presence of high blood pressure or diabetes are all part of a well-balanced attack on the disease. The emphasis you place on each is an individual matter and will depend on your own particular weaknesses. It's not much use smoking fifty cigarettes a day and then bragging that you have trained your wife to buy skim milk and trim the fat off your meat!

Smoker's Heart

The link between cigarette smoking and coronary heart disease has been verified in several large epidemiological studies carried out in the United States, Canada, Great Britain and elsewhere. Male smokers under the age of 65 have twice as high an incidence of heart disease as non-smokers, and a similar, though smaller, risk exists in female smokers. Furthermore, smokers seem to suffer from a more severe form of the disease; crippling angina is more frequently encountered, and the incidence of sudden death is four times as great. It's as though smoking decreases the heart muscle's threshold for electrical failure, or fibrillation. The heavier one smokes, the higher the risk. Cigar and pipe smokers resemble non-smokers in incidence — provided they are not ex-cigarette smokers; this is possibly because of the cigarette smoker's inability to forsake the habit of inhaling.

Actually, the ill effects of smoking have been demonstrated in a very concrete way. Post-mortem examination of the hearts of smokers has found a marked thickening of the walls of the coronary arteries and also a thickening of the small arteries which course through the substance of the heart muscle. These appearances are so distinctive and so characteristic of smokers that the investigator, Dr. Auerbach, has labelled them "smoker's heart."

Smokers are not only at high risk for that first heart attack; if they continue to smoke, they are more than likely to have a second one. Our own experience is that among heart attack survivors twice as many smokers have a recurrence as non-smokers. An Irish study published in the *British Medical Journal* in 1983 showed that the post heart attack fourteen-year survival rate for those who stopped smoking was 80 per cent compared with a dismal 20 per cent for those who could not forsake the weed. An appalling indictment.

A word of consolation to the long-term cigarette smoker who would like to quit but is discouraged by the thought that it is probably too late to gain any benefit. I can assure you that stopping smoking promptly reduces the liability of coronary artery disease to the level of that for non-smokers — provided, that is, the ex-smoker does not have a plethora of other risk factors. In reality, he often has a high blood cholesterol, is hypertensive, and out of shape physically. Misery loves company!

Diabetes

Atherosclerosis takes a more severe form in diabetic patients, involving a greater number of the smaller blood vessels than usual. The clinical course of coronary heart disease, therefore, is likely to be more severe and the progression more rapid. Both the young and middle-aged diabetic male have a high mortality rate from myocardial infarction, four times higher than the non-diabetic, and the female diabetic loses her immunity and becomes six times more prone to heart attack.

It is imperative, then, that diabetics, especially young diabetics, adhere strictly to their treatment regimen, striving to keep their disease under control at all times.

Heredity

A study by Gertler and his co-workers showed that twice as many fathers of coronary patients had died of a heart attack as had the fathers of an equal size non-coronary group; 10 per cent of mothers had succumbed to a myocardial infarction as opposed to 7.7 per cent in the control group, and 9 per cent of the brothers and sisters compared with 1 per cent in the controls. Thomas, in another study, demonstrated that when both parents have heart disease, their sons have a five times greater chance of developing the same disease than if both parents were healthy. When only one parent has the condition the risk is only two-fold.

Nevertheless, it seems doubtful that there is a specific genetic factor for coronary disease. The familial tendency is more likely explained by the predisposition for other risk factors to run in families — for example, hypertension, diabetes, high blood lipids, smoking — and some of these are probably the result of environmental background and training rather than genetic traits.

Obesity

This factor above all others has been considered the major villain of the piece. A series of studies in the past has associated overweight directly with an increased incidence of heart disease, which goes to show how carefully you must interpret the epidemiological "evidence." Recent researchers have demonstrated that, in the majority of cases, obesity is associated with other well-proven risk factors such as diabetes, hypertension and physical inactivity; consequently, obesity has been blamed for the ill-deeds of the company it keeps. On its own (a rare enough occurrence, admittedly), it appears to be blameless. On the other hand, obesity may be the cause of high blood pressure and high blood cholesterol.

Coronary-prone Personality

Of all the factors considered to be associated with the increased incidence of heart disease, emotional stress is the hardest to evaluate. Workers such as Buell and Russek in the United States have found a correlation between stressful work habits and coronary artery disease.

Against their findings is the study of Hinkle, who followed 270,000 employees of Bell Telephone Company over five years, and found a lower incidence of heart disease in senior executives with heavy responsibility. Theorell, in Sweden, studied a group of heart attack victims in Stockholm and compared them with a matched control group who were free from coronary disease. The control group actually carried greater responsibility at work, were more involved in supervision, and spent more of their free time in committee work of various types. The patients differed from the control group mainly in that they took less time to relax at home and took less physical exercise.

Friedman and Rosenman have described a "Type A" behavioural type who is, they say, particularly susceptible to heart disease. This individual is characterized by competitiveness, excessive ambition, impatience with delay, and irritability. He is very time-conscious and has a compulsion about punctuality. He is constantly setting goals just beyond his reach, is never satisfied with any achievement. "Type B" behaviour is the opposite; low ambition, no desire to compete, and a phlegmatic approach to problems. According to Friedman, the Type B individual rarely, if ever, sustains a myocardial infarction.

I have always believed that this is too simplistic an approach. If the over five thousand patients referred to the Toronto program are anything to judge by, the heart disease population is anything but homogeneous. Furthermore, a significant proportion of these individuals clearly fulfil all the criteria for Type B personality. There are other arguments against the theory. For instance, cigarette smoking is a clearly proven risk factor for heart disease. Since Type A personalities are frequently heavy smokers, is it not more reasonable to assume that it is the smoking and not the personality which is the culprit? Then again, how can we explain the failure of Type A behaviour to exert any influence prior to the 1920s. After all, the history of politics and business would make dull reading indeed were it not for the superabundance of Type A's. Probably a more cogent reason for rejecting the personality-heart disease connection is that, tenuous at best, it grows weaker when applied to populations other than the mid-Western middle-class white-collar Americans in whom it was first described. Japanese and Israeli investigators have found Type A subjects to have the same or even less heart disease than Type B individuals. In one hundred patients from a London teaching hospital who were separated into Type A and Type B, and who then underwent X-rays of their coronary arteries, no correlation could be found between severity of coronary disease and personality type. Indeed, if anything there were more Type A's in the group who had normal coronaries than in the group who had evidence of disease! Finally, in following up thousands of post-heart attack patients over the last seventeen years, I have not found that individuals with the so-called Type A personality have had any more fatal or non-fatal recurrences than the rest. This has also been the experience of other physicians in the field of cardiac rehabilitation.

Environmental Stress

I believe that there is far too much misconception about stress, the effects of stress, and its connection with heart disease. Somehow the term stress has become synonymous with "the system," and I use that term in the derogatory sense. When someone tells you that his heart attack was brought on by stress, he is often laying the blame on his employer, or his immediate boss, or his spouse. In short, on some individual or some set of circumstances beyond his control. "They" (that convenient anonymous source of all rumour and all evil) are responsible. How convenient. Nothing to do with smoking too much, eating too much, exercising too little. But where does stress fit into the picture?

Actually, the term stress as we know it in today's context was first used by Dr. Hans Selye some thirty years ago. He borrowed the word from physics, and used it to describe the body's responses to a variety of physical and emotional harmful stimuli such as extreme cold, chronic sleep deprivation, etc. These bodily responses are ingrained, involuntary, and an integral part of our heritage. Primitive man's reaction to danger was one of instant physical action — fight or flight. In our modern society such simple solutions are rarely permitted. Talk of fighting or running away is inevitably metaphorical, not literal. The human body, however, still reacts in the age-old primitive manner. Chemicals which we now refer to as stress hormones (cortisol, adrenaline, and noradrenaline) are released from the brain and suprarenal glands. Their purpose is to mobilize those resources which would be required for vigorous muscular action. Blood levels of sugar and fat, the two major muscle fuels, rise appreciably as they are freed from the storage depots. Blood circulation is accelerated by an increase in heart rate and blood pressure. Quickened breathing augments oxygen supply. Finally, in the event of wounding and possibly blood loss, the blood itself becomes "stickier," and clots more readily. In short, the body is now like a newly charged battery, poised and ready for physical action (see diagram). Assuming one is able to cope quickly with the provocative situation, then the state of readiness subsides, and all is well.

Our response to distressful situations is primitive. Adrenaline-like substances prepare us for muscular action, i.e., fight, or run. Regular exercise puts these responses to the use for which they were intended by burning oxygen, fats, and sugars, and reducing blood stickiness.

What, however, if the individual is unable to overcome the problem and it becomes a chronic worry. The normal everyday stress of living (*eustress*, as Selye called it) has now become *distress*, and leads to feelings of frustration, desperation, and hostility. There is prolonged and exaggerated secretion of adrenaline and noradrenaline (referred to collectively as the catecholamines) maintaining elevated blood fat and blood sugar levels, high blood pressure, and an augmented clotting tendency. The ominous implications of all this for a cardiovascular system which is already the site of atherosclerosis are, I think, quite obvious.

When looked at in this fashion, not only is it easier to understand how a heart attack or sudden cardiac death can be triggered by continued emotional stress, but also how regularly repeated bouts of physical exercise can help in "defusing" the situation.

CHAPTER TWO

Physical Activity and Heart Disease

The early years of this century saw the development of an invention which was destined to have a profound effect on the lifestyle of all of us. I refer, of course, to the internal combustion engine. Cheap, efficient and effortless transportation became the order of the day. For those of us who could not afford an automobile, there was always the bus, motor-driven by sixteen horse-power instead of hauled by two. And if Henry Ford's Model T symbolized the height of personal driving luxury, England's unique double-decker bus became equally famous as the modern city's answer to the now-universal demand for mass transportation.

Herein lies a most interesting paradox, for that same double-decker bus was to figure prominently in an article written by Professor Jeremy Morris of the British Medical Research Council, which appeared in the medical journal, *The Lancet*, in 1953. The title was "Coronary Heart Disease and Physical Activity of Work." It compared the occurrence of heart disease in two groups of workers in the London Transport Department: the bus drivers and the bus conductors. The conductors were found to have one-third less heart disease than the drivers, and they sustained only one-half the number of fatal and non-fatal heart attacks.

The likeliest explanation of this seemed to lie in the different nature of their jobs. Driving is a sedentary activity requiring a low expenditure of energy; the conductor, on the other hand, has to collect fares, and in a double-decker this necessitates making an average of up to twenty-four trips an hour up and down the winding staircase of the moving vehicle, in addition to walking back and forth along the aisles of the upper and lower compartments. Over an eight-hour shift, the energy expenditure is considerable, equal to walking from the basement to the top floor of a sixty-storey skyscraper twice a day.

Morris and his colleagues were quick to point out that this very significant association between physical activity and immunity from heart disease was precisely that — an association; there was no proof of cause and effect. For instance, it might be that a process of self-selection was at work; the coronary-prone individual might be more likely to seek employment as a driver than as a conductor. Nevertheless, despite this very legitimate caution, Morris' pioneer work was quickly recognized as being of the utmost importance, and soon other researchers in the field set about trying to duplicate his findings.

The results almost invariably were the same. In the United States, Zukel showed that sedentary workers had six times the incidence of heart disease as did individuals who engaged in heavy work. Taylor compared active U.S. railroad switchmen and sedentary ticket clerks; he found the latter had one-third higher death rates from heart attacks. Kahn, also in the United States, as well as Morris in England, looked at postal workers, comparing mail carriers and sorting clerks; the active carriers had one-third to one-half less heart disease than the sedentary clerks and even greater protection against rapidly fatal heart attacks.

Israel has a high prevalence of heart disease, which is likely why its doctors have carried out so much excellent research on the subject. Probably the best known to physicians is the work of Dr. Daniel Brunner. In pursuing Morris' findings, Dr. Brunner made use of a unique feature of Israeli life, the existence of the kibbutzim. In these communities, people live in a uniform environment, eating the same food, experiencing the same climate, and largely subject to the same stresses. Their standard of living is not influenced by their occupations. Obviously a study carried out in such a setting eliminates many sources of error. In analyzing the causes of death of ten thousand residents of a kibbutzim over a period of fifteen years, Brunner ascertained that "the incidence of anginal syndrome, myocardial infarction and fatalities due to ischemic heart disease was found to be 2.5 to 4 times greater in sedentary workers than in non-sedentary workers." That same study contributed a further significant piece of information: no difference could be found in the serum cholesterol values of sedentary and non-sedentary workers. An argument against the confirmed "cholesterol watchers"?

In talking to Dr. Brunner a few years ago, I found that he ranked physical inactivity much higher on the list of risk factors for a heart attack than either blood fat levels or racial origin. We discussed the incidence of coronary heart disease in Jews of European and Oriental origin, and he was forthright in stating that this was much more likely due to their level of daily physical activity than to any racial or psychological characteristics.

Closer to home, Dr. Curtis Hames, a family physician practising some sixty miles from Savannah, Georgia, was intrigued by the apparent selective manner in which heart disease attacked his patients. Whites seemed to suffer more heart attacks than blacks; yet the black population not only had a higher incidence of hypertension, but also consumed a high animal fat diet. Determined to seek the answer to this anomaly, Dr. Hames instigated a series of epidemiological studies which commenced in 1960 and continued throughout most of the decade. The Evans County Study, as it came to be known, confirmed Dr. Hames' clinical impression; heart disease was found to be four times more prevalent in whites than blacks.

And yet this difference could not be explained on the basis of any known risk factors such as hypertension, smoking, obesity, or high blood fat levels. However, it was noted that the incidence of heart disease varied inversely with the nature of the job. The harder a man laboured, the less heart disease he suffered, irrespective of his race or colour. Since the majority of the black people were manual labourers and field workers, they showed an immunity to coronary disease. As if to underline this point, it was further found that the white of lower socio-economic status who shared the toil of his black brother, also shared that immunity. During the 1960s, Evans County became more industrialized, and this brought with it an upward mobility for the poor white. At the end of the decade, fewer and fewer whites could be found resistant to heart disease; the only ones remaining immune were those who, for various reasons, had not made it in the race for affluence — in other words, the sharecroppers, who still worked hard and long in the fields.

These are only some examples of the studies which have been

carried out since Morris' article first appeared in 1953. With a few exceptions, they have all demonstrated that those who are physically active have a significantly reduced incidence of morbidity and mortality from heart disease. As for studies which have not shown the protective benefit of heavy physical work, the answer is to be found in modern technocracy which has reduced the energy cost of so-called "heavy" jobs to very modest levels. As one European expert in the field has said: "The discrepancy can be explained by the fact that nowadays work labelled as 'heavy' is not heavy at all, so that the study population was not divided into appropriately different categories of physical activity, but rather into different categories of physical *inactivity*."

This is borne out by the work of the American epidemiologist and physician, Dr. Ralph Paffenbarger of Berkeley, California, who over a period of twenty-two years has studied the incidence of heart disease in some 6,351 longshoremen living in the San Francisco Bay area. Paffenbarger's work is noteworthy in showing the encroachment of modern methods on this traditionally heavy labouring field. He has been able to stratify his subjects into light, moderate and heavy workers. He found that the light workers had two and one half times the incidence of fatal heart attacks and three times the incidence of sudden death from cardiac causes as did the heavy or moderate physical workers.

Interestingly, this benefit persisted even when the ill effects of high blood pressure, obesity, previous heart disease and cigarette smoking were taken into account. According to Paffenbarger, analysis of the figures showed that the effect of heavy work was to reduce the chance of a fatal heart attack by 54 per cent; he estimated that stopping smoking or reducing high blood pressure would cut the risk by 27 and 29 per cent respectively. The charge of pre-selection (that is, that individuals who are genetically endowed with healthy hearts automatically tend to choose vigorous pursuits while those prone to atherosclerosis are more sedentary in nature) is countered by the fact that union rules require that all longshoremen work in physically demanding jobs as cargo-handlers for at least five years; in point of fact, the majority continued in this heavy work for many more years than that.

Another approach has been to use insurance company statistics. The Health Insurance Plan of New York was able to categorize its members into those who had a high level of both on- and off-the-job physical activity and those who had a low level. The low-level individuals had twice the number of heart attacks as the high-level members; there was also a striking difference in the two groups with regard to death within the first 48 hours after the attack —48 per cent death rate in the sedentary as compared with 22 per cent in the active.

In recent years, there has been increasing interest in off-the-job physical activity, since heavy physical work has become increasingly rare. Once again, the pioneer Jeremy Morris was first to look at this aspect of the problem. In February 1973 he published a preliminary report in *The Lancet* which dealt with the beneficial effect of leisure-time exercise in a group of 17,000 British civil servants. He found that those who reported carrying out vigorous recreational activities in their leisure time such as brisk walking, swimming, digging in the garden, and other similar vigorous activities in excess of thirty minutes, had about one-third the incidence of coronary disease as those whose behaviour was similar, except that their recreational activities were of a more sedentary nature. The more vigorous the exercise, the lower the incidence of coronary disease. Light exercisers, on the other hand, had no greater immunity than non-exercisers. In this particular report, the vigorous exercisers did not seem to differ significantly from the rest of the group with regard to other coronary risk factors (e.g., family history of heart disease, high blood pressure, high cholesterol levels or Type A/B personality). This suggests that one of the ways exercise exerts its beneficial effect is by blocking the other risk factors. A further source of comfort for those of us who are past our prime is Morris' finding with this group that the beneficial effect of exercise did not fade with advancing age. Morris concludes: ''Habitual vigorous exercise during leisure time reduces the incidence of coronary heart disease in middle age among male sedentary workers.''

In addition to looking at heart disease in longshoremen, Paffenbarger has also studied the effect of vigorous physical activity in leisure time. In following 17,000 Harvard University male alumni aged 35 to 74 for a ten-year period, he recorded a 64 per cent greater incidence of heart attacks in those with sedentary recreational habits as compared with vigorous exercisers. The difference applied at all age levels (35-44, 76 per cent; 45-54, 32 per cent; 55-64, 47 per cent; 65-74, 31 per cent). The charge of ''pre-selection'' is largely forestalled by the fact that college athletes who became sedentary in adult life showed no protective effect, while academicians who had taken up vigorous sports after leaving school did. A further refinement of this particular experiment was the emergence of a "threshold" of exercise at which the maximal degree of protection pertains. This worked out to be 2,000 kilocalories a week — or 20 miles of jogging a week. Finally, it was estimated that if all the alumni had been free from the risk factor of high blood pressure then the number of heart attacks would have been reduced by 16 per cent; if none had smoked, the heart attack rate would be reduced by 25 per cent; if all had exercised regularly at the level of 20 miles of jogging a week, the heart attacks would have been reduced by 26 per cent.

It must be realized that the perfect epidemiological observation is impossible; all the investigations which associate inactivity with heart disease can be faulted on some score of other, as Morris himself was the first to point out. Nevertheless, it has been estimated that to provide even minimal statistical proof of the exercise theory, you would have to set up a prospective study involving some 8,000 individuals randomly allocated to an exercise and a non-exercise group and follow up for a minimum of five years to see how many in each group suffered a heart attack. The project would be a major undertaking, and a costly one. For argument's sake, let's say that the organization of the whole scheme, including recruitment, follow-up, provision of exercise facility, etc., amounted to $1,000 per annum per subject. You are looking at a $40 million bill. When you consider that attempts to measure the effects of differing lifestyles on mortality and morbidity are fraught with innumerable intangibles, all of which can affect your result, it's understandable that there have been no takers.

Despite the lack of such totally conclusive statistical evidence, the following facts emerge from an analysis of the various reports which have been published to date:

1. The published studies are highly consistent in showing that the physically active, either at work or in recreation, are less liable to fatal myocardial infarction or sudden death, the difference in risk being two- to three-fold.

2. Such protection does not apply to other causes of death.

3. Sophisticated methods of statistical analysis, as well as taking into account the previous employment history and scho-

lastic athletic habits, have refuted beyond all reasonable level of doubt the charge of pre-selection.

4. Physical inactivity (or, as Paffenbarger refers to it, "low energy output") has been shown to act as a separate risk factor variable for ischemic heart disease, acting independently of other known risk factors such as cigarette smoking, high blood pressure, elevated blood fat levels, abnormalities in the electrocardiogram, diabetic conditions, age, or race. Indeed, in his study of university alumni, Paffenbarger has calculated that physical inactivity accounted for a greater number of heart attacks than either high blood pressure or cigarette smoking.

5. Even in the presence of other known and established risk factors, physical activity continues to confer a benefit, the sedentary risk-bearers sustaining about twice the number of heart attacks compared to their more active counterparts.

In the face of the above statistical, observational, and circumstantial evidence, it seems eminently reasonable and sensible to accept that physical activity confers a degree of protection from fatal heart attack and sudden cardiac death.

LESSONS FROM PRIMITIVE PEOPLE

Would you like to live to be one hundred? For years, we have heard tales of communities where centenarians are commonplace; not only that, but are healthy and alert enough to work until they are past 80. Lately, scientists and gerontologists (physicians who specialize in the treatment of the aged) have become particularly interested in these reports. The three regions of the world most renowned for longevity are the Ecuadorian Andes, the Karakoram mountains in Kashmir, and the Abkhazia region of the southern Soviet Union. On-the-spot research in these areas verified that ages of one hundred years and up are not unusual. Heart attacks are extremely rare. Why is this so?

The inhabitants of high Ecuador and Kashmir eat sparingly of a diet low in animal fat; conversely, the Abkhazians eat well, with meat and dairy products as regular items. Smoking is common in all three areas, and many of the old people enjoy their wine, vodka and local spirit. Researchers have remarked that in all three areas, the lifestyle is characterized by lack of stress, contentment with one's station in life, and heavy involvement of the aged in both family and civic affairs. People expect to live to a ripe old age, and assume they will work for as long as they are capable. Any or all of these factors may be important contributions to their longevity. A more objective finding, however, is their high degree of cardiovascular fitness. This is due to the nature of their work: heavy physical labour interspersed with a great deal of walking, not infrequently over hilly terrain. Dr. David Kakiashvili, a Russian cardiologist who is intensely interested in this subject, is convinced that it is this active lifestyle, commencing in early childhood and continuing for eighty years or more, which confers the high degree of cardiac health and results in such lengthy lifespans. In other words, if you have a fit cardiovascular system, then the odds are that you will live for a long time.

Two features always considered to be an inevitable consequence of aging are a deterioration in the blood flow to the brain, and a reduction in the body's ability to utilize oxygen. The former results in apathy, forgetfulness, depression, and many of the other mental hallmarks of senility; the latter in a decline in physical vigour. A United States Department of Health study cast a new light on the matter. A large number of elderly males from an Old Age Home were medically examined and from these were selected twenty-seven men aged 65 and over who were completely free from atherosclerosis. Further comprehensive tests revealed that these favoured individuals had the same cerebral blood-flow and oxygen consumption as a group of 21-year-olds. It is not chronological aging *per se*, then, which is responsible for many of the stigmata of aging, but rather the presence of diseased arteries. Which is probably why some Abkhazians are able to work efficiently into their nineties and older, and reportedly sire children while in their late eighties! In a recent television program dealing with this subject and shot on location, one of the attractive female directors commented that a resident in his late eighties made a very determined pass at her. So, if we can keep atherosclerosis at bay, we may have more to look forward to than just the old age pension!

However, to return to the question of physical activity. Dr. Alexander Leaf, an American cardiologist who has made a study of these people in their own environment, repeatedly found a high level of endurance fitness in the aged and was obviously impressed with their capacity for heavy work. He wrote of "Markhti Tarkil, who walks half a mile downhill to his daily bath in the river and then climbs uphill again. Surely any day a man can do this he must be too fit to die. The next day he repeats this physical activity and so on, day after day while the years roll by, and at 104, Tarkil is still much too fit to die!'' On one occasion, Dr. Leaf toiled up a steep mountain side to interview a 106-year-old shepherd. The journey took him six hours, and the going was so rough that two of the four-man party, including the interpreter, had to turn back. The cardiologist's pride on making it to the top was, however, short-lived; it turned out that the ancient shepherd did the journey regularly in three hours!

Dr. Leaf truly took the lesson to heart, for on his return home, he commenced jogging as a hobby. At a recent meeting of the American Medical Joggers Association (a group of physicians dedicated to jogging, which I shall talk about later), it was reported that he continues to jog regularly and still feels very enthusiastic about the beneficial effects of regular endurance-type exercise.

Man has become domesticated only within the last ten thousand years; for one million years before the discovery that we could grow and eat grain (provided we stayed around long enough to reap it), man was a nomad, a hunter. He moved with the game, walking, running, stalking, and constantly setting up and breaking camp. Is ten thousand years long enough to extinguish the needs of his body for activity and motion? If it were, why is the child still afraid of the dark? Why does our hair stand on end and our pupils dilate in preparation for fight or flight when we are startled? We are closer to our stone age ancestors than we sometimes choose to admit.

Wherever pockets of primitive peoples are still to be found, they are relatively free from heart attacks (recognizing the fact that some may not survive to the age at which heart attacks become common). The Australian aborigine, the Kenyan Masai tribesman, the Mexican Tarahumara Indian, the peoples discussed previously in this chapter, all rely mainly on their legs for locomotion. The Tarahumara call themselves the Raramuri, which literally means runner, and part of their culture rites consists of a one-hundred-mile foot race over rugged terrain at 7- to 8-minute mile pace, at the same time kicking a small hand-carved wooden ball! Their freedom from cardiovascular disease is well documented.

To sum up, there is a substantial volume of evidence indicating that regular physical activity carried out over many years protects against a heart attack. The degree of protection is considerable, with about one-third the incidence of fatal and non-fatal myocardial infarctions among active as opposed to non-active workers. Furthermore, evidence is now accumulating that sedentary workers who indulge in vigorous physical pastimes of an endurance type have a similar degree of immunity.

But if regular exercise, either as part of work or play, protects us from heart disease, do we know how it accomplishes this? Not precisely. Exercise physiology, or the study of the effects of short- and long-term physical activity on bodily mechanisms, is a relatively new subject. It has made great advances in the past twenty years or so, but it still hasn't got all the answers. Nevertheless, there is sufficient known for us to be able to consider a number of the beneficial effects of physical fitness, and from this, choose the likeliest contenders for the honour of "heart disease antagonists."

To follow the discussion fully, however, we must understand something about the mechanism of physical activity itself; we must know how our lungs, heart, blood stream, and muscles work to counteract gravity and move our skeletal form around. In short, we must look at the manner in which our body functions during exercise.

CHAPTER THREE

The Physiology of Exercise

We all know that man is an aerobic creature; that is, he requires a constant supply of oxygen to survive. A few short minutes without oxygen, and the cells of his body begin to die, starting with the most sensitive in the brain. The environment of this planet is, as far as we can tell to date, unique within our own solar system in that its atmosphere consists of a mixture of gases containing 21 per cent oxygen. Our bodies are designed to utilize that fact, and the specific mechanism concerned is referred to as the "oxygen transport system." This provides a steady supply of oxygen to the muscles, and is obviously heavily taxed when we exercise vigorously. It works as follows. A series of "feedback" systems throughout the body keep the brain constantly supplied with information as to the level of oxygen in the blood stream and the tissues. When the oxygen content falls below a critical level, the brain, acting through a relay of nerves, causes the diaphragm and other chest muscles to contract. The chest cavity expands, the lungs follow suit, and air passes down through a sequence of ever-smaller air passages—the bronchi and then the bronchioles, finally reaching the myriad of tiny terminal air sacs known as the alveoli. The walls of the alveoli contain fine hair-like capillary blood vessels which are part of the lung's blood circulation. In accordance with the laws of physics, oxygen passes from the region in which it is in the highest concentration to that where it is in the lowest, that is, from the alveoli to the capillary blood vessels. Here, the major part of the oxygen combines with red cells in the blood stream: more specifically, with a protein substance in the red cells known as hemoglobin. In this form, it is carried away from the lungs to the left side of the heart. From here, it is pumped through the arterial system. The arteries branch and subdivide, becoming smaller and smaller, until eventually they form capillaries again, this time in the muscles. Thus, oxygen-rich blood is carried to active muscles. Once in the muscle tissue, the oxygen separates from hemoglobin, under the influence of various environmental conditions such as the heat of muscle contraction, acidity, and the presence of myoglobin, a protein substance in the muscle fibre, which has a greater affinity for oxygen than hemoglobin. The net result is that the oxygen-poor muscle receives a fresh supply of oxygen from the capillaries. The de-oxygenated blood is then returned to the right side of the heart through the great veins, from where it is pumped once more to the pulmonary capillaries, and the whole cycle starts again (Figure 9).

Muscle Contraction

We must now take a closer look at what happens in a muscle when it contracts, and the precise manner in which it uses oxygen. The invention of the electron microscope has enabled us to examine the minute cells which make up the various tissues of the body, with the result that we now know that our muscles consist of bundles of partially interlocking strands of protein. These strands, or filaments, are two in type; one is composed of the protein actin, and the other, the protein myosin (Figure 10). When a muscle contracts, it shortens in length and, by an interlocking action, the actin fibrils slide over the myosin fibrils to produce an overall reduction in length; expressed chemically, the two proteins combine to form actinomyosin (Figure 10). Energy is required to start and continue this process. The immediate source of energy is a chemical substance known as adenosine triphosphate or, more commonly, ATP. Each muscle fibre contains small quantities of ATP which are ready for use when a message from the brain calls for muscle action. The message passes down the spinal cord, and then along a nerve to the muscle. When it arrives at the muscle, it releases minute particles of calcium. The calcium triggers off the breakdown of ATP to a lesser substance known as adenosine diphosphate (ADP), with the simultaneous release of energy—energy to

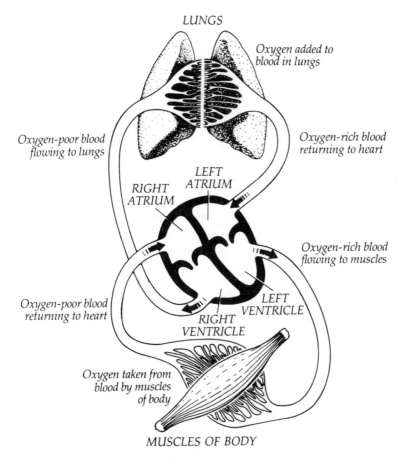

LUNGS

Oxygen added to blood in lungs

Oxygen-poor blood flowing to lungs

Oxygen-rich blood returning to heart

LEFT ATRIUM

RIGHT ATRIUM

Oxygen-rich blood flowing to muscles

Oxygen-poor blood returning to heart

LEFT VENTRICLE

RIGHT VENTRICLE

Oxygen taken from blood by muscles of body

MUSCLES OF BODY

Figure 9   Your Heart is a Pump

initiate the sliding movement of actin and myosin. Hence the muscle shortens, or contracts.

It should be noted that ATP is the only immediate source of energy acceptable to the muscle. Therefore, the body must be able to replace the muscle's local store of ATP quickly, and for as long as the muscle contraction requires it. The ultimate source of all our energy is the food we eat. In terms of ATP formation, the major short-term energy resource is the breakdown of a substance known as glycogen—the principal form in which carbohydrate-type foods

**Figure 10   The Sliding Action of Your Muscles' Actin and
Myosin Filaments**

(starches and sugars) are stored in the muscles and the liver. So
you see, it's what you eat that makes you go!

By a process known as glycolysis, glycogen is broken down to
glucose and then oxydized into simpler compounds, i.e., carbon
dioxide and water. But—and this is a big but—a plentiful supply
of oxygen is needed if the process is to continue to its ultimate
end, which is the formation of carbon dioxide and water. In the
absence of sufficient oxygen, breakdown of glycogen halts part-
way and less ATP is synthesized. Furthermore, an undesirable substance known as lactic acid accumulates both in the muscles and
in the bloodstream. High lactic acid levels block the formation of
more ATP, are associated with the sensation of fatigue, and eventually lead to cessation of muscle contraction. The exercising subject is forced to rest. Depending upon the intensity of effort, this
point may be reached in anywhere from 20 seconds to a minute.
The type of exercise which leads to this state of affairs is known
as *anaerobic* activity—that is, an effort that deliberately outstrips
the rate of oxygen supply. It occurs when we swim underwater,
or if we run for a bus at our maximum pace.

Work which is carried out anaerobically gives rise to an oxygen debt, and like all debts, this must be paid back after the spending spree is over. The accumulated lactic acid must be removed from the system; some is burned by the heart and inactive muscles, but the majority is changed to glucose. This takes place in the liver, by a process which also requires oxygen. Thus, we can appreciate why the sprinter is breathless for some time after he has stopped running — he needs additional oxygen to rid him of his excess lactic acid. For the same reason, the heart continues to beat at a faster rate than normal following a race, for, as we have seen, the heart has a major part to play in supplying oxygen to the muscles.

Some individuals have a greater ability than others to sustain a high level of anaerobic work. World champions, whether sprinters or distance performers, are born rather than made. Training can improve both speed and the ability to incur large oxygen debts, but this acquired improvement is not sufficient to make the difference between an indifferent performer and a record-holder. The potential record-holder in the anaerobic events such as sprinting probably possesses not only larger muscles but also muscle chemical systems and/or a type of muscle fibre which adapt easily to the process of operating efficiently in oxygen debt.

Let us return to the mechanism of muscle contraction. If the rate of muscle contraction (that is, the intensity of exercise) is such that it does not outstrip the supply of oxygen, then the breakdown of glycogen proceeds without interruption to the production of carbon dioxide and water. This *aerobic*, or "with oxygen," process is altogether more efficient than the anaerobic route; twice as much energy is obtained from a given amount of carbohydrate, and thirteen times more ATP is produced. If the degree of muscle activity is moderate, then a fine balance is achieved between the rate with which the muscle uses oxygen, and the speed with which it is supplied to the muscle: thus there is little tendency for lactic acid to accumulate.

Endurance Fitness

From what has been said, it is apparent that the ability to sustain muscle contractions of moderate force is dependent upon a steady supply of oxygen to the muscle tissue: in other words, an efficient oxygen transport system. A good long distance runner or swimmer possesses such a system. Exercise physiologists usually measure this in terms of the maximum volume of oxygen an individual can utilize per minute (litres of oxygen per minute or, to take into account the factor of body weight, millilitres of oxygen per kilogram of body weight per minute). The more oxygen one can use per minute, the higher is one's oxygen consumption, and the higher is one's ability to perform aerobic-type or endurance-type work. We shall be particularly interested in this measurement when we come to discuss the details of exercise training in post-coronary rehabilitation.

Thus, other factors being equal, the individual with a maximum oxygen consumption (vo$_2$ max.) of 80 ml/kg/min (that is, 80 millilitres per kilogram per minute), will also perform better in a 5,000 metre race than a competitor with a vo$_2$ max of 70 ml/kg/min. This does not tell us precisely how the two individuals differ. By definition, the oxygen transport system of one is superior to that of the other, but this is merely a label which leaves us no wiser as to the true basis for that superiority. We must look at each of the links in the oxygen transport system and see which is the most important in terms of increased or decreased fitness.

Provided there is no evidence of chest disease such as chronic bronchitis or emphysema, the ability to get air into the lungs is not a critical factor in oxygen transport. While the first-class athlete may have a large lung capacity, this is often a reflection of body build and muscle strength. Lung capacity in itself should not account for any great difference in performance since it does not limit the healthy individual's capacity to exercise. The same applies to the rate of breathing. The ability to breathe quickly and deeply is not a fundamental index of high-level performance. Blood leaving the lungs is almost always fully saturated with oxygen, and no additional quantity of oxygen can be carried as a result of more vigorous breathing.

However, when there is a reduction in the content of blood hemoglobin, fully saturated arterial blood has a relatively low oxygen content. Hemoglobin molecules contain iron, and their formation requires adequate body stores of that metal. Chronic blood loss (from, say, excessive menstrual bleeding or a bleeding ulcer), leads to a depletion of body reserves of iron and, unless this is compensated for by an increased dietary intake, the subject becomes anemic and, therefore, less efficient in transporting oxygen to the tissues. There is some evidence that athletes occasionally suffer from anemia, but this is not a limiting factor in the average healthy individual, male or female.

Exercise stress testing: bicycle ergometer and treadmill

At the other end of the oxygen transport chain, we have to consider the process by which oxygen is given up to the active muscles by the blood. The delivery of oxygen depends both upon the speed of local blood flow and amount of oxygen extracted from the bloodstream by the muscle (the arteriovenous oxygen difference or avO_2). Exercise usually increases local muscle blood flow and also avO_2 difference by causing a rise in muscle acidity, temperature and waste products. There is some evidence that a trained and physically fit individual has a greater ability to extract oxygen from the blood in his muscle capillaries. This is probably due to the development of a more efficient muscle chemical system of oxygen extraction which can be a definite factor in characterizing the individual with an efficient oxygen transport system. However, it does not play a fundamental role in determining oxygen supply.

Which leaves us with our remaining link, the heart pump. It is here that an individual's ability to transport oxygen is ultimately decided. The quantity of blood pumped by the heart each minute is known as cardiac output. It is the product of the amount pumped per beat (stroke volume) and the number of beats per minute (heart rate). Each individual has a characteristic maximum heart rate, and this maximum rate decreases with age. Similarly, there is an upper limit to an individual's stroke volume. From a practical point of view, therefore, we can say that one's maximum oxygen consumption is mainly a measure of one's maximum cardiac output. We can also conclude that fitness is determined very largely by the body's ability to transport and utilize oxygen.

Finally, an efficient oxygen transport system implies efficient lungs, an adequate hemoglobin level and blood volume, an efficient distribution of cardiac output and an efficient chemical system within the muscles, but above all, an efficient heart.

CHAPTER FOUR

Exercise, Training and the Cardiovascular System

We have seen how regular physical activity protects against a heart attack. However, most of the studies quoted dealt with occupational exertion — with people who work as bus conductors, farmers, mailmen. The mechanism by which such work could have protected the heart was deduced from the results of scientific investigations carried out on trained athletes. Are we justified in concluding that the effects of heavy work and heavy sports training are comparable? The answer is yes.

One way to measure the amount of effort expended on a physical task is to estimate the amount of calories the body burns to accomplish it. The active and heavy workers in the studies mentioned averaged between 400 and 900 calories per day over and above the sedentary worker; this was the effort required to evoke the mechanism which gave them a high degree of protection from heart disease. An international endurance athlete trains seven days a week, often a twice a day, burning around 1,000 calories in each session. Small wonder that long distance runners and cyclists and the like, provided they remain active, have almost total immunity from heart attacks. However, such dedication may not be necessary. Even the 170 lb. "hobby" runner expends 700 calories if he goes for a one-hour jog. You will note that the physical worker's effort is more likely to be spread over an eight-hour day, so that his work costs him an extra two calories per minute. The jogger, on the other hand, concentrates his effort into 60 minutes, burning around 10 calories per minute. This seems to make little difference although, as we shall see later, there is a critical intensity of exertion below which cardiac benefits fail to occur.

For practical purposes, we can divide all exercise into two types— aerobic and anaerobic (see Chapter 3, pp. 60-62). The latter consists of short, sharp bursts of activity lasting only a matter of minutes, and leaving us gasping for breath in order to pay back the oxygen we ''borrowed'' to accomplish the task. Sprint runners and cyclists, weight-lifters, hockey players, are typical examples of anaerobic performers. Aerobic exercise, on the other hand, is less intense, more prolonged, and is carried out without any, or only slight, breathlessness. There is no need for the muscles to function without oxygen because the task required of them is well within the capacity of the oxygen transport system. It is this type of long, steady endurance exercise which is associated with benefits to the cardiovascular system and which will, therefore, be of primary interest to us. Running, cycling and swimming for long distances, cross-country skiing, canoeing and rowing are all sports in which a high degree of aerobic effort is needed. Active participants in these activities, if they are to be successful, must be capable of using large quantities of oxygen. By definition, this is synonymous with a highly efficient oxygen transport system—in other words, a healthy and effective heart pump.

We have now progressed to the crux of the whole situation. If all successful aerobic performers possess such superior cardiovascular systems, can the bulk of the sedentary population attain equal benefits by the regular practice of similar activities? Exercise physiologists and physical educators now think that this is so. Neither the physical labourer nor the long distance runner chooses these activities *because* he has a healthy cardiovascular system; he is healthy *as a result* of the activity. Admittedly, individuals such as Roger Bannister, the Englishman who first broke the four-minute mile, and mythical figures such as John Henry of American railroad fame, likely have to thank their forebears for a proportion of their legendary ability. But that does not alter the fact that the bulk of their greatness came from regular practice and training.

Thus, if we wish to see our children grow up with healthy cardiovascular systems, we will ensure that they are introduced to endurance type sports in their early school days, and we will provide the facilities and motivation for them to continue with these activities into adult life.

All the evidence suggests that the beneficial exercise-induced cardiorespiratory changes which occur in the young also take place in the individual who starts to train for the first time in his (or her) middle years. However, there are some differences in the reaction of the middle-aged heart to effort, and these are more evident when the heart is the site of coronary artery disease. Thus, if we are going to advocate exercise for the 30-year-old and over, we must examine these differences more closely. Exercise can help us beat heart disease, but if we are to employ it, we must use it like any other medication. We must be familiar with its indications and contra-indications, its optimal dosages, its side effects, and its adverse reactions. We must also be able to measure its effects in an objective manner so as to be able to adjust the dosage accordingly. Like any potent medicine, exercise does wonders when used wisely but can be useless or even dangerous when dispensed with ignorance.

ACUTE EXERCISE AND THE NORMAL MIDDLE-AGED HEART

We must distinguish between the physiological changes caused by acute exercise and by chronic exercise. The former refers to an isolated bout of activity, and it is the effects of this on the normal heart that we will discuss under this heading.

An increase in physical activity requires an increase in the supply of oxygen-carrying blood to the muscles. The heart responds with a higher output. As we have seen, it can achieve this in three ways: either by an increase in the number of strokes per minute, in the amount of blood ejected with each stroke, or by a combination of both. In the untrained, the oxygen requirements of casual exertion are largely met by a speed-up in heart rate. This accounts for the extremely rapid heart beat which accompanies even mild exertion in the sedentary. The trained heart increases its output largely by stepping up the stroke volume.

Our blood pressure depends upon three factors: the force with which the blood is pumped into the general circulation by the heart; the elasticity or "give" of the arterial walls; and the resistance to flow experienced by the blood as it courses through the vessels in the muscles, skin and internal organs. During endurance-type exercise there is a rise in blood pressure, probably because the vigorously contracting muscles squeeze the blood vessels in the legs and arms, thus necessitating an increase in the force required to move the blood around the body. The more intensive the exercise becomes, the more the blood pressure rises.

The *middle-aged heart* suffers to some extent in terms of these adaptations. It is a physiological fact that each of us possesses a maximum heart rate. Furthermore, the maximum heart rate declines with age. The net result is that the older exerciser has a smaller potential increase of heart rate. Also, the middle-aged heart contracts more slowly, and this has the effect of lengthening the phase of systole at the expense of the phase of diastole. However, as we have seen previously (page 16), it is during diastole that the blood flows through the coronary arteries, and therefore a shortening of diastole means less time for coronary blood flow. Finally, middle-aged muscles are often flabby from disuse, and so have to work closer to all-out effort in order to achieve a given workload; thus, for any given effort, the rise of blood pressure is much more marked.

Despite these differences, the normal middle-aged heart is perfectly capable of sharing in the benefits of an exercise program, provided that these differences are borne in mind when the exercise regime is designed.

ACUTE EXERCISE AND THE ATHEROSCLEROTIC HEART

So far, we have been considering the response of the healthy heart to acute activity, with some allowance made for age. We will now look at the effects of an acute bout of exercise in the presence of coronary artery disease. This is of supreme importance to the heart attack patient who becomes involved in an exercise rehabilitation program. It also has value for the middle-aged exercise neophyte who, without knowing it, may already have significant atherosclerosis of his coronary arteries — which probably includes most of us over 40!

Severe coronary disease may be complicated by an irregular heart rhythm, weakening or stiffening of the wall of the heart from previous scarring or, if an actual heart attack has taken place, weakness and debility as a result of a period of sustained bed rest following the attack. For this reason, a great deal more caution must be used when prescribing exercise in these individuals.

In the normal individual, there is a close relationship between the increase of heart rate and the increase of intensity of effort. However, occasionally the heart rate of the atherosclerotic patient may not rise in such a linear manner. This may be due to a narrowing of the artery which supplies blood to the heart's primary rhythm regulator, the sino-atrial node. Thus, there is a sluggish response to the body's demand for an acceleration of heart rate. In extreme cases, this can be dangerous, and Dr. Ernst Jokl of the University of Kentucky has ascribed some unexplained sudden ''exercise'' deaths in apparently healthy individuals to a deficient blood supply to the sino-atrial node. The condition may reveal itself during an exercise stress test when it is found that an increase in workload does not bring about the anticipated increase in pulse rate. Vigorous exercise is contra-indicated in such individuals.

Atherosclerosis may equally affect the blood supply to other parts of the electrical conducting system of the heart. This may cause different portions of the heart to beat out of phase, giving rise to so-called ''dropped'' or ''skipped'' beats (see page 97). These are readily recognized on the electrocardiogram, which will also indicate to the physician which part of the heart is contracting irregularly. There seems to be an innocent form of this irregularity which is present at rest and clears up during exercise. Such cases are often discovered in youth and are probably due to excessive adrenalin release in the highly strung individual. In the absence of other signs of heart disease, they are not considered by physicians to be harmful. However, when irregular beats are induced or increased by exercise, they are more serious in import, and can well be a manifestation of coronary atherosclerosis. If frequent, they can reduce the quantity of blood being pumped around the body.

In the absence of damage to the pacemaker or the rhythm-conducting system, the heart rate and stroke volume will usually increase normally in response to exercise, despite disease of the coronary arteries. On the other hand, subsequent to a heart attack, pumping may be sustained with the scarred part of the muscle wall contributing nothing to the squeezing action, or even bulging outwards and thus absorbing part of the force developed by the healthy muscle. This may affect the stroke volume, which in some cases may actually decrease in response to demand for higher output. Pressures inside the heart may rise excessively, with a consequent abnormal increase in ''back-pressure'' both in the general circulation and also in the lung capillaries. In such cases, exercise will cause swelling of the legs and feet, or excessive breath-lessness. Blood pressure may rise excessively, and this will increase the cardiac workload and possibly induce angina pectoris. The patient becomes anxious, his blood pressure rises further, the pain increases, and a vicious circle is established.

"Asynergy" of cardiac muscle, or inability of all parts of the wall to contract together as one, may result from either an electrical conduction defect or fibrous scarring. It also gives rise to a less effective pumping force. The valves of the heart may be involved in the atherosclerotic process, and may not function efficiently when the heart is beating rapidly, thus decreasing the amount of blood being delivered around the body.

Finally, there is the emotional aspect of exercise. The average post-coronary patient may see a bout of exercise as a threat to his health. Excessive stress hormones (adrenalin and noradrenalin) are secreted, the heart muscle becomes more irritable and liable to "skipped beats," the heart rate and blood pressure increase, and the workload of the heart rises. Thus, while many patients with coronary artery disease apparently respond to exercise in the same manner as normal, healthy middle-aged individuals, some will react in an abnormal and potentially dangerous manner. The more serious and extensive the disease, the greater the likelihood that the heart will respond abnormally. Therefore, the post-coronary patient should approach exercise with due caution. Neither exercise stress tests nor post-coronary exercise classes should be undertaken lightly. Why then, you may ask, take the risk at all? Do the benefits of training outweigh the possible hazards?

A study carried out in conjunction with Dr. Roy Shephard showed that of 203 consecutive cases referred for post-coronary rehabilitation, 60 were engaged in vigorous physical activity at or shortly before the time of their heart attack. The breakdown was as follows:

Heavy domestic chores	14	Baseball	1
Walking	13	Soccer	1
Snow-shovelling	9	Basketball	1
Running	8	Hockey	1
Curling	4	Squash	1
Tennis	2	Gymnastics	1
Sexual intercourse	2	Dancing	1
Ice-breaking	1		

If acute exercise can cause a heart attack, how can chronic exercise be a suitable form of therapy? The answer is that an acute bout of unaccustomed physical activity merely reveals the presence of a diseased coronary artery system which is already highly susceptible to physical and mental stress. This is largely unavoidable; most of us face excessive activity at some time or another. Training prepares us for such emergencies and reduces the danger of such episodes.

CHRONIC EXERCISE (TRAINING) AND ITS BENEFITS

Constant repetition of an acute bout of activity constitutes chronic exercise, or training. There is now a good deal of data available on the beneficial effects of training on the heart as well as on the other body systems which influence the heart. We will now examine the information under the headings of psychological and physical effects, and further subdivide the latter into a discussion of changes that occur within the heart, and changes that occur in the body as a whole. Needless to say, such a division is arbitrary and artificial since, as with all human performance, considerable overlap and interplay occurs between all three.

Psychological Benefits

As we have seen earlier, the survivor of a heart attack frequently

	AVERAGE REDUCTION IN DEPRESSION SCORE (%)
ADHERENTS TO JOGGING PROGRAM (N = 38)	*13%*
NON-COMPLIERS	*NO CHANGE*

Table 1 Four Year Follow-up of Depression in 44 Post Heart Attack Patients on Jogging Program

	% CHANGE
TENSION/ANXIETY	SIGNIFICANTLY REDUCED BY 19%
DEPRESSION/DEJECTION	'' '' BY 23%
ANGER/HOSTILITY	'' '' BY 14%
VIGOUR	INCREASED BY 16%

Table 2   Change in Mood after One Year on an Exercise Program (317 patients)

suffers from mental depression. Even after physical recovery is apparently complete, this may continue to be a major problem. Psychological evaluation of patients referred to the Toronto program has consistently shown that between one-third and one-half of these individuals can have quite profound depression. Fortunately we have found a considerable improvement over one year of training. A four-year follow-up of 44 of our most severely depressed subjects showed a very significant and substantial benefit, and we were also able to report that this was related directly to compliance with our exercise program (Table 1). Recently, we have also reported that 317 male post-heart-attack patients who have completed one year of training on the Toronto program have less tension and hostility as well as more confidence and increased feelings of vigour (Table 2).

The explanation for this training-induced improvement in mood could well be chemical. Recently scientists have isolated from the brain and other nervous tissue a number of naturally occurring substances called peptides which have opium-like qualities. One of these, beta-endorphin, has been reported to increase significantly in the blood after bouts of exertion. Furthermore, it has also been shown that regular training augments this response. While we still need to do considerably more work in this area, evidence at the moment is highly suggestive that the physical "high" experienced by those who work out regularly, as well as the post-training session feelings of relaxation and physical gratification, are due to release of these natural opiates. The value of such training-induced improvements in mood and self-esteem cannot be over-emphasized. The patient with heart disease who exercises on a regular basis is not only more health conscious, but has greater fortitude to give up cigarette smoking, maintain an ideal body weight, avoid a high fat diet, and choose a prudent balance between work and recreation. In short, avoid many of the lifestyle risk factors associated with coronary artery disease.

Training and the Heart

One must be careful not to apply conclusions drawn from animal studies to humans; nevertheless, I think it is fair to say that this type of investigation does demonstrate that regular training brings about beneficial changes in the structure, function, and circulation of the heart.

It has been known for some considerable time that the wild animal has a larger heart than its domestic equivalent. We can argue forever whether this difference is due to the presence or absence of regular physical activity, or whether it is due to a trait of heredity. More to the point, however, are the experiments in which coronary artery disease and its clinical manifestations (heart attack and sudden death) are induced in animals, thereby allowing study of various treatment procedures, including exercise.

The classical example of this latter approach is the study carried out by Dr. Richard Eckstein. This scientist took a group of ninety dogs and, using surgical thread, artificially narrowed their coronary arteries to give them varying severities of non-fatal heart attacks. He then divided them into two groups, one group being confined to cages and the other put on an exercise program consisting of 20 minutes of running on a treadmill, five times weekly. At the end of a six- to eight-week period he measured blood flow through the coronary arteries, and noted that the exercised dogs had compensated for their narrowed blood vessels by developing new branches; these new branches are known medically as collaterals. The sedentary dogs, on the other hand, showed no such effect. Eckstein concluded that "the judicious use of early and continued physical exercise may reduce the clinical manifestations of coronary disease."

Potentially fatal heart attacks can also be induced in the animal, and exercise has been shown to reduce by one-half the incidence of sudden death in dogs who have had one of their major coronary arteries tied off. One of the most relevant investigations in this area has been carried out by Dr. Tim Noakes of South Africa, whose sophisticated study demonstrated that the hearts of rats who had been subjected to an intensive distance-running type of training (running on an inclined treadmill two hours a day) developed a significantly greater resistance to electrically induced cardiac arrest after a main coronary artery had been tied off than did the hearts of a sedentary control group.

Monkeys are probably considered closer to man than other animals, which is one of the reasons why I find the work of Dr. Dieter Kramsch using Macaca monkeys particularly exciting and provocative. He reported a study which involved feeding a diet very high in animal fat to a sedentary control group of monkeys and also to a group conditioned by an exercise program "comparable to jogging in human beings" (one hour of running on the treadmill, three times a week, for three and a half years). At the end of the study, the exercisers were found to have substantially larger hearts and significantly less disease of the coronary arteries. Not only that, but they had wider coronary arteries than even those sedentary animals that were fed on a normal monkey diet. It is also of interest to note that the exercise group had significantly higher blood levels of "good" (HDL) cholesterol, and much lower levels of "bad" (LDL) cholesterol and triglycerides.

The human heart responds to exercise training by changes in dimension and performance. It is nearly one hundred years ago since the first observation was made that fit long distance skiers had large hearts, and the fitter and more successful the skier, the larger his heart. This led to the coining of the term "athlete's heart," meaning a heart which as a result of regular training was healthy, efficient, and powerful. Unfortunately, in later years the paradox arose in that "athlete's heart" came to be synonymous with a diseased heart. How could such a situation arise?

The explanation was as follows: the physician (who, incidentally, rarely gets the opportunity to examine and study superlatively healthy subjects) has always equated an enlarged heart with disease. A failing heart will dilate, and thus increase in size. A heart which is working for years against the pressure of a defective valve or a malformation of the large blood vessels will develop enormously thickened muscular walls, and this will also increase its size. Small wonder then that the examining physician, used to dealing with disease rather than health, is inclined to look with some suspicion on the athlete with a big heart, despite the fact that he cannot find any evidence of the diseases which customarily cause the pathological enlargement. Even when the subject is a world champion in his sport and can out-perform practically all his competitors, some doctors are still not convinced that the enlargement in this particular case goes hand-in-hand with the very opposite of disease — that is, positive health. And where numerous investigations fail to unearth any evidence of danger, they may still murmur dire warnings of future ill-health, reduced longevity, and even sudden death.

With the advent of better methods to observe, delineate, and measure the exact nature of the heart enlargement which comes with training, we have been able to allay these fears. X-rays and, in the last few years, the use of echocardiography (a form of x-ray using sound waves to picture the heart and its movements) have shown that the ventricles or pumping chambers of the endurance athlete's heart possess increased volume and capacity. This volume enlargement is physiological, not pathological, and rarely attains the exaggerated sizes found in the heart grossly dilated by disease. Further studies have confirmed that these changes result from a good training program; furthermore, it has been found that the heart reverts to normal size after discontinuance of training for a period of time. Where the training is commenced in youth and continues through to middle age, this beneficial enlargement may persist for many years.

I think by now that the old bogey of "athlete's heart syndrome" (syndrome being the collective term used for the clinical signs of a disease) has been well and truly laid to rest. Most modern physicians recognize that endurance athletes have larger hearts; that the enlargement is associated with health rather than with disease, and that the enlargement rarely exceeds a safe physiological level, which is in direct contrast with the excessive enlargements seen in patients suffering from certain disease. Not only this but the healthy size increase is accompanied by a proportionate increase in the size and number of blood vessels of the coronary artery tree.

So far we have been discussing cardiac changes which occur in normal individuals as a result of training. Can they also occur in

middle-aged subjects with coronary artery disease? It is understandable that to date reports of such cardiac responses to training have been sparse. After all, only in recent years have healthy
middle-aged individuals become involved in regular exercise on
a mass basis. The involvement of heart disease patients in such
regimes is an even later innovation. Alternatively, it could be that
the training methods used with patients have been inadequate in
terms of intensity and duration, or that such patients adhere less
faithfully to the training methods or finally, that the procedures
used to discover and measure changes in heart size have been
too crude. Some support for all these might be inferred from two
recent reports which appeared in the medical literature. The first,
using radioactive dye to visualize the ventricles of the heart,
demonstrated increase in the volume of these pumping chambers in fourteen patients with coronary artery disease who completed six months of a jogging program which required them to
work out for 30 minutes, five times weekly. Similarly, echocardiography recorded similar significant size increases in the ventricles of eight post heart attack patients who faithfully complied
with a twelve-month jogging program which worked up to one-
hour training sessions, five times weekly. In my opinion, as more
and more coronary artery disease patients are involved in worthwhile exercise programs, we can expect to see an increasing
number of similar reports in the medical literature.

Of course, heart size is one thing, performance is another. How
does training affect cardiac performance? The most characteristic
result of regular exercise is a drop in the resting and exercising
heart rate. This is referred to medically as bradycardia (Greek for
slow heart). It is so characteristic of fitness that if it does not occur
in the individual who is on a training program, you can be sure
that the subject is either not adhering faithfully to that program,
or that the training regime is badly designed.

Since the heart is now beating more slowly at rest and at all
levels of exertion, it compensates for this by expelling more blood
per beat. This increase in stroke volume is another characteristic
of the trained heart. The bottom line is a more efficient cardiac
pump.

The trained heart brings with it another advantage. There is
a limit to the maximum speed or rate at which the heart will pump.
This figure is age-related, reducing from about 200 per minute
when we are in our teens to about 170 or 160 per minute when we

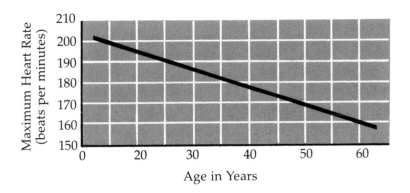

Figure 11   The Older You Are the Lower Your Maximum Heart Rate

are in our sixties and seventies (Figure 11). As far as we can tell, training will not increase one's maximum heart rate. Thus, if that were the limiting factor then there would appear to be no way in which we could improve our performance in any of the endurance type sports or games if we are in the older age groups, since these activities require a highly efficient and copious supply of blood to the exercising muscles. And yet experience teaches us that sedentary middle-aged individuals who begin to train for the first time when they are in their forties or even their fifties are capable of vast improvements in physical condition and performance. The answer is, of course, that maximum cardiac output is enhanced by an improvement in maximum stroke volume.

This increase in stroke volume and cardiac output has always seemed a logical explanation for improvement with training. However, demonstrating it experimentally in humans has been difficult. Experimental work done in the 1960s and 1970s gave us strong presumptive evidence of improved stroke volume, but it was not until the 1980s that echocardiography clearly demonstrated superior heart muscle performance in experienced long distance runners, as well as previously sedentary male and female subjects who had satisfactorily completed a period of jogging training.

It should be noted that in evaluation reports covering the effects of training on the heart function of coronary patients, we should not overlook the type, duration and intensity of training employed, for this may explain some of the apparent contradictions. For instance, Dr. Robert Bruce of Seattle reported no increase in stroke volume improvement in cardiac performance in a group of twelve post heart attack patients who were trained for three months on a regime of calisthenics, walking, jogging, and running, each workout lasting for 45 minutes and repeated three times weekly. On the other hand, a scientific study carried out on forty-six patients enrolled in the Toronto Rehabilitation Centre's program demonstrated stroke volume had increased by some 10 per cent in those patients who were assigned to the exercise group. This was not apparent, however, until after twelve months of high-intensity jogging workouts. Indeed, the findings after the first six months were similar to those of Dr. Bruce, the improvements in heart performance not becoming apparent until after one year. In a similar vein, Dr. Ali Ehsani of Washington University also found a five-days-a-week jogging routine lasting one year was required to produce echocardiographic evidence of improvement in cardiac performance of his post heart attack patients.

As we have seen, increase in heart size is paralleled by a proportional increase in the diameter and number of branches of the coronary vessels, together with an increase in the tiny capillary blood vessels which course through the substance of the heart muscle. In this way, blood supply keeps pace with demand. Clarence de Mar, a famous American long distance running champion, died of cancer in his seventies; an autopsy of his heart revealed that his coronary arteries were unusually large. While this may be the result of natural endowment, it seems more likely to have been brought about by his many years of intensive training. Large coronary arteries are a distinct advantage in that they are unlikely to be blocked by even a lifetime's deposit of fatty atheromatous material. Maybe this is why myocardial infarction is a rare occurrence in active marathoners, even though a significant number of these men are middle-aged. In the previous chapter we noted that oxygen-rich blood flowed through the coronary arteries to supply the heart muscle between beats (that is, during the resting phase, or diastole). Thus, the higher the heart rate, the shorter the time between beats. Conversely, the slower the heart rate, the greater the proportion of time spent in diastole. Fitness bradycardia, therefore, is synonymous with a lengthening of diastole and an increase in coronary blood flow.

As if an improved blood supply to the heart were not enough, the fit exerciser has a further advantage over his sedentary counterpart. Fitness brings with it a reduction in the blood supply requirements of the heart. The slowly beating heart muscle uses oxygen more sparingly, and so the blood flow does not need to be so vigorous. It is a case of living well within one's cardiac budget. The oxygen income is potentially high, while at the same time the expenditure is low. Obviously, this affords a high measure of safety, with adequate protection from the vicissitudes of modern life, including disease.

All of the beneficial changes described above are very impressive, and they go a long way towards explaining why the fit heart is a healthy heart. But if we do not possess the exotic equipment required to measure such changes, we would still be left with the simplest and yet one of the most important observations of all — the effect of training on the heart rate. We have already seen that training reduces the resting and exercising heart rate. It has a similar effect on blood pressure. We can obtain a very accurate index of the amount of work being done by the heart at any given time by *multiplying the heart rate by the blood pressure*. The result of this simple mathematical calculation is known as the *Double Product*, or, as some people call it, the Rate Pressure Product. Thus, if while sitting quietly reading this book your heart rate was found to be 72/min. and your blood pressure 120mm Hg, then the work being carried out by your heart would be represented by a double product of 8,640 (72 × 120 = 8,640). Assuming you were to put this book down, stand up, run vigorously on the spot for a few minutes so as to bring your heart rate up to 102/min. and your blood pressure up to 140mm Hg, then you would have increased your Double Product, and therefore the amount of work your heart would have been required to do, to a figure of 14,280 (102 × 140 = 14,280). Obviously, if training gives you a lower heart rate and a lower blood pressure for a given intensity of exercise, then this results in a lower Double Product and thus a reduced workload on the heart. Physiologically, you are getting more for your money.

Since the Double Product measures the work of the heart, it can be used as a benchmark for the onset or development of angina pectoris. You will recall that angina is the chest pain resulting from cramp of heart muscle, which is in turn due to reduced coronary blood supply. The level of cardiac work at which the patient experiences angina is known as his angina threshold. This threshold can be expressed in terms of the Double Product. It is usually constant for any individual angina sufferer.

We now come to the crux of the matter. Since training reduces the heart rate and the blood pressure, both at rest and during exercise, it therefore reduces the Double Product for all levels of activity. The net result is to raise the angina threshold.

Let us suppose that an individual develops angina at a Double Product of 18,000. This is his angina threshold, and, if he exercises vigorously enough to bring his heart rate up to 120/min., and his blood pressure to 150 mm Hg, he will experience symptoms. If, after training, the same bout of exercise increases his heart rate only to 100/min. and his blood pressure to 130 mm Hg, then his Double Product would be only 13,000, he would not have reached his angina threshold, and consequently he would not have any problems. The fitter he gets, the more work he can do without symptoms. Thus, even if the reduction or elimination of angina which results from the training program were not due to increased blood supply to the heart, it could still be explained on the basis of a reduced Double Product.

As the angina improves we often see improvement in the exercise electrocardiogram. Again, this can be explained either on the basis of an increased coronary blood flow, or a reduced Double Product at that workload. We have shown that post-coronary patients can be brought to a high level of fitness through an intensive training program. Evidence to date suggests that these fortunate individuals not only get relief from chest discomfort at a given workload, but also push their angina threshold higher and higher, until they can perform even maximum exercise tests without developing subjective or objective evidence of cardiac ischemia. These are the men who have attained jogging distance of four miles or up, averaging twenty-five or more miles a week for over two years or more.

But why is it that some post-coronary exercisers are unable to attain such intensity of training? Is it a question of being less motivated? Or is it that they are physiologically incapable of meeting the demands of the program, either because of age, or because of the severity of their disease? These are questions which we cannot as yet answer, but hopefully we will be able to do so as our research progresses.

Other Benefits

Most of these benefits have been referred to elsewhere under the appropriate sections. However, for completeness' sake they will be outlined here again in point form.

1. The large muscles of the leg and trunk (the so-called skeletal muscles) develop a greater blood supply, as well as an increase in the size and function of the specialized cells (mitochondria) which extract and utilize the oxygen from the blood. This improvement at the delivery end, as it were, of the oxygen transport chain means less effort is required at the source, i.e. the pumping heart. The fact that these peripheral gains are possible and, indeed, inevitable in a good endurance training program explains why individuals whose initial cardiac status is quite poor can nevertheless benefit from a carefully prescribed training program.

2. We have seen that emotional stress releases epinephrine and norepinephrine, raising blood pressure, increasing heart rate, and elevating blood sugar and blood fat levels. The body is prepared for physical action. However, in the absence of such action, and in the presence of atherosclerosis, these responses are unnecessary and harmful. Regular physical activity combats the situation. The working muscles burn off the excess fat and sugar and, by demanding an increased blood supply, provide a "run-off" for the enhanced cardiac output. Not only that, but increasing fitness leads to a reduction in the stress-induced secretion of epinephrine and norepinephrine.

    We have seen earlier that coronary thrombosis may be due to increased stickiness of the small, disc-like blood cells called platelets, and that both stress and smoking-induced epinephrine will exaggerate platelet stickiness. Again, there is evidence to suggest that physical training has the opposite effect. A group of 69 healthy men and women who were put on a ten-week jogging program were found at the end of the training period to have augmented the clot-dissolving property of their blood by 50 per cent. Even more exciting is the report that a small group of patients who had survived a heart attack and who spent six months on a walk-jog training program showed a 40 per cent reduction in epinephrine-induced platelet stickiness.

Research into the effect of training on blood content and blood behaviour is still in the early stages, but the results already are highly thought-provoking.

3. Since the 1960s there has been increasing scientific evidence showing an inverse relationship between ''good'' or high density lipoprotein (HDL) cholesterol and the risk of developing coronary artery disease. Subsequent reports indicated that those who participate in regular jogging programs have a high percentage of HDL cholesterol. Not only have these gains been reported in healthy individuals, but also in survivors of heart attacks (see pages 34, 36).

4. A number of studies show that physical training improves sugar tolerance in the mild diabetic. Interestingly enough, exercise was a main form of therapy for diabetes before insulin was discovered, but it seems to have been neglected by physicians since then. The active diabetic requires less insulin, and it is well known clinically that the sedentary diabetic requires to increase his insulin dosage. The precise mechanism by which this comes about is uncertain, but it seems to be connected with the development of a more efficient carbohydrate metabolism. There may also be an indirect connection between certain high blood fats and a tendency to diabetes, and so reduction in the former could be of benefit to the latent diabetic. Weight control is an important feature in the management of diabetes and so a reduction in weight due to physical activity may be yet another aspect of the problem.

If we consider the benefits discussed above, it seems fair to argue that the task of training post-coronary patients is no mere academic exercise. In particular, the reduction of the Double Product at a given intensity of work is unquestionable. There is no shortage of evidence that training is physiologically beneficial. But can it increase the lifespan of the heart attack victim by reducing the frequency and severity of recurrent attacks? And if it can, what is the optimum intensity, duration and frequency of exercise sessions required? Are men who devote themselves to the demanding program of 20 or 30 miles of jogging each week going to gain a more decisive advantage over those who remain content with one or two weekly sessions of calisthenics?

These and similar problems will be discussed more fully in the second part of this book which deals with the inception and operation of a post-coronary exercise rehabilitation program over the past sixteen years. However, before closing this section, we must examine the method by which response to training is measured. This is a vital part of any exercise program, providing feedback not only for the exerciser, but also for the trainer, be he coach or physician.

CHAPTER FIVE

Exercise Testing

In recent years, exercise physiologists and physical educators have become increasingly interested in the measurement of endurance fitness, leading them to invade areas long regarded as the province of the physician. Laboratory testing of high-performance endurance athletes has shown that the most valid measurement of superiority is maximum oxygen consumption (VO_2 max) which is another way of saying efficiency of the oxygen transport system. The most vital link in this system, of course, is the heart, which pumps the oxygen-rich blood to the muscles.

In principle, measurement of the amount of oxygen an individual can utilize is easy. The air we breathe in contains 21 per cent oxygen. Analysis of the air we breathe out (the technical term is "expired gas") will show a reduction in this figure; the difference represents the amount of oxygen consumed by our muscles. The more vigorously the muscles contract, the more oxygen they require. Ultimately, however, the point will be reached where the oxygen transport system can no longer cope with the increasing demand of the muscles for oxygen. Heart rate and stroke volume have reached their zenith. So far, and no further, they say; or to use a modern analogy, the engine has run out of gas.

Maximum Exercise Test with Measurement of Oxygen Consumption

Posed with the task of measuring someone's maximum oxygen consumption, you would need to estimate the oxygen consumed in carrying out increasingly vigorous physical tasks until exhaustion supervenes, taking the final figures as the VO_2 max. Expressed in scientific jargon, what you have done is progressed the subject through multi-stage standardized workloads while continuously measuring oxygen intake; the end point is reached when the subject cannot continue because of exhaustion.

A discerning reader may detect a weakness in this description. What if the subject voluntarily quits before his muscles have reached the limit of their performance, before they are totally exhausted? It may be that his threshold for physical discomfort is low and that he is not prepared to push himself to this limit. There is no doubt that motivation plays a large part in the successful accomplishment of a maximum test, and this is one of its drawbacks. It is, however, possible to tell if the maximum level has been reached. Analysis of expired gas samples will show that the amount of oxygen consumed has plateaued, despite an increase in the final workload. For example, increasing the speed of walking will increase the amount of oxygen consumed in a linear fashion until eventually the walking speed will outstrip the muscle's ability to function aerobically. At this point, anaerobic muscle contraction will take over; but, as we have seen, this is a wasteful and self-limiting process, building up lactic acid and forcing matters to a halt within sixty seconds or so. Measurement of the oxygen content of the expired gas will now show that it is the same or only fractionally more than that for the speed immediately preceding it. Professor Roy Shephard has recommended that an increase in oxygen consumption of less than 2 millilitres per minute per kilogram body weight for a 10 per cent increase in workload intensity can be accepted as proof that the subject has attained maximum effort; this is the standard used in our laboratory. Another indication of supreme effort is the high level of lactic acid in the blood as a result of the final few seconds of anaerobic activity. Of course, there will also be the more usual signs of acute exhaustion, such as leg fatigue, staggering gait, facial pallor, nausea, gasping for breath and extremely high heart rate.

It will now be obvious that measurement of endurance fitness by maximum testing is a somewhat arduous procedure. It is usually carried out in the exercise laboratory on a treadmill, a piece of equipment which consists essentially of a moving belt, approximately three feet wide, on which the subject walks or runs. The speed and/or elevation of the belt is increased in a step-like man-

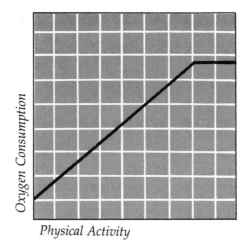

Physical Activity

Figure 12   The More Vigorous Your Physical Activity, the More Oxygen Your Body Uses.

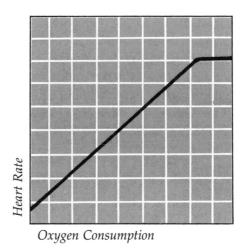

Oxygen Consumption

Figure 13   As You Use More Oxygen in Physical Activity, Your Heart Rate Increases Accordingly

Age	Maximum heart Rate	75% Maximum Heart Rate
20	197	148
25	195	146
30	193	144
35	191	143
40	189	142
45	187	140
50	184	138
55	182	137
60	180	135
65	178	134
70	176	132
75	174	131
80	172	129
85	170	128
90	168	126

Table 3   Age-Related Maximum Heart Rates

ner every two or three minutes. The treadmill is bulky, noisy and frightening to subjects who have never been on one before. At high speeds, it is potentially dangerous, especially when the subject has become unco-ordinated as a result of maximum effort. In general, then, the sedentary middle-aged and the elderly are unsuitable candidates for maximal testing. How then can we assess the cardiovascular fitness of these individuals?

Sub-maximal Exercise Test with Measurement of Oxygen Consumption

Fortunately, there is a method which is based on two very convenient facts. One is that oxygen consumption increases in a straight line in response to augmentation of effort (Figure 12). The second is that heart rate and oxygen consumption are related in the same fashion (Figure 13). And since everyone has a maximum heart rate which decreases with age, this has led to the construction of tables containing average values for the population at large (Table 3). A little reflection will enable us to put these three pieces of information together and come up with a method of predicting an individual's maximum oxygen consumption from the measurement at a sub-maximal level of exertion. For example, having determined from the tables that the maximum heart rate for a 45-year-old subject is 187/min., one can take 75 percent of this, i.e., 140/min., and aim to attain that figure in the test—provided, of course, that no adverse signs or symptoms occur prior to that level.

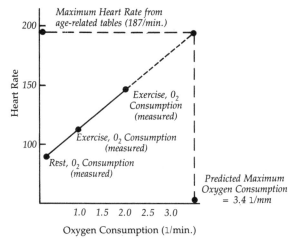

Figure 14   Oxygen Consumption

The principle of sub-maximum exercise testing is as follows. The 45-year-old subject's heart rate and oxygen consumption are measured at rest and at two sub-maximum levels of effort. These values are plotted on a graph, the points joined, and the resulting line extended to intersect the upper horizontal axis (the subject's maximum heart rate as read from the age-related tables). The maximum oxygen consumption is then read off from the lower horizontal axis.

In order to predict the maximum oxygen consumption from the sub-maximal test, one measures heart rate and oxygen consumption at rest and then at two or three workloads, the final workload being gauged so as to achieve the 75 per cent target of 140/min. These are plotted on a graph, and then, since the relationship between heart rate and oxygen consumption is linear, the points can be joined and extrapolated to the maximum heart rate figure of 187/min. The oxygen consumption of 3.4 litres per minute is then read back from the other axis (Figure 14).

It usually takes a few minutes for the heart rate and oxygen consumption to stabilize at any given workload, and the test protocol calls for the subject to work a minimum of three minutes at each load to ensure the so-called "steady state" as being reached.

The validity of sub-maximal testing is dependent upon the accuracy of the maximum heart rate tables, and while purists will prefer to establish the actual figure by maximum testing, by and large the tables are correct to within a range of 10 per cent. For practical purposes, this is quite adequate, and is a reasonable trade-off for the inherent difficulties and dangers of maximum testing. When measuring the fitness level of patients who are suffering from coronary heart disease, one has to be particularly careful, and submaximal testing has obvious advantages.

Some physicians argue that the maximum heart rate is frequently reduced in coronary artery disease and that the use of heart rate maximum tables is not justified. However, I have compared the results of maximum and sub-maximum tests on a group of heart attack patients, and found that their maximum heart rates are frequently within normal limits, and that the predicted values for VO_2 max are close enough to the actual measurements to be perfectly acceptable from a clinical point of view.

There is one important situation, however, in which the tables will not be correct. Certain cardiac medications, particularly the beta-blockers such as Inderal, tend to drop the heart rate. Patients on these drugs, therefore, will have lower maximum heart rates than shown on the tables. Because the reduction is linear—i.e., if the resting heart rate is reduced by ten beats per minute, the maximum rate is reduced by the same amount—some allowance can be made for this. However, prediction of maximum oxygen consumption from a sub-maximal heart rate becomes much less accurate a procedure. In these cases, the practice of collecting and analysing the patient's expired air is very valuable. It not only allows us to directly measure the oxygen consumption of the body at each workload, it also alerts us as to when the patient is approaching his maximum effort. For example, if we were to assume that our patient's maximum heart rate was 184/min. when in fact it had been reduced to 150/min. by the use of Inderal, then were we to rely on heart rate alone, we might inadvertently push him to maximum effort, when in fact our aim was a sub-maximal test.

This use of direct oxygen measurement is facilitated by modern computerized equipment which permits us to analyse the expired air almost on a breath-to-breath basis. Thus, we can literally watch the patient's oxygen consumption increase as we step up the resistance of the bicycle pedals (or increase the speed of the treadmill) and so force him to work harder and harder. Instant graphs of oxygen consumption and carbon dioxide production plotted against workload and rate of breathing also allow us a further bonus—the identification during the test of another level of effort intensity known as "anaerobic threshold" (AT). This is the point at which working muscle begins to produce dispropor-

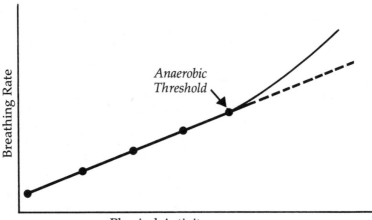

Physical Activity

Figure 15   Anaerobic Threshold
The anaerobic threshold is the point at which the relationship between breathing and exercise becomes non-linear. This is an appropriate level of exertion for endurance training.

tionately more carbon dioxide than was needed at lower work-loads. The increased carbon dioxide is blown out through the lungs, resulting in a sharp increase in the breathing rate. Graphically, the anaerobic threshold is seen to occur at the point where the breathing rate line becomes steeper (Figure 15).

The AT occurs at about 40 to 70 per cent of maximum effort, and so can be determined without having recourse to a maximum test. Its importance lies in the fact that it occurs at about the intensity of effort required for endurance fitness training. However, in contrast to heart rate, the AT is unaffected by beta-blockers.

A further simplification of the exercise test, maximal or submaximal, is the use of tables which relate workload to average oxygen consumption. These tables have been developed from samples of the normal population at large and provide an alternative to actually collecting and analysing the air.

This is the approach most frequently adopted by hospital cardiology departments, where exercise testing is used more to detect and diagnose coronary artery disease than to determine fitness level or prescribe an exercise training program. The emphasis here is on observing the effects of physical effort on symptoms, heart rate, blood pressure, and electrocardiogram. Newer developments have been the use of echocardiography and also radioactive ''scanning'' to observe effort-induced abnormalities in cardiac appearance or performance. However, more of that later.

Exercise Testing Equipment

Exercise testing can be performed on a treadmill, a set of steps, or a stationary bicycle. Steps are awkward if the subject is expected to breathe into a gas collection apparatus. The stationary bicycle is the most convenient, provided the thigh muscles are not so weak that they give out before the heart rate has achieved the desired level—an occasional occurrence in North Americans who are unaccustomed to cycling (actually, this is one of the major reasons for choosing the treadmill over the bicycle in maximal testing). The type of bicycle used delivers a measured workload by applying resistance to the drive-wheel either mechanically by means of a friction belt, or electrically by a variable magnetic field. The resistance must be constant, and accurately reproducible from test to test. Incidentally, the home exercise bicycle which uses a crude screw and tension spring arrangement to adjust workload is useless for this purpose. The great advantage of the stationary bicycle is its cost ($500 to $1,000 as opposed to $5,000 and up for a motor-driven treadmill), and the fact that it allows the upper portion of the body to remain relatively free from movement during the test. This makes for greater convenience in collecting expired gas and obtaining blood pressure readings and good quality electrocardiograph tracings.

Use of the Electrocardiogram in Testing

So far, we have only considered the application of exercise testing to the measurement of maximum oxygen consumption. This requires the recording of heart rate and, in most cases, the collection of expired air for analysis. A heart rate may be counted manually by feeling the pulse at the wrist or in the neck, or it may be obtained by the use of a cardiotachometer, an instrument which picks up the heart beat from an electrode applied to the chest and transmits it by a solid wire lead to the dial of a counter. The more normal method, however, is to connect the subject to an electrocardiogram so that a simultaneous ECG tracing is obtained throughout the test. This has two advantages: it allows the physician to count the number of electrical complexes every few seconds, thus obtaining a very accurate heart rate count; it also permits detection of irregularities in the rhythm and shape of the electrical signals indicative of cardiac stress.

As a matter of fact, it is this simultaneous recording of the ECG tracing during exercise which has interested the cardiologists most, ever since it was discovered that latent coronary heart disease could frequently be detected in this manner. A patient with advanced atherosclerosis of his coronary arteries and consequent impairment of blood supply to his heart will often show evidence of this in his resting (or static) ECG. But what if the atherosclerotic narrowing is not so severe, and the myocardial blood supply only becomes inadequate when the heart has to work hard? In such cases, the static ECG might well be normal. Only an ECG recorded during exercise (a dynamic ECG) will demonstrate the abnormality. The milder the degree of disease, the higher the intensity of exercise needed for its detection.

In the final analysis, sub-maximal or maximal exercise testing can be used to diagnose hitherto unsuspected heart disease in an individual who has no apparent evidence of any abnormality. By the same token, the completion of a maximum exercise test without the development of ECG irregularities is highly indicative of freedom from coronary disease.

The work of Robb and Blackburn has indicated that such testing may be able to predict whether or not the subject will have a heart attack in the future. Over a twelve-year period, they subjected a group of 1,659 life insurance applicants to an exercise test which involved stair-stepping followed by immediate post-exercise electrocardiograms. All of the applicants were free from impairment which would call for rejection of their applications. The cardiac response to exercise testing was abnormal in 269 individuals (16.2 per cent), and when followed over the years, these subjects had a death rate from heart attacks two and a half to thirteen times higher than those with normal exercise tests, the frequency increasing with the abnormality of the exercise response. Furthermore, even in those subjects who were considered on the basis of pre-test medical evidence to have probable or definite coronary heart disease, the dynamic electrocardiogram proved to be a significant forecaster of mortality; a positive exercise response in these people was followed by a five-fold increase in coronary death rate; a negative response meant a more benign outlook despite the previous poor history.

While underlining the diagnostic value of the step-exercise test, the authors in their report went on to postulate that there may have been some cases of heart disease undetected ''because they were not exercised enough to make it manifest.'' Hence, the increasing interest by cardiologists in maximal and high sub-maximal treadmill and bicycle tests, with simultaneous dynamic electrocardiogram recordings.

Thallium Exercise Test

This is a non-invasive procedure involving the use of a small amount of radioactive tracer substance, thallium (similar to potassium), which is injected into the forearm vein in the final minute of a maximum exercise test. The thallium is carried in the blood stream through the coronary arteries to the heart, where it can be visualized by a highly sensitive "Gamma" camera and converted into an image on a film. An area of the heart which is scarred from a previous heart attack will not have as profuse a blood supply as the surrounding healthy heart muscle, and so will outline only faintly on the film. If the size of this defect remains fixed on a series of pictures taken for the two-hour period following exercise, this verifies that it is indeed due to an old scar. On the other hand, if it is maximal at peak exercise and gradually diminishes in size as the heart rate slowly returns to resting level, then it indicates that the coronary artery supplying that segment of heart is narrowed and can only maintain adequate circulation at low work levels. The thallium exercise test, then, does not provide us with a picture of the coronary arteries, but it allows us to make inferences about the state of the arteries from radioactive pictures of the regions they supply.

The test is quite painless, and the amount of radioactive exposure is no greater than that one would get from a normal x-ray. The test is only carried out in specialized medical centres, since the equipment used is both expensive and complex. Furthermore, because a series of pictures may have to be taken at about half-hourly intervals after the exercise test, the procedure can be rather time-consuming.

Echocardiography

This method has been refined considerably in recent years. High-frequency sound waves are generated by an ultra-sonic machine, "bounced" off the heart, and these sound echoes converted into electrical energy to be displayed visually on an oscilloscope. From the resultant image, one can determine the size of the heart's chambers, the thickness of its walls, and the efficiency of its performance. If the examination is done before and immediately after exercise, one is even better able to detect abnormalities in pumping capacity. There is no radioactivity involved, and the patient feels nothing during the examination. The whole process takes approximately half an hour. The technique has still to be developed to the stage where the procedure becomes routine.

WARNING SIGNS IN TESTING

In recent years, a number of objective criteria for labelling an exercise test "abnormal" or predictive of ischemic heart disease have emerged. They are: (1) ST segment depression, (2) irregular heart action, (3) inappropriate blood pressure response to exercise, and (4) inappropriate heart rate response to exercise. Since this requires some explanation, we will deal with each separately.

ST Segment Depression or "Silent Angina"

The beating heart muscle produces minute amounts of electricity which, when amplified, can be recorded on a piece of moving graph paper (Figure 16). Each spike on the tracing is labelled by a letter for convenience of reference, and represents electrical activity in a different portion of the heart. The P wave is caused by the upper chamber of the heart, the atrium, contracting. The QRS complex is caused by the ventricles "discharging" as they squeeze blood out of the chambers. The T wave marks the recovery phase when the ventricles "recharge" their electrical energy. The portion of the tracing between the S and the start of the T wave is known as the ST segment.

You will notice that in the normal heart each labelled deflection of the tracing returns directly to the mid-line, or "iso-electric" line, as soon as it has reached its peak. The iso-electric line represents electrical neutrality. When the ventricle has completed its contraction (the S point of the QRS complex), it has discharged its electricity, and so the trace returns quickly to neutral before commencing to recharge again (T wave). In other words, the ST segment ascends vertically and without delay to the iso-electric line. In cases of ischemic heart disease, however, this prompt ascent may be delayed, in which case, the moving graph paper will show a "depression" of the ST segment (Figure 17).

The greater the degree of depression (measured as x in the diagram), the more severe the degree of ischemia. Actually, this change in the ST segment merely tells us that the heart muscle is short of oxygen; it does not tell us why. For instance, the patient may be anemic, or may be suffering from a form of thyroid disease,

Figure 16   Normal Electrocardiogram

Figure 17   Electrocardiogram Showing Depression of the S-T Segment Indicating Reduced Blood Flow Through the Coronary Arteries

or may be taking a type of medication which results in a similar picture. However, since coronary heart disease is by far the most common cause of heart muscle ischemia these days, depression of the ST segment has become characteristic of that condition. Obviously, the physician will know if the patient is on the sort of medication which gives a "false" ST segment depression.

In practice, the electrocardiogram tracing at the beginning of the test may well be normal. Only as the level of work increases does the ST segment begin to sag. Sometimes this may not occur until the patient is exerting himself to 85 per cent or more of his maximum. Not infrequently the depression will revert to normal almost immediately on stopping the exercise — hence the insistence of some physicians on obtaining concurrent tracings during the test rather than relying on immediate post-exercise electrocardiograms. By international agreement, a depression of the ST segment measuring more than 2 mm is considered abnormal. It is highly likely that such a response is evidence of coronary heart disease, and the greater the depression, the higher the likelihood of a heart attack in the future. That is not to say that a positive test is an irrevocable portent of tragedy. No test is one hundred per cent certain. Nevertheless, the evidence favours acceptance of a high degree of predictability—enough to make the individual with a positive exercise test take steps to avoid future trouble by altering his lifestyle in such a way as to reduce his risk factors. Similarly, while a negative test carried out to maximum intensity does not absolutely guarantee freedom from myocardial infarction in the future, it makes such an event unlikely.

In some subjects with clearly established atherosclerosis, exercise-induced ST segmental depression is not accompanied by typical anginal pain. We know that the ST changes are an indication of shortage of blood to the heart muscle, but unfortunately the patient cannot feel anything wrong. In discussing this type of situation with a patient, I usually tell him that his exercise electrocardiogram has shown evidence of "silent angina"; in other words, we know from his electrocardiogram that at a given level of exertion he develops myocardial ischemia, but for a number of reasons this does not give rise to the usual cramp-like pain. We therefore prescribe a level of exertion below that at which the electrocardiogram changes appear. This helps him to understand why we are asking him to walk or jog at a slower pace than he feels capable of.

Finally, ST segment response to exercise may change, some individuals regressing from a negative test to a positive test, others progressing from positive to negative; in my experience, the latter is a fairly common result of an exercise rehabilitation course.

Irregular Heart Rate

In a healthy heart, the electrical events follow a relatively fixed time sequence. The P wave, representing atrial contraction, rarely lasts more than 0.08 seconds; the QRS complex, representing the ventricular contraction, also takes 0.08 seconds; from the beginning of the P wave to the start of the Q wave is never more than 0.2 seconds. These intervals, together with many others, can be quickly read off the electrocardiogram paper by the physician, using the standard graph paper (1 mm squares) and standard paper speed (25 mm per second), so that each of the squares corresponds to 0.04 seconds. Not only are the events within the cardiac

Figure 18 Electrocardiogram Showing an Irregular Beat, Normal Heart Rhythm Interrupted by One Irregular Beat

cycle on a time and sequence basis, but the intervals between each cycle, or heart beat, are also regular. Obviously, as the heart beats quicker or slower, these inter-beat intervals will change, but the alterations will occur evenly in the same manner as a well-tuned automobile engine accelerates and decelerates. However, if the heart is starved of blood, then an increase in tempo will result in a shortage of oxygen to the myocardium, with resultant "misfiring" which gets worse as the rate accelerates. These irregular beats are known as "ectopics" or "extrasystoles" and we have referred to them earlier as "skipped beats" (Figure 18).

Note that the extra complex is followed by a prolonged pause; the heart is recovering from the unexpected interpolated effort, and the recharging process takes a little longer. The shape of the ectopic beat is abnormal, as is the sequence and timing of each event, so that the P wave is missing altogether, and the QRS complex lasts longer than 0.08 seconds.

The development of such ectopic beats during exercise and their increasing frequency as the intensity of the exercise is raised, is considered to be an adverse sign. Very frequent irregularities can be dangerous and, by general agreement, the exercise test is terminated when they exceed 3 in every 10 normal beats.

It should be pointed out that there is an innocent form of irregular heart beat which occurs at rest, is often present from childhood, and which disappears as the heart rate increases with exercise. There is no evidence that these types of extra beats are due to, or are even a forerunner of, heart disease.

Another variant of benign ectopic beats is sometimes found in very fit individuals whose resting heart rates, as a result of training, have fallen to low levels, such as the 50s or the high 40s. Here, the gap between beats is so long that the muscles of the ventricles become impatient for the electrical impulse to arrive from the sino-atrial node, and so they "escape" from the influence of the vagus nerve and initiate an early contraction on their own.

Inappropriate Blood Pressure Response to Exercise

The increased demand imposed by exercise on the pumping ability of the heart is evidenced by a rise in blood pressure. If for some reason the ventricles are unable to pump vigorously, then the blood pressure will fail to rise concomitantly with the workload. Even worse, it may fall, signifying a serious state of affairs in which the heart is the seat of so much damage that it gives up the struggle to keep pace with the demand. This may be because previous heart attacks have caused so much scarring that healthy contraction is no longer possible.

So far, we are considering the systolic blood pressure, or pressure in the arteries during the heart's pumping phase. When the heart is resting between beats, or in its phase of diastole, the diastolic pressure obviously remains steady, being unaffected by exercise. If the diastolic pressure starts to rise, it means that the pressure within the chambers of the heart is rising abnormally due to increasing back pressure or damming up of blood from ineffectual onward pumping. A stationary or falling systolic pressure then, and/or a rising diastolic pressure during the exercise test, is a signal for the physician to halt the procedure. While not characteristic of coronary disease, it does denote pump failure, and in the context of today's incidence of atherosclerosis, probably means ischemic heart disease.

Inappropriate Heart Rate Response to Exercise

In 1972, Hinkle and his associates noted that a sluggish heart rate response to an exercise test in middle-aged men was often the forerunner of a later heart attack. Dr. Myrvin Ellestad has observed a similar relationship. In a study published in 1975, he reported that of 2,700 patients with and without evidence of heart disease who were subjected to a maximum treadmill test, those with normal ST segments but with a low heart rate response to exercise went on to develop the same incidence of coronary events (sudden death, myocardial infarction, angina pectoris) as patients who had an ischemic ST segment depression. While there is no doubt that *failure* of the heart rate to increase with workload is a dangerous sign, and probably indicates damage to the pacemaker or electrical conduction system of the heart, *slowness* of response is more difficult to define. Dr. Ellestad has established standard heart acceleration rates for his particular test protocol. Sufficient data have not as yet been accumulated to permit their application in other test procedures. Various medications, as well as a high fitness level will affect rate of response. For the time being, then, although this sign has intriguing possibilities, it does not have the same degree of predictability as the previous three described.

Before leaving the matter of adverse criteria, mention should be made of maximum oxygen consumption. Dr. Robert Bruce of Seattle, using maximum treadmill testing, has ascertained that the maximum oxygen consumption is reduced in coronary artery disease; he believes that this is due to a drop in maximum heart rate. The amount by which maximum oxygen consumption is reduced represents, he believes, a measure of the disease's severity. He refers to the patient's "functional aerobic impairment," and has constructed tables to calculate this parameter from the result of his treadmill test.

We have now come full circle, tracing the use of exercise testing in the evaluation of fitness, the diagnosis of latent coronary heart disease, and the combination of both. In recent years, additional uses have developed. These include the guidance of normal individuals who wish to undertake an exercise program, the determination of suitability for entrance to rehabilitation exercise programs, and the prescribing of safe and suitable training activities based on individual requirements.

Needless to say, exercise testing carried to maximum or even sub-maximal levels can be hazardous in patients with heart disease and, for this reason, should never be carried out on such individuals by unqualified personnel, or without a physician being present. Furthermore, it is not enough for the physician to play a passive role in the proceedings, being prepared to act only if resuscitation is required. He or she should be thoroughly conversant with the testing protocol. In addition to observing the patient's reaction, reading the simultaneous electrocardiogram, and taking the blood pressure at regular intervals, he should designate successive increments in the workload and halt the test at the first evidence of untoward signs or symptoms. The experienced physician will rarely have to take emergency measures; his handling of the test will not infrequently prevent the need arising.

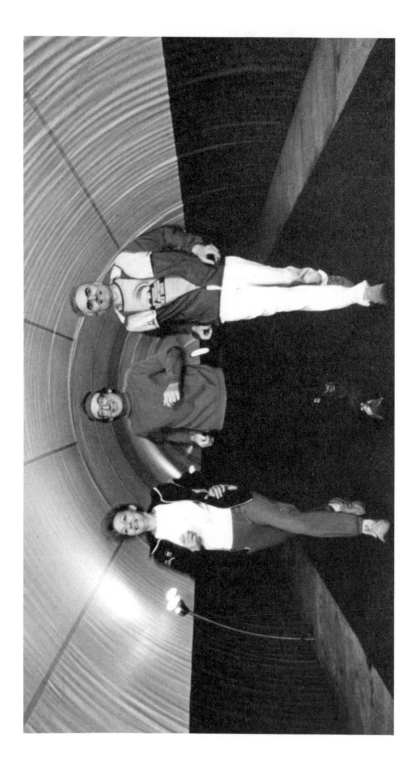

Part Two

A REHABILITATION PROGRAM

Better to hunt in fields, for health unbought,
Than fee the doctor for a nauseous draught.
The wise, for cure, on exercise depend;
God never made his work for man to mend.
John Dryden

CHAPTER SIX

The Rehabilitation Program

"There is no way you can go back to your old job," said the physician.

Bill H., a 39-year-old construction worker, stared across the desk in disbelief. "What can I do?" he said. "I don't know any other trade. How will I get by?"

Firmly, the doctor reminded him of the facts. Bill had just been discharged from hospital having sustained his second serious heart attack. The first was a year previous. Both attacks had been severe, and an additional factor to take into account was the family history. Bill's father had died at the age of 42 from a heart attack. One older brother had died, again in his 40s, from a heart attack, and another brother had sustained a heart attack at the age of 38.

It was essential, said the doctor, that Bill take all sensible precautions to see that he had recovered completely before exposing himself once more to the stress of heavy physical effort. His wife would have to go out to work, and he would have to stay at home to look after their two children, preparing their meals and carrying out the routine housework.

This "role reversal" is a familiar rehabilitation technique, used primarily when the male breadwinner is so incapacitated from disease or accident that he is no longer employable. To Bill, however, this approach was hard to take. His common sense told him that his doctor was right; he was not in fit shape to withstand the physical strain of his old job. On the other hand, it was difficult to see himself as disabled. He looked the picture of health, as do many convalescent heart attack patients. He felt that he was essentially a strong and healthy individual who had merely had a stroke of bad luck.

Thus, as the months went by, Bill became more and more morose. Never what you would call an abstainer, he began to drink heavily. His tenseness and anxiety increased, and instead of benefiting from the enforced rest from work, he became worse. He would wake up in the night restless and sweating. In the daytime, he began to notice chest pains, some of which he thought were angina and others he thought were "nerves." He was irritable with the children and downright ugly to his wife.

Fortunately, his doctor was astute enough to realize that things weren't working out the way he had hoped. He still felt that return to work was not the answer, and yet neither was sitting all day at home.

"The less I do, the flabbier I get," said Bill, plaintively. "At this rate, I'll never work again."

Doctor and patient gazed speculatively at one another, each trying to find a solution.

Then Bill had a thought. "Why not send me to one of the "Y's" fitness classes? Wouldn't that build up my strength again?" As he spoke, his voice became more enthusiastic. Already he was seeing himself active and vigorous again, participating in the games and sports he had enjoyed at school.

The physician was torn. There was no doubt of the morale-boosting effect of a fitness program, but what of the safety factor? How could he entrust Bill and his damaged heart to a fitness class geared to the needs of essentially healthy individuals? Then, a half-awakened thought stirred in his mind. Hadn't he read somewhere recently that a local rehabilitation centre had just started a post-coronary rehabilitation program? He promised Bill he would enquire further, and let him know the outcome the next day.

He was true to his word and the following week, Bill was waiting in the lobby of the Toronto Rehabilitation Centre. It was 1968, and he was one of the first patients to be referred to the new exercise rehabilitation program for heart attack patients.

Stuart K. was 54 years old. He had "had it with doctors." This was largely because his doctors had almost "had it" with him. A highly successful executive, Stuart was a prime example of the unco-operative patient. He was also a magnificent example of a type of patient seen all too often in the coronary care unit.

He had just been discharged from hospital after recovery from his second heart attack. The first was only three months earlier, and his reaction at that time had been most businesslike—keep a stiff upper lip and stay in there fighting. In Stuart's terms, this meant denying that he was suffering from anything other than a minor setback, and dispensing with medical assistance as soon as possible. Accordingly, he took his own discharge from hospital one week earlier than his cardiologist advised, and then returned to work the following week. Shortly after this, he put himself on an exercise training program as outlined in a popular book on fitness. Naturally, he considered himself already a rather fit individual, and so quickly skipped through the precautionary chapters of the book, written for "old guys and crocks," and started half-way up the training table at a level suitable for those whose fitness rating was good.

In short, Stuart did all the wrong things. Small wonder that six weeks later, while on a business trip and shortly after attempting to run a seven-minute mile through Stanley Park in Vancouver, he experienced severe chest pain. On his return to Toronto, he was diagnosed as having sustained another and this time more extensive heart attack. He was lucky enough to survive, and one would have thought that after that experience he would have adopted a more cautious approach. Obviously, this was not his nature; if nothing else, one has to give him A for persistence. He was still determined to work, worry and play at his customary pre-attack level.

He presented his hapless cardiologist with an ultimatum: "Tell me how to get fit and strong again, or send me to someone who can."

His physician, feeling that Stuart had had a great deal more luck than he deserved, and anxious to protect him from further excesses, recalled reading of an exercise rehabilitation program that was being carried on in the city. He recommended that Stuart attend this program.

"My God," said Stuart. "Rehabilitation! You mean basket weaving?"

"Not quite," said his doctor, but feeling that maybe he might have scored a point in that encounter!

Harold D. was thoroughly depressed when he came out of hospital. He had been taking part in a curling championship play-off five weeks earlier when he had felt intensely nauseated and sweaty. Within minutes, he developed intense, crushing pain in his chest, and an hour later found himself in the emergency department of the local hospital. A myocardial infarction was diagnosed, and he was admitted. Four weeks later, he was discharged. His progress had been uneventful and free from complications. On the day of his discharge, his wife came to help him pack and drive him home. He felt weak, and unsure of himself. Would he be able to go back to his old job? Would he be able to curl again? What restrictions and limitations would the doctors place upon him in the future?

Unwittingly, one of his wife's first actions as they left the hospital seemed to reinforce all his fears. "Don't carry that, dear," she said, lifting his suitcase. "It's too heavy for you."

As they walked across the lobby, he deliberately fell behind, ashamed of his weakness in not being able to carry his own case.

The following day, his doctor phoned him. He was going to be referred to a post-coronary exercise program which had been instituted in a nearby rehabilitation centre. His feelings were mixed. Such places were for the severely disabled, the handicapped. Well, if that is what he had become, he might as well accept it. But hadn't he read somewhere that a group of heart attack patients had recently taken part in a two-mile demonstration run? Maybe they were from the same program. Well, he'd have to see. There was no sense giving up now.

The rehabilitation program to which these men were referred was unique in that it stressed prolonged endurance exercise. If Stuart expected basket weaving, he was in for a shock. From the outset each participant would be asked, depending on his condition, to walk or jog for half an hour, five times a week. Within a matter of weeks, the time would be increased to one hour. His immediate goal would be to jog four miles in 48 minutes; ultimately, he could look forward to jogging six miles in 72 minutes (were he under 45, his prescription would amount to six miles in 60 minutes).

His starting level and rate of progression would depend upon the results of rigorous cardio-respiratory fitness testing. His exercise plan would be carefully tailored to accommodate his two-fold need: developing endurance fitness, and doing so with minimal risk to his already damaged heart. He would be given an individual prescription specifying duration, intensity and frequency of exercise: in short, the distance he would have to jog, the time it should take, and how many times a week it should be carried out.

He would be expected to attend exercise classes regularly until he achieved his fitness potential. During these supervised sessions, he would be observed by physicians, therapists and physical educators to see how he performed. If he developed cardiac symptoms he would be examined again, or his electrocardiogram monitored while he exercised. He would be instructed in the art of taking his own pulse, reading a stop watch, pacing himself, and jogging in an easy and relaxed manner so as to avoid minor injuries to his muscles, tendons and joints.

Physician-led discussions would deal not only with the physiological and medical aspects of endurance training, but also the significance of exercise-induced symptoms associated with coronary heart disease. Individual advice as to whether or not he should participate in other sports such as squash, weight-lifting, tennis or curling, would be available to him. The value or otherwise of vitamins, low-fat diets, soft water versus hard water would be some of the topics relevant to his disease which would be covered in the short pre-exercise discussions.

In point of fact, he was in for the experience of a lifetime. For the first time in his life, he was going to be subjected to a systematic, medically directed, scientifically designed onslaught on his deplorable and heinous state of unfitness. In the process, some of his long-cherished beliefs and prejudices about training were going to be exploded; he was going to discover that many of the sports he had taken part in, under the impression that they were good for his health, were actually of little value in attaining true worthwhile fitness; and that a set of singles tennis played on odd occasions throughout the year to a perspiring, gasping, knee-trembling finish did more harm than good. But more important, he was going to find that he was expected to work constantly and assiduously on his own, changing his lifestyle to accommodate to five one-hour sessions of exercise every week. His reward? Something that money cannot buy. The attainment of a quality of life far surpassing anything he had experienced before: the relaxed, confident satisfaction that only regular exercise can bring. He would experience the sheer physical elation of being fit.

Not only that, there was an additional bonus. At the initial induction lecture it had been carefully pointed out that the outlook for an individual who had already had a heart attack was somewhat gloomy. This statement in itself had been a bit of a revelation, in more ways than one. First, he had not fully realized this sombre fact; and secondly, he was accustomed to his physician wrapping unpalatable news in a more attractive package. To be told that the recurrence rate among heart attack survivors was high, that in fact some 20 to 25 per cent are dead from a second attack within five years of the primary one, had been quite a jolt. Yet the physician (who incidentally was clad in a track suit and seemed curiously jocular about such bad news) produced the results of a series of different studies to back his statement. He put the case bluntly:

All of you here listening to me have to face the fact that your life expectancy is less than normal. I tell you this for one reason only: so that you understand right from the outset that the task facing us in post-coronary rehabilitation is a formidable one. Our job is to try to increase your life expectancy, by reducing the incidence of fatal recurrences.

Can we do that? We offer no guarantees, but the evidence is highly suggestive that we can. Regular exercise has been found to be a powerful factor in the primary prevention of fatal heart attacks. Individuals who have been engaged in heavy work before their attacks have a higher survival rate (two to three times as high) both immediately and over a five-year follow-up. It is not unreasonable, therefore, to theorize that an exercise program instituted *after* your heart attack will have a similar protective effect. Furthermore, there is enough presumptive evidence now to say that it does. Of course, if you want more definitive proof, you can wait another ten years to get it — but that might be a bit late for some of you.

The work of Drs. Hellerstein, Gottheimer, Brunner and Rechnitzer, as well as our own studies, has shown as much as a three-fold reduction of fatal recurrences in patients who attend a rehabilitation program which contains an exercise component. Our own experiments have also led us to prefer walking and jogging as the mode of training, and LSD (long, slow distance) rather than ''speed.''

So that's it in a nut shell. We offer hard facts, hard work, and hard-line direction. In return, you get a second chance at life, and an opportunity to live it in a high state of physical fitness. But remember, your new lifestyle can only be maintained by constant effort. You can't build up a store of exercise or fitness that can be used over later months or years of sedentary living. Deterioration sets in within weeks of stopping training. So if you can't hack it, then don't bother starting. Exercise must become an integral part of your daily routine. The only way out is to obtain the letters R.I.P. after your name, and we don't intend to be handing out too many of those types of diplomas!

Stuart, Bill and Don, like many others, responded to the challenge. They entered the program, and began a new way of life.

THE ORIGINS OF THE PROGRAM

The remarkable escalation in the incidence of heart attacks, together with the realization that the survivors were still in peril from a fatal recurrence, led the author and his colleagues to the realization that something more than routine physician follow-up was required. If all the risk factors were to be covered, then a change in lifestyle was indicated. This cannot be achieved by a 30-minute visit with a physician every six months. Granted, such risk factors as high blood pressure, diabetes and high blood levels of cholesterol can be controlled by the regular visit to the physician, but the latter is only too ready to admit his failure in advising on such matters as diet, increasing physical activity, avoidance of excessive stress, and giving up smoking.

For most sedentary workers, increased physical activity can only be attained by an exercise program carried out in their non-working hours. To obtain advice from the physician on such a program is, as many patients will attest, notoriously difficult. The plain fact of the matter is that most physicians have not been trained to prescribe exericise. Increasing public and government interest in physical fitness programs is improving this situation slightly, but it is safe to say that the vast majority of physicians are still ignorant of this area.

Nevertheless, studies have shown that post-coronary exercise programs can be very effective in increasing cardiac efficiency by decreasing heart rate and myocardial oxygen consumption at a given workload. The training permits the muscles to extract more oxygen from the blood, thus reducing the amount of blood the heart has to pump for a given task. The trained heart muscle is more resistant to such unfavourable conditions as shortage of oxygen (a situation which arises when the narrowed coronary arteries are unable to supply an adequate amount of blood to a rapidly beating heart), or excess stress hormones (catecholamines) which are liberated into the blood stream in response to situations of high urgency. There is an increased feeling of well-being and a lessening of depression. There is often an improvement in chest pain, with many patients reporting relief from angina as they become fitter. These, and other benefits, are what one would expect to see in any individual who embarks on a training program. The encouraging thing is that having had a heart attack doesn't prevent you from obtaining these advantages.

A number of workers have reported that exercise programs reduced the incidence of fatal and non-fatal recurrent heart attacks in their patients. One of the longest studies has been carried out by Dr. Hermann Hellerstein in Cleveland, who found that deaths among his exercised post-coronaries amounted to only 1.9 per hundred patients per year. This compares favourably with the figure of 5.1 per hundred which he calculated for the non-exercising post-coronary population.

Dr. Daniel Brunner compared a group of 64 patients in his exercise program with another group of 65 post-coronary patients who had not followed any exercise regime. Over the period of a year, there were four recurrences and two deaths in the exercise group; the non-active group had nine recurrences and seven fatalities.

In a similar study by Dr. Peter Rechnitzer of Ontario, a group of exercise subjects were compared over a five-year period with a group of non-exercisers. The exercisers had a 1.3 per cent recurrence rate and a 3.9 per cent death rate, while the control group had a 27.9 per cent recurrence rate and an 11.8 per cent death rate. Dr. Gottheimer reported a 3.6 per cent death rate in a group of 1,100 male Israelis with coronary disease who followed an exercise plan; again, this is in marked contrast to a 12 per cent rate in a non-exercised group. Finally, Dr. Weinblatt reported no recurrences and no deaths over a five-year period in his exercise group, as opposed to a 4.6 per cent recurrence rate and 3.1 per cent death rate in a control group.

In terms of medical proof, we can only say at this stage that the work of these physicians is promising. Larger groups of patients, a longer follow-up, and more tightly controlled experimental factors are needed in order to satisfy all of the criteria necessary to come to a definitive conclusion. Once again, however, with coronary heart disease accounting for 40 to 50 per cent of the death rate in advanced countries, it does not seem unreasonable to examine this work and take from it whatever advantage may be offered to the current victim.

It was with this background in mind that my post-coronary program at the Centre was started. The aim was to offer positive advice and help, and by regular attendance to instill a set of health habits which could only do good. A pattern of exercise would be the main thrust, with additional factors being brought in as the program progressed.

As Medical Director of the Centre and prime mover of the project, I was convinced that its success would depend largely on the enthusiasm and quality of the initial treatment team. I was extremely fortunate in this regard. From my own staff came Johanna Kennedy, R.N., who assumed the role of co-ordinator. Professor Robin Campbell was loaned from the University of Toronto to work in the exercise testing laboratory.

Consultants were Professor Roy Shephard from the Department of Preventive Medicine and Biostatistics, University of Toronto, and Dr. Art Chisholm, Director of Cardiovascular Services at the University of Toronto's Sunnybrook Hospital. We were fortunate indeed in having Roy Shephard, an internationally recognized authority in exercise physiology, assume consulting responsibility for the exercise-testing protocol. Art Chisholm, a cardiologist with a long-standing interest in exercise rehabilitation, provided not only expertise in his field but also those vital first few patients without which our plans would never have materialized. Johanna Kennedy brought to the position of co-ordinator outstanding organizational ability and also, as a result of her involvement as an administrator with the Canadian Track and Field Association, an intimate knowledge of the trials and tribulations and vicissitudes of the aspiring runner.

For we had decided to use running—or more correctly jogging —as the exercise of choice. It was ideal for our purpose in that it required little in the way of equipment or expensive facilities, could be accurately prescribed in terms of intensity, duration and frequency, and was an excellent builder of endurance fitness. Today, sixteen years later, the treatment team has increased six-fold, and includes physicians, physiotherapists, occupational therapists, and physical educators; but happily the original founder members continue, more active than ever, and in expanded roles.

Post-coronary exercise programs are plagued by poor attendance and high drop-out rates. The patient's first flush of enthusiasm for exercise is often short-lived. He begins to find that regular attendance at the classes disrupts his social and business commitments. This problem is compounded in a large city, where he often has to travel long distances on traffic-clogged roads and highways. The answer is to reduce the number of weekly medically supervised sessions to the minimum compatible with training effectiveness and safety, and then have the individual work out on his own the rest of the week. After all, if he cannot be taught to exercise prudently when he is away from the watchful eye of the physician, how can he be expected to cope with the inevitable sudden physical stresses and strains of normal everyday living? Then again, if safe exercise rehabilitation programs are to become universally available, the logistics of the situation make it mandatory that medical staff be used for the maximum good of the maximum number; physicians, nurses and therapists are in short supply, and their services should be deployed carefully.

Thus it was decided that the group would exercise at the Centre under medical supervision only once a week. Since a greater frequency of training is needed for attainment of endurance fitness, four additional home workouts would also be required. This approach has worked very well, despite the opinion of many physical education authorities that at least two and probably three supervised exercise sessions a week would be necessary. The fact is that our patients have become fit and attend the weekly session with great regularity; indeed, the program has one of the lowest drop-out rates recorded.

Our program requires that all patients be referred by a physician. The referral documents, together with hospital reports and electrocardiograms, are carefully studied by the Centre's doctors to see if there are any absolute contra-indications to exercise. The patient is then brought in to the Centre for a complete examination. His height, weight, muscle power in arms and legs, and the thickness of the fat layers over various parts of his body are recorded. A medical examination, which includes a routine electrocardiogram, is carried out. Finally, the patient performs a sub-maximal exercise stress test as described in Chapter 5, either on the bicycle ergometer or the treadmill. The electrocardiogram is monitored continuously during this test, and expired gases are analyzed in

The post-coronary program in action. *Above,* the pre-exercise discussion; the warm-up; *opposite*: patients exercising under supervision on the Centre's 200-metre track in summer; the track covered in preparation for exercising during the winter months.

order to estimate the patient's maximum oxygen consumption.

As a result of this test, the patient is placed in one of two categories: "uncomplicated" or "complicated." An uncomplicated test means that he has continued through to an estimated 75 per cent of his maximum heart rate without developing angina or any serious abnormalities in his electrocardiogram. The complicated case is one in which the subject did not finish the test because some evidence of cardiac ischemia supervened. A walking/jogging exercise prescription is now prescribed on the basis of the test result, the complicated cases being handled somewhat differently from the uncomplicated. The prescription states the specific distance to be covered and the time it should take. It calls for five workouts a week, one of which is carried out under supervision at the Centre.

In effect, then, each patient has an individual prescription based on his particular response to the exercise test. Repeated stress tests show whether or not there is any improvement in fitness, and if there is, this leads to a new prescription; in this way, the patient progresses safely and at a rate based on his increasing level of fitness. Not infrequently, the complicated case, which initially may have a low starting level compared with the other patients, improves his performance on subsequent stress tests to the degree that he can transfer to the ranks of the uncomplicated.

Initiation into the program proper takes place after the first exercise test. The patient attends the Centre for a series (approximately ten hours in all) of introductory lectures and discussions on coronary heart disease, common risk factors, recognition and interpretation of cardiac signs and symptoms, and the rationale of exercise training. Interspersed with the talks are practical sessions dealing with the art of reading a stop watch and taking a pulse count. Both of these procedures are of vital importance to the post-coronary patient who intends to exercise. If he is to interpret his prescription correctly, he must not only measure out the distance that he has to walk accurately, but he must also time his walk or jog equally precisely. An ordinary watch is not good enough for this purpose, and we always insist that before starting the program our patients purchase and become proficient in the use of a stop watch, which is also used to time the pulse count. Without a stop watch for guidance the patient tends to go too fast.

A most important part of the induction procedure is the "field trial." Under the supervision of a therapist, the patient carries out a one-mile walk on the Centre's track. The pace is prescribed, and is based on the results of the exercise test. This enables us to check the accuracy of the prescription. If the trial workout results in the desired training heart rate, and does not cause symptoms, then the prescription is confirmed. On the other hand, if the post-workout heart rate is too high or too low, or symptoms occur during the walk, then the prescription is adjusted accordingly.

After attending the initiation sessions, patients are streamed to one of eight weekly exercise classes. At least two physicians supervise each class, and there is one nurse or therapist for every ten patients. A typical supervised session starts with a 20-minute discussion in which patients are encouraged to discuss problems they may have encountered with their home prescription. This affords an opportunity to educate the group into the do's and don'ts of exercise, the significance of various cardiac signs and symptoms, the importance and action of certain medications, and the trends of modern research into heart disease. There is a deliberate attempt to establish a free-wheeling type of atmosphere, and this enables full and frank discussion of various topics which would otherwise be suppressed in a more structured discussion: for example, sexual problems following the heart attack, the use of various "fad" diets, and the value of the current "cure" for heart disease constantly being reported in the lay press.

The discussion is followed by a 20-minute warm-up to music. The emphasis here is on simple flexibility exercises designed specifically for the middle-aged, and interspersed with walking and jogging. The group circle the exercise leader and at regular programmed intervals the music is interrupted by a 10-second characteristic low-pitched hum — a signal for the class to take a 10-second pulse count. These counts are then called out, thus giving the leader a "feel" for the individual's exercise response. Throughout the warm-up, and after each pulse count, an inquiry is made as to whether anybody is experiencing chest discomfort, skipped beats, vertigo or any other symptom. Again, this gives the supervising group an awareness of the individuals who are prone to ischemic symptoms. Marked problems during the warm-up will be an indication for a discussion with the patient, and possibly further medical assessment, including electrocardiograms. Opportunity is also taken during these warm-ups to teach the newcomers the style and technique of jogging.

It frequently surprises visitors to the program to find that I act as exercise leader in the warm-up. They seem both amused and intrigued at the spectacle of a middle-aged physician, clad in a baggy sweat suit, acting as a pseudo physical educator. My reasons are both medical and psychological. There is no better way to become familiar with your patient's responses to exercise than to take him through a warm-up. Untoward symptoms can be personally observed and noted. After two or three sessions of personal involvement you are in a better position to distinguish between the symptom-sufferers and the symptom-claimers — an important division when one is dispensing exercise therapy on the large scale. The "denier" of symptoms, the inept pulse-taker, the timid and frightened exerciser, the competitive type, are all stock characters in any post-coronary exercise class, and can be identified with more assurance by a trained physician — provided he is located where the action is, which in this case is on the floor of the gymnasium. Of course, he could stand and watch somebody else put his patients through their paces. But then how much more encouraging it is for the newcomer to take his first jogging steps "on medical orders," and from a physician who is not embarrassed to be attired as ridiculously as himself. Obviously not all doctors have the time or indeed the inclination to cavort around the gym with their patients; but I suspect more would be willing to do so if the benefits were drawn to their attention. Besides, what a splendid opportunity to get fit while on the job!

Patients are encouraged to discuss their problems openly rather than trying to corner the physician or nurse for a private tête-à-tête. We have found that most problems and symptoms are common to a large number of people, and therefore open discussion not only helps the individual who brought the problem up, but the many others who are having the same difficulty but are, at least in the early stages of their attendance, too shy to mention them. After the warm-up is over, the patients then proceed to carry out their individual prescriptions under the observing eye of the medical team.

All patients are required to keep an exercise log which they hand in every two weeks. This records their current prescription, the distance and time of each workout, and their pre- and post-workout heart rates. Once a month they record their resting heart rate; this is taken before they get out of bed in the morning, and the average of three morning counts is entered. The log also has space for noting any adverse symptoms experienced during a particular workout. The logs are read carefully by the treatment staff, and the distances, speeds and heart rates are carefully charted for each patient. In this way, progress can be easily gauged at a glance. Adverse symptoms are underlined in red and immediately passed through to the physician for his attention. If necessary, the physician will phone the patient to clarify some remark or even to suggest that the rate of exercise be reduced until he is seen at the next supervised session.

Our studies at the Centre have shown that the patient often feels a great improvement in mood and morale within weeks of starting the program. Nevertheless, a period of at least a year is required for more objective physiological benefits to appear. Ideally, two years is needed. However, while one is reluctant to discharge individuals from the program, the number of referrals has increased steadily over the years. This problem has been solved to a large degree by "promoting" patients when they have reached the satisfactory level to a group which attends the Centre only once every fourth week, and still later to another group which attends only every other month. These "post-graduates" are still expected to complete and return their exercise logs every two weeks, however, and these are reviewed as assiduously as those from the weekly attenders.

Due to the steady demand from out-of-town physicians, we have also instituted a home exercise program. The patient travels into the Centre for testing, is instructed in the execution of his prescription, and reports his progress by means of mailed-in exercise logs. Progressively heavier training workouts are prescribed as he gets fitter, and he returns for re-testing at six monthly or yearly intervals.

This book represents the final extension of the program. It is an attempt to reach the individuals with coronary heart disease who want to go on an exercise program but lack expert guidance. Obviously no book, no matter how well written, will substitute for personal supervision and contact, but it can help in the avoidance of the more dangerous pitfalls.

Over the years, the two commonest questions asked of me by doctors and patients alike are: what is a safe starting level of exercise, and how does one safely increase this to improve the training effect? Obviously, there is no single answer to either question. The starting level will vary with the individual, depending upon his initial state of fitness, the severity of his heart attack, his age, and the presence or absence of symptoms. Any increase in his training prescription will depend upon his response, expressed subjectively in his feeling of well-being and objectively in his heart rate response to the workout and to repeated stress tests. However, over the years, we have learned to streamline our exercise-prescribing technique and have developed a series of tables especially designed for cardiac patients. These, together with a set of progressing nomograms, should provide safe and effective guidelines for the intelligent layman. Used with the accompanying remarks on training techniques, they constitute a home version of the Centre program.

CHAPTER SEVEN

So You Want to Exercise?

Most coronary heart disease sufferers will benefit from a sensible exercise program. This includes individuals who have had a heart attack as well as those who experience anginal pain with exertion even though they have never actually had an attack. It also includes the middle-aged who exhibit any of the risk factors previously described (and that means most males over 40) or who have a high incidence of heart disease in their family. There are, however, some cases in which exercise is positively contra-indicated, either on cardiac or non-cardiac grounds. In others, there are relative contra-indications to exercise: situations in which exercise is possible, but must be modified and adjusted so as not to be harmful.

CARDIAC CONTRA-INDICATIONS TO EXERCISE

As I have said, these are few, and your physician should be your final guide. I shall, however, include a brief checklist here.

1. Recent myocardial infarction: Since the infarction scar takes six weeks to become firm, vigorous activity prior to that time may well result in an aneurysm, or bulging of the damaged area. This bulging occurs with each heart beat and, if large, constitutes in itself another contra-indication to exercise,

    Arthur P. is a case in point. He was discharged from hospital three weeks after his heart attack, and was advised to restrict his activities to casual walking for a further month before returning to his doctor for a check-up. Unfortunately, he became overly enthusiastic about the benefits of exercise and, through a combination of misinformation and misinterpretation, began to follow a self-devised running program. By the seventh week, he was forcing himself to jog between one and two miles over hilly terrain. Shortly after, he was re-admitted to hospital with another attack. Fortunately, it was not fatal, but when he was later referred to me to ensure that any future exercising would be under supervision, he was found to have a large aneurysm of the heart wall. There is a strong likelihood that this was due to his premature vigorous running. One of my most depressing experiences was having to tell this man, who was still keen to exercise, that exercise therapy was now out for him, that anything more intense than a casual walk would be too dangerous.

2. There is no role for exercise in acute heart failure. In this condition, the heart is unable to pump the blood efficiently around the body. If the right side of the heart is affected, the blood tends to back-up in the general circulation, with resultant swelling from retention of fluid (edema) in the feet and legs. Left-sided heart failure causes the blood to back-up in the lungs, and this leads to excessive breathlessness in response to even the mildest physical activity. No matter which side of the heart is affected, exercise training aggravates the situation. Heart failure is a rare complication of coronary artery disease, but when it does occur, it is usually only in association with a severe myocardial infarction. Even then, healing of the infarct is often accompanied by complete recovery in pump efficiency, at which time exercise again becomes permissible.

3. As we have seen, a large aneurysm of the heart wall is a bar to exercise. Aneurysms may also occur in the walls of the large blood vessels (for example, the aorta), and their presence here also precludes vigorous training. There are, of course, cases in which small aneurysmal bulges are detected; here the question of whether or not to exercise becomes a matter of fine judgment. The benefits to look for may be psychological rather than physiological. In general, such individuals should not attempt to regulate their own program, and skilled supervision by a physician is essential.

4. Patients with rapidly progressing anginal pain should not exercise. A marked change for the worse in the pattern and incidence of exertional pain may well be the warning of another heart attack. To exercise under these circumstances may well be to invite disaster.

5. The heart muscle can sometimes be involved in generalized infections, giving rise to a condition known as myocarditis, or inflammation of the myocardium (the medical ending "-itis" means "inflammation of"). This can occur in acute rheumatic fever or in diphtheria; viral infections such as poliomyelitis, influenza, and even infectious mononucleosis (glandular fever) can also affect the heart. Since exercise is always contra-indicated in acute infections, it is obviously even more dangerous when the infection involves the heart. While your physician will be the one to diagnose myocarditis and will certainly ensure that your physical activity is limited until the condition has cleared up, it should be stressed that mild subclinical myocarditis may be common in association with a number of viral-type infections. For this reason, I insist that all individuals on an exercise program stop training whenever they develop a heavy cold or an influenza-like illness. Exercise should never be performed in the presence of a fever, and to be on the safe side, the temperature should have returned to normal for a full seven days before working out again. Colds or flu which are accompanied by muscle pain and tenderness and a heart rate higher than normal are features suggestive of heart muscle involvement.

6. Grossly irregular heart action which is accentuated by exertion is a deterrent to training, especially if the electrocardiogram shows that the ectopic beats are emanating from more than one area in the heart. These "multi-focal" ectopics, which are aggravated by strenuous exertion, can on occasions lead to fatal ventricular fibrillation and exercise should not be undertaken until the condition has been controlled by suitable medication. Lesser degrees of rhythm irregularity can be compensated for by modifying the training regime; indeed, an increase in fitness will often reduce the incidence and severity of the condition. The occasional severe form will not respond satisfactorily, even to medication, and with these cases, regular exercise can do nothing but aggravate the situation.

It should be stressed at this time that there are two types of irregularities that are benign. In the first, the condition is often present from youth. The irregularity, or skipped beat, is present at rest but disappears as the heart rate increases with exercise. The subject may or may not be aware of the occasional missed beat, and if he is, he usually describes it as a "palpitation" or a "hollow pause" felt in the chest. The second harmless type of irregularity occurs in the highly trained individual whose resting heart rate has fallen to very low levels because of the increased influence of the nerve which slows the heart, the vagal nerve — that is, training bradycardia due to increased vagal activity. This may be an indication of over-training (see later), and usually clears up in a week or two when the intensity of the work-outs is reduced.

7. In certain types of valvular heart disease, especially those which lead to narrowing in the region of the aortic valve, exercise training is not advisable. Coronary heart disease does not affect the valves in this manner; rheumatic fever in childhood is the usual offender. Occasionally, the two conditions coexist, in which case one has to be guided by the severity of the valvular difficulty.

8. Recent cases of blood clots occurring either in the lungs (pulmonary embolism) or in the peripheral arteries or veins (thrombophlebitis) should not be exercised. Physical activity may bring about further clots, or extension of the existing ones.

9. Repeated bouts of heart failure may, in the long run, give rise to a dilated enlarged heart. This will show up on the x-ray and, where the enlargement is gross, there will be no benefit from training. The stretched heart muscle has no reserve left and so is incapable of benefiting from even measured small doses of stress.

10. Many experts feel that exercise therapy is of little value in the condition of complete heart block. Here, the electrical conduction system between the upper and lower chambers of the heart is non-functioning, with the result that the two portions beat independently. Furthermore, an increase in heart rate does not occur when the subject exercises. In such a condition, a pacemaker, or artificial rhythm conductor, is inserted. This brings the heart rate up to a set level and may

also, depending on the type and design, permit it to accelerate in response to exercise. Although our experience with pacemaker patients is still limited, we nevertheless have dealt with enough of them to know that they can indeed obtain a training effect from the exercise program.

11. Most patients with high blood pressure do well on an exercise program. However, if the hypertension is very marked, and cannot be controlled by medication, then vigorous exercise is harmful in that it drives the pressure up even higher and may even contribute towards brain hemorrhage.

12. Certain forms of congenital heart disease, especially those which are associated with bluish discoloration of the face and limb extremities (cyanosis) are bars to exercise.

NON-CARDIAC CONTRA-INDICATIONS TO EXERCISE

1. If you suffer from severe uncontrolled diabetes, you are best to avoid undue physical exertion. Milder forms of the disease are usually not a hindrance to training; in fact, the individual with marginal or latent diabetes may find that blood sugars approach normal levels with the attainment of fitness.

2. Exercise brings the body to a state of "arousal," and this may have untoward effects on the sufferer from epilepsy — on occasion increasing the frequency of attacks. The same applies to the related but much rarer condition of narcolepsy, in which the patient's seizures take the form of sudden uncontrollable bouts of sleepiness. One such individual was referred to my program but had to be refused when close questioning revealed a clear relationship between physical exercise and increased frequency of attacks.

3. Sustained exercise makes increased demands on the lungs, kidneys and liver. Therefore, certain chest conditions — for example, recent tuberculosis or recurrent spontaneous pneumothorax (entry of air into the chest cavity from rupture of a small "bleb" on the surface of the lung)—as well as severe kidney or liver disease are obvious contra-indications to exercise.

4. The acute stage of various types of arthritis, such as rheumatoid arthritis or gout, are treated by appropriate medication and rest. Exercise will do more harm than good. However, during the quiescent phase, and provided the disease has not caused too much deformity by destroying bones and joints, suitably modified exercise programs will be beneficial. The

more crippling type of osteoarthritis may be aggravated by running or jogging, and activities where the impact of body weight on joints is reduced, such as swimming, are more suitable. However, it is interesting to note that long distance runners have been shown to have a lower incidence of osteoarthritis in their hip joints than the population at large; this is due to the fact that movement keeps the protective cartilaginous lining of the joint surfaces healthy and well nourished. Our legs were meant for walking and running — not sitting and lying!

5. Chronic low back trouble is often exacerbated by jogging or calisthenics. Aggravating factors include obesity, running on an uneven surface, unsuitable running shoes, and sudden twisting movements of the spine. If a careful watch is kept for flare-ups, and activity is slowed with any suspicious symptoms, back strength should develop to the stage where a full program of jogging can be sustained without problem.

6. Anemia is a condition in which a lack of the protein hemoglobin in the blood causes an inadequate supply of oxygen to the organs and muscles of the body. In severe cases this results in fatigue, breathlessness, and sometimes anginal type pain on exertion. There are many causes for anemia, but among the most common are chronic loss of blood from a bleeding ulcer, bleeding hemorrhoids or excessive menstrual loss. Until the appropriate medical measures are taken to raise the blood level of hemoglobin to normal, exercise training is bound to be ineffective, since a vital link in the oxygen transport chain is defective. There is little point in the heart learning to pump blood more efficiently around the body if the blood itself contains an inadequate supply of oxygen.

7. There are a number of conditions, in addition to the above, in which exercise may be ill-advised. These include various neurological, muscular and glandular diseases which are relatively rare and, for practical purposes, need not be outlined here. In any event, the physician must be the final judge in these matters, and his advice and permission are essential for any patient with coronary heart disease who wishes to embark upon the training system outlined in this book.

PRINCIPLES OF ENDURANCE TRAINING

We have described the cardiovascular benefits of endurance training. Maximum oxygen consumption increases, the heart rate drops while its stroke volume improves, blood pressure falls, the oxygen-carrying capacity of the blood increases, and the muscles extract oxygen more efficiently from the blood stream. The endurance athlete's heart develops a greater blood supply and volume size. With all of these advantages (as well as such peripheral ones as reduction in the percentage of body fat, a drop in the level of circulating blood fats and stress hormones, and decrease in blood stickiness) is it any wonder that the long distance runner, swimmer, or cross-country skier rarely suffers from heart disease or sustains a heart attack? If you wish to develop the same degree of protection, then you must train in the same manner as these athletes — although not, of course, to quite the same degree. After all, you are not aiming to enter the Olympics, just to get some of the bonuses in terms of health and long life.

Training for endurance fitness requires the use of the large muscles of the legs or the trunk in a rhythmic fashion and on a regular basis. For our purposes, walking and jogging are the ideal activities. While I have no intrinsic objection to cycling, swimming, cross-country skiing or other similar endurance exercise, I feel that jogging gives as great, if not greater, returns of endurance fitness for a smaller investment of both time and money. The skill required to jog is minimal; the technique will be described later and can be learned in a matter of minutes. Special equipment is limited to a pair of good shoes and, if you want to go first-class, a sweat suit. You can jog almost anywhere — through parks, along roads or sidewalks, around neighbourhood school tracks. In cold weather, you can use the local Y gymnasium or you can try covered shopping malls, or even underground apartment garages. Opportunities are legion; the only basic requirement is motivation.

Although the principles of training are simple, we have to examine them more closely if we are to achieve success with our jogging program. It is generally accepted that in order to produce a minimal training effect in an unfit person, the intensity of training must be high enough to ensure that the heart rate reaches a certain level. How is this level established? Our own work and that of others have shown that endurance fitness results from training intensities equal to 50 or 60 per cent of your maximum oxygen consumption.

You may be interested in the manner in which this research is carried out. Large numbers of subjects are tested on the treadmill in order to establish maximum oxygen consumption, and also ascertain the running speed necessary to achieve it. It is a simple matter to calculate various percentages of this maximum speed, and note the heart rates for each speed. Training sessions resulting in heart rates less than those obtained at treadmill workouts that are below 50 per cent of maximum oxygen consumption are found to be relatively ineffectual in improving fitness. Ideally, an intensity of between 50 and 70 per cent of maximum oxygen consumption is needed to make a substantial gain; an intensity of jogging which is equivalent to only, say, 30 per cent of one's maximal oxygen consumption will likely be valueless in training the heart. Are there any upper limits to the desired intensity? Surprisingly enough, the answer is yes. To run at a speed which is 95 or 100 per cent of maximal oxygen consumption seems also to be relatively ineffective, largely because the activity cannot be sustained long enough to stimulate the development of endurance.

Thus, the optimum band of training speeds is narrow and, unless well advised, many individuals will jog at a pace which is either too slow or too fast for attainment of endurance fitness. The art of designing an efficient training program is to be able to match training speed to the immediate fitness and health status of the individual.

For the post-coronary patient, an even more important factor is the question of safety. While an activity level equal to 60 per cent of maximal oxygen consumption might be highly desirable from a training point of view, it could well, especially in the early stages of the program, exert excessive strain on a heart which is already suffering from an impaired coronary artery circulation. Not only that, it will probably prove too much for muscles, joints and bones weakened by years of inactivity. Most of us are grossly out of shape — even those who should know better! Recently a physician patient, when given his initial prescription requiring him to walk one mile in 20 minutes, admitted shamefacedly that he probably hadn't walked more than a quarter of a mile a day in over 25 years.

To sum up, then, the intensity of exercise must be sufficient to obtain a training effect, but care must be taken to see that it is within the tolerance of both the heart and the musculoskeletal system.

There are two other components to be considered in designing a training program: the length of the training session, and the number of times it should be carried out per week. With intensities in the order of 60 to 70 per cent, the duration of a workout should be at least 30 minutes, and our goal should be a 60-minute session. More intense levels of activity — say 80 or 85 per cent of maximum — may achieve the same training effect with shorter sessions, but the individual with coronary heart disease is better to hasten slowly.

There is another reason for preferring the one hour workout. The energy for short bouts of high intensity exercise comes almost entirely from the starches stored in the liver and muscles. Sprinters, football players, and ice hockey players, are "sugar athletes." Their bursts of physical effort are measured in seconds or minutes, and the fuel for their high-speed action comes from the quickly mobilized glycogen stores. The long distance runner, on the other hand, cannot rely entirely upon sugar stores, which begin to drop within 5 or 10 minutes of starting to run. By 30 minutes, glycogen provides no more than half the energy required, and from then on, the body begins to draw more and more on its fat stores (Figure 19). Have you ever seen an obese long distance runner? You probably never will. The duration of his training sessions are such that he burns all excess fat, with the result that his percentage of body fat is amongst the lowest of all athletes. It is duration rather than intensity, then, which burns off calories.

The implications for the patient with coronary heart disease are obvious. Not only will "long slow distance" keep his weight down, I have often thought it is not beyond the bounds of possibility that it could also reduce the size of the fatty plaques in his arteries — provided, of course, that these plaques have not become calcified so that the fat is inaccessible.

As for the frequency of training, five times a week is ideal. Nowadays, the competitive athlete trains seven days a week, and not infrequently twice a day. Such draconian measures may well pay off in a situation where only yards and seconds separate the world's best and the third-rater. However, by the law of diminishing returns, one must expect a smaller improvement for every hour spent in training over and above a certain level. Individuals who train less than three times a week make minimal progress; those who average four or five times a week seem to do much better, and those with the time and motivation to train seven times a week show maybe an additional 1 or 2 per cent increase over that. Five times a week seems to be the answer, in terms of fitness payoff for time invested.

Time (minutes)

Figure 19 The Longer You Exercise, the More Fat Your Body Burns

THE TRAINING TABLES

I have developed these tables over the past seven years; they are the result of practical experience in the training of hundreds of patients with heart disease. Used sensibly, and in accordance with the instructions which follow, they will provide safe and effective exercise for the development of endurance fitness.

However, let me start with a word of warning. The aim is to provide a personal exercise plan. But you must remember that circumstances and individuals vary. Mindless adherence to these or, indeed, any other set of training tables, no matter how intrinsically sound they may be, could have unpleasant consequences in the presence of coronary heart disease. While improvement in general health and cardiac function is the usual response to a fitness program, from time to time the disease may become unstable. The warning signs and symptoms of such deterioration will be described elsewhere in this book; if they become apparent, the exercise prescription should be reduced immediately. Similarly, if you are having difficulty completing a prescribed workout, even though the guidelines indicate that you should be able to accomplish that particular level of activity, then do not hesitate to modify the requirements to suit your tolerance. If in doubt, consult your physician. Prudence takes precedence over enthusiasm when you are training a damaged heart!

With these precautions in mind, we will now take a closer look at the training tables reproduced in the Appendix on pages 304-305. They consist of three phases, each of which will be described in detail.

Phase 1

This relates your fitness level, in terms of maximum oxygen consumption, to a "starter prescription." Allowance is made for age; if you are over 45, your general physical condition is probably poor and the possibility of atherosclerosis more likely.

If your initial maximum oxygen consumption (VO_2 max) is less than 16 ml/kg/min. (and we will see later how to measure this), then you should carry out a preliminary phase which lasts eight weeks. Actually, if you are overweight, or have been sedentary for many years, or suffer from musculoskeletal problems such as low back pain or mild osteoarthritis in your knees or hips, then it is not a bad idea for you to adhere to the eight week breaking-in period — even though your initial fitness may be higher than the specified level.

If your VO_2 max is higher than 16 ml., then the table will call for a three-mile walk, at a speed which varies with your level of fitness. The three miles should be approached in stages, walking one mile for two weeks, then two miles for two weeks, and finally the three miles, all at the prescribed speed. After that, of course, progression is made to the next level by walking the full three miles distance at a faster pace.

You should work out five times a week, and take two days' rest. It is immaterial whether these rest days are taken together, or split through the week; the choice is a matter of personal convenience, as well as the avoidance of cumulative fatigue.

It should be noted that the predicted maximum oxygen consumption levels used in Phase 1 were derived from the program's customary sub-maximal exercise stress test (see Appendix, p. 305). Ideally, your own initial level of fitness should therefore be estimated in the same manner. However, if this is not possible, a comparable test should be used; the step test described elsewhere in this book is a rough equivalent suitable in most cases.

Phase 2

This table progresses you through a series of steps which increase the intensity of the workout to a desired pace (10 minutes per mile if you are under 45, 12 minutes per mile if you are over 45). When you achieve your desired pace, then the distance is lengthened to four miles, while maintaining the same speed. This is a crucial phase and may take many months to complete. If you have heart disease, you should be particularly attentive to the possible development of such adverse symptoms as chest pain, extreme breathlessness, skipped beats, and light-headedness during the workout. These symptoms will be discussed again in the next chapter. If the condition of your heart is unstable, it is more likely to reveal itself at the faster speeds. In general, walking at a pace quicker than 15 minutes per mile tends to develop into an awkward gallop, and becomes excessively strenuous. In order to prevent this, we introduce short jogging segments when the prescription calls for 14½ minutes-per-mile pace. This is done gradually through each of five stages until one attains 12 minutes-per-mile pace, at which time the entire distance is jogged.

Patients attending the Centre are taken through the jogging transition stages in terms of distances on the Centre's 200-metre track. The instructions given to them are as follows:

> Please note that in the following exercise prescriptions, walking is done at 15 minutes-per-mile pace, and jogging at 12 minutes-per-mile pace. All speeds for the mile and three mile distances are rounded off to the nearest minute or half-minute. It is essential to try and keep as closely as possible to the 15 minutes-per-mile pace for walking and the 12 minutes-per-mile pace for jogging. The 13½ minutes-per-mile pace is repeated in the tables so as to effect a smoother transition from half-lap (100-metre) jogs to whole-lap (200-metre) jogs.
>
> 1) 14½-minute-mile (43½ minutes for three miles). Walk first 3½ laps, jog the next half-lap, and repeat five times to give three miles.
> 2) 14-minute-mile (42 minutes for three miles). Walk the first 1½ laps, jog the next half-lap, and repeat eleven times to give three miles.
> 3a) 13½-minute-mile (40½ minutes for three miles). Walk the first half-lap, jog the next half-lap, and repeat twenty-three times to give three miles.

3b) 13½-minute-mile (40½ minutes for three miles). Walk and jog alternate 200-metre laps for total of twenty-four laps to give three miles.

4) 13-minute-mile (39 minutes for three miles). Walk the first ½ lap, jog the next 1½ laps, and repeat eleven times to give three miles.

5) 12-minute-mile (36 minutes for three miles). Jog the entire distance.

For those of you who do not attend the Centre, you may still have access to a 200- or 400-metre track, in which case the above instructions should be adhered to. However, if you are using the sidewalk or park as your training course, you will have to use a slightly different approach. The first and most important task is for you to thoroughly familiarize yourself with the 15-minutes-per-mile walking pace and then with the 12-minutes-per-mile jogging pace. The latter is equivalent to jogging 100 metres in 45 seconds. Having mastered this, then the five stages outlined above can be expressed as follows:

1) 14½-minute-mile (43½ minutes for three miles). Walk for 6½ minutes (700 metres at 15-minute-mile pace) and jog for 45 seconds (100 metres at 12-minute-mile pace). Repeat five times to give three miles.

2) 14-minute-mile (42 minutes for three miles). Walk for 2 minutes, 45 seconds (300 metres), and jog for 45 seconds (100 metres). Repeat eleven times to give three miles.

3a) 13½-minute-mile (40½ minutes for three miles). Walk for 56 seconds (100 metres) and jog for 45 seconds (100 metres). Repeat twenty-three times for three miles.

3b) 13½-minute-mile (40½ minutes for three miles). Walk for 1 minute, 53 seconds (200 metres) and jog for 90 seconds (200 metres). Repeat eleven times for three miles.

4) 13-minute-mile (39 minutes for three miles). Walk for 1 minute (100 metres) and jog for 2 minutes, 15 seconds (300 metres). Repeat eleven times for three miles.

5) 12-minute-mile (36 minutes for three miles). Jog the entire distance.

As you can see, you will need a good sense of pace and an accurate stop watch for the jogging transition phase, but the effort is worth it in terms of safety and avoidance of minor but irritating injuries to muscles and tendons.

The jogging technique will be described in detail later, but at this stage it is sufficient to say that it should be relaxed, flat-footed and with short strides; the speed should be a little above that of a walk. Actually, I feel that the term "plodding" is more descriptive than jogging.

Phase 3

Here, you will progress to jogging six miles in 60 or 72 minutes, depending on your age. This goal requires about twelve months, and is well worth achieving. It puts you into the class of the long distance jogger, and brings all of the benefits we have previously discussed. Anyone who has managed to progress through the first two phases and is free from symptoms and signs should certainly attempt to finish Phase 3. Jogging for an hour a day five times a week may be time-consuming, but it pays off in terms of high-level cardiorespiratory fitness. From the ranks of the "one hour joggers" have come the post-coronary marathoners who so amply demonstrated the rehabilitative power of physical exercise.

HOW TO USE THE TABLES

Determining your Starting Level

How fit are you? The only way to answer this accurately is to undergo a maximal or sub-maximal exercise stress test, as outlined in Part One of this book. This will give you a figure for your maximum oxygen consumption, expressed as the number of millilitres of oxygen your body burns each minute for every kilogram you weigh. Not only that, but the test will also show whether or not you develop electrocardiographic abnormalities during training sessions. Such a test is, of course, highly desirable for individuals with coronary artery disease who wish to start exercising. It is mandatory for all patients entering my exercise rehabilitation program. If you are a would-be exerciser, and have a heart problem, then you should ask your physician to arrange an exercise test. If he doesn't do this procedure himself, then he should refer you to a physician who does.

What if there aren't any facilities for exercise testing in your area? There are a number of do-it-yourself tests, but these should only be carried out if you have had prior clearance from your physician to do so. They are a lot more strenuous than they look, and may even be dangerous for the middle-aged sedentary individual suffering from symptomless and so far undetected atheroscle-

Table 4

Legend: Rate of Stepping (steps per min.) / Energy Cost of Stepping (millilitres of oxygen)

How to Estimate Your Rate of Stepping, the Resulting Energy Cost, and Target Heart Rate from Your Weight and Age.

MALE

Weight lbs. (kg.) / AGE	110 (49.9)	120 (54.4)	130 (59.0)	140 (63.5)	150 (68.0)	160 (72.6)	170 (77.1)	180 (81.6)	190 (86.2)	200 (90.7)	210 (95.3)	220 (99.8)
20 – 29	120 / 1570	120 / 1690	120 / 1813	126 / 2018	126 / 2143	126 / 2273	126 / 2398	126 / 2524	126 / 2653	126 / 2779	126 / 2908	126 / 3034
30 – 39	108 / 1437	114 / 1618	114 / 1734	114 / 1848	114 / 1962	114 / 2079	114 / 2192	114 / 2307	114 / 2423	120 / 2658	120 / 2781	120 / 2901
40 – 49	96 / 1304	96 / 1400	96 / 1498	102 / 1679	102 / 1781	102 / 1885	102 / 1987	102 / 2089	102 / 2193	102 / 2295	102 / 2400	102 / 2502
50 – 60	78 / 1105	78 / 1183	78 / 1262	78 / 1340	78 / 1418	78 / 1498	84 / 1679	84 / 1763	84 / 1849	84 / 1933	84 / 2018	84 / 2103

FEMALE

Weight lbs. (kg.) / AGE	80 (36.3)	90 (40.8)	100 (45.4)	110 (49.9)	120 (54.4)	130 (59.0)	140 (63.5)	150 (68.0)	160 (72.6)	170 (77.1)	180 (81.6)	190 (86.2)
20 – 29	96 / 974	102 / 1125	102 / 1229	102 / 1331	102 / 1433	108 / 1616	108 / 1724	108 / 1832	108 / 1942	108 / 2050	108 / 2158	108 / 2268
30 – 39	96 / 974	96 / 1070	102 / 1229	102 / 1331	102 / 1433	102 / 1537	102 / 1639	108 / 1832	108 / 1942	108 / 2050	108 / 2158	108 / 2268
40 – 49	84 / 877	84 / 961	84 / 1047	90 / 1198	90 / 1288	90 / 1380	90 / 1469	90 / 1560	90 / 1652	90 / 1742	96 / 1932	96 / 2038
50 – 60	60 / 684	60 / 744	60 / 805	60 / 865	60 / 925	60 / 986	60 / 1046	60 / 1106	60 / 1163	60 / 1228	60 / 1288	60 / 1349

(age-related) after 3–5 minutes of stepping

Age (Years)	Heart Rate (Beats/min.)
20–30	160/min.
30–40	150/min.
40–50	140/min.
50–60	130/min.
60–70	120/min.

Table 5   Target Heart Rates

and let us say, for illustrative purposes, it comes to 150 beats per minute. Then, from nomogram E (p. 302) you read off a predicted maximum oxygen intake of 2200 millilitres per minute (a line joining 1885 on the right column and 150 on the left column intersects the centre sloping line at 2200). You now divide your predicted maximum oxygen consumption of 2200 by your weight in kilograms (72.6 kg) and you obtain your VO_2 max. corrected for weight, i.e. 30.3ml/kg min. Applying this to the training tables would mean that you could start at Level 7 of Phase 1, or three miles in 45 minutes.

Sounds complicated: It isn't really, but if you find it a chore even to contemplate, then skip it and start at the Preliminary Phase, Level 1.

What if you develop chest pain or discomfort, extreme breathlessness, light-headedness, or other adverse symptoms before the five minutes are up? If this occurs, then stop immediately, and note your pulse rate. This will represent your maximum heart rate for training purposes. For safety's sake, you should obtain your doctor's permission before you start the exercise program. If he agrees that exercise can help you, then start at the preliminary conditioning stage of the tables, and be sure that your pulse rate during the workout remains at least 10 beats per minute below the symptom-producing level.

Two very important points! Your stepping rate must be as accurately timed as possible. The best way to do this is to use a simple metronome, the sort that piano teachers used to use. If you don't want to invest, I'm sure you can borrow one from one of your musical friends. Just set the scale to the desired stepping rate, and merely keep in time with the beat. Secondly, pulse rate should be obtained *immediately* on stopping. Ideally, it should be taken during the last minute of the test, but this is very difficult to do. Instead, as you stop, take a ten second pulse count, and then multiply the result by six to give a full minute's count. Remember, the heart rate begins to drop pretty rapidly with the cessation of exercise, and if you delay as little as even 30 seconds in finding and counting your pulse, the result will not truly represent your heart rate in the final minutes of the test.

You may find that after two minutes or so of stepping you feel that you cannot continue for the plain and simple reason that your legs are too tired. This means that you are even less fit than the average sedentary person of your age and weight, i.e., the rate of stepping prescribed for you in Table 4 represents more than 75 per cent of *your* maximum oxygen consumption, and so you can't keep the pace up for more than a few minutes. If you take your pulse rate at the time that you have to stop, you will find that it is already well above target rate. Don't despair, try again the following day, but this time choose the tempo listed next lowest in the table, e.g. 96 instead of 102 steps per minute.

Finally, at the risk of being unduly repetitive, let me once again warn you against attempting this or any other self-administered test without the permission of your physician — especially if you have any of the symptoms of coronary artery disease. Paradoxically, those most curious to know their fitness level are the overweight, sedentary, obviously unfit members of the population — precisely those in whom atherosclerosis is likely to be present. Beware that curiosity doesn't kill the fat cat.

You are now in the position to choose a suitable starting level from Phase 1. If you do not know your fitness level, and suffer from heart disease, then start from Level 1 of the Preliminary Phase. If your fitness level has been measured, then it is a simple matter to use the calculated maximum oxygen consumption and apply it to the tables. For example, assume you are age 40, and were found to have a fitness level of 25 ml/kg/min. This would place you in Phase 1, Level 5 of the training tables, and would give a starting prescription of three miles in 48 minutes, five times weekly. You would start by walking one mile in 16 minutes for two weeks, and then increase this to two miles in 32 minutes for a further two weeks. At the end of this time, provided that you are not suffering any cardiac or musculoskeletal problems, you would proceed to your three miles in 48 minutes.

A unique meeting in Boston, 1975: Dr. Roger Bannister (*left*), the first man to run a mile in less than four minutes, and Herman Robers, the first man to be an official entrant in the Boston Marathon after having had a heart attack.

HOW TO PROGRESS THROUGH THE TABLES

Having chosen a suitable starting level, we must now consider how you are to progress through the higher levels of Phase 1, through Phase 2 and then Phase 3, preferably without frequent repetition of time-consuming and relatively expensive laboratory exercise tests. We can achieve this by using our knowledge of the effect of training on heart function.

We have seen that endurance fitness is attained by exercising regularly at an intensity of about 50 to 70 per cent of maximum oxygen consumption. The problem is, oxygen consumption is not something which can be measured readily. Fortunately, however, there is a relationship between oxygen consumption and heart rate. Provided we know our resting heart rate and also our maximum heart rate, we can calculate a training heart rate which, as a practical field guide, corresponds to 70 per cent of maximum oxygen consumption.

Resting heart rate is easy to obtain. You merely take your pulse rate immediately on awakening in the morning, and before you get out of bed. As before, count the number of beats in 10 seconds and then multiply by six. This is much more accurate than obtaining a resting pulse after sitting still for five or ten minutes; too many extraneous factors such as a recent meal, emotional excitement, or recent physical activity can give a false result.

Maximum heart rate decreases with age, and varies substantially from one healthy person to another. The only way to assess maximum heart rate accurately is to carry out a maximum exercise test. However, since this requires all-out effort, it poses problems both in terms of motivation and safety. A more practical alternative is to use tables of average values for maximum heart rates at different age levels. Such tables are sufficiently precise for the safety of the post-coronary patient who is free from symptoms (See Table 5).

Thus, we have available the two essential pieces of information necessary to control progression in the training program: the actual resting heart rate, and the age-related maximum heart rate. Remember, however, that as you become fitter, you develop a training bradycardia; that is, both resting and working heart rates become slower. Eventually, the intensity and duration of the prescribed workout is ineffectual in obtaining the 70 per cent training heart rate. When this stage is reached, progression to a higher level is indicated.

The above basic principles have been used to devise a simple nomogram (A) which relates resting heart rate and age to a progressing heart rate. When the prescribed workout consistently fails to achieve the progressing heart rate for a period of two weeks, then the time has come to move up to the next level on the table. Say, for instance, that our 40-year-old who started at Level 5, Phase 1 (three miles in 48 minutes) had a resting heart rate of 68 beats per minute. To use nomogram A, he would take a piece of black

NOMOGRAM A
To Be Used for Calculating Your Progressing Heart Rate
For those who have completed a stress test without adverse symp-
toms or who are free from heart disease.

| Age | Progressing Heart Rate (beats per minute) | Resting Heart Rate (beats per minute) |

A line joining your resting heart rate and your age will intersect the centre column at your progressing heart rate. Resting heart rates below 72 beats per minute should be charted at 72.

To obtain your heart rate (pulse rate) and resting heart rate see pages 139, 141-2.

thread and place it so as to join 72 on the resting heart rate column (values less than 72 can, for the purposes of the prediction, be ignored) and 40 on the age column. Where the thread crosses the centre line is his progressing heart rate: 130 beats per minute. Thus, when his pulse count in the 10 seconds following his three-mile walk is at or below this level consistently for a period of two weeks (an average for ten successive workouts), he would be ready to progress to Level 6 (three miles in 45 minutes). The use of the nomogram, therefore, enables safe and effective progression without constant retesting. It gives you an element of objectivity in your training regime; instead of stepping up your program because you feel good, you can apply a physiological measure to validate your enthusiasm.

For the nomogram to be of maximal value, however, it must be used correctly. Not only must the post-workout heart rate be at or below the progressing heart rate *consistently* for ten or more exercise sessions but, moreover, progression to a higher level of effort should not be attempted in the presence of any of the signs of over-training such as excessive tiredness, palpitations (premature ventricular beats) or muscle aches and pains. (The latter will be discussed in more detail in the next chapter.) Your heart rate must be charted at the end of each exercise session in order to keep an accurate record.

Of course, the nomogram contains two other variables, age and resting heart rate. The majority of patients reach the end of Phase 2, or attain their maximum fitness potential, within a two-year period; therefore, once started on the program it should not be necessary to change their age level on the left-hand column. As for resting heart rate, this also drops with training but, as we have seen, the change is more variable than with exercise heart rate. For patients on a supervised program a new resting heart rate can be established at the time of each laboratory exercise stress test; failing this, you can obtain your resting heart rate every six months and adjust the right-hand column accordingly.

Obtaining Your Pulse Rate

It is essential that the pulse rate be correctly obtained. So far, this has been taken for granted, but is such an integral part of a home exercise program that we will take the time now to discuss it in more detail. The pumping heart imparts to every large blood vessel an impulse which coincides with the heart beat. Physicians traditionally measure heart rate by timing the pulse of the radial artery in the front of the wrist just below the base of the thumb. The vessel is easily accessible in this position, lying just beneath the skin, and is easily felt because it can be steadied against the underlying wrist bones. Exercise physiologists tend to use the carotid pulse, the large artery in the front of the neck which can be felt on either side of the Adam's apple; this vessel pumps very vigorously during exercise, and for that reason is easer to obtain (except in short, thick-necked individuals when there may be some difficulty).

Whether you use the carotid or the radial pulse is probably unimportant, and will depend on whichever you find the easiest. If you use the carotid, then be careful not to press too hard with your palpating fingers, otherwise you will press on a structure known as the carotid sinus, and this will artificially slow the heart rate momentarily. (As a matter of fact, simultaneous firm pressure on both sides of the neck over the carotid sinus may slow your heart rate to such a degree that consciousness is lost — a well-known tactic in karate!) Even though it may be more difficult to obtain the carotid pulse in some people, I usually try to train my patients to use this method of pulse counting; once mastered, it allows you to operate a stop watch in the other hand and so get an accurate count. If you are having difficulty in feeling the carotid pulse, it may be that you are instinctively throwing your head back, a movement which causes the carotid arteries to retract away from the front of the neck. If you want to feel the carotid pulse easily, then hold your head in the normal position, or even slightly tilted forward.

Having found the pulse, you must now count it accurately. Since you are only counting for 10 seconds, and multiplying by six, accuracy is essential. If you are as much as one beat out, then your one minute reading will be substantially in error. For uniformity's sake we have always told our patients to start counting zero, one, two, three, etc., the zero marking the commencement of the ten second count. Actually, I find it easier to repeat the word "five" a number of times as I watch the second hand of my watch approach the start point, thus: five, five, five — zero, one, two, three, etc. Somehow or other it gives me the correct rhythm for counting.

Why count for only 10 seconds? Ideally, we want to know what the heart rate is *during* the exercise session. As soon as you start to work out, your resting heart rate climbs, and within two or three minutes reaches a plateau which remains steady for as long as you exercise — provided, of course, that you maintain the same pace. It is the level of heart rate during the exercise session which we need to know. Since it is impractical to take the pulse rate while jogging, or even walking, we utilize the fact that it takes 10 or 15 seconds to drop from the plateau as soon as the exercise stops. Pulse rates, then, taken within 10 seconds of stopping jog-

Figure 20   When to Take Exercise Heart Rate

ging or brisk walking, are a fairly accurate measure of the heart rate during the workout. Thereafter, the rate drops off rapidly, and if you wait as little as 20 seconds to take your count, it will no longer be representative of the rate during exertion (Figure 20). Hence the need to be speedy and well-practised in this technique.

THE INDIVIDUAL WITH ANGINA PECTORIS OR RELATED SYMPTOMS

So far, we have been discussing the use of the nomogram to check the progress of the individual who, while he has heart disease, does not suffer from symptoms such as angina pectoris. In my program, I refer to him as the "uncomplicated exerciser." What of the individual who suffers from symptoms, especially when exercising? He falls into the category of the "complicated exerciser" and for him there is a special nomogram. Into this category also fall those patients who have had a formal exercise test which has revealed the presence of such ECG abnormalities as severe ST segment depression or increasing extrasystoles. Here, our interest is not so much in fitness level as in determining the level of activity at which adverse symptoms or signs occur, and then formulating a training prescription which takes this factor into account.

This is no problem in a hospital-type program where regular stress testing can be carried out and an exact figure specified for the level of exertion at which cardiac problems develop. Such repeated testing is impractical, however, in a community-type home program. On the other hand, the use of average tables of maximum heart rates does not ensure enough accuracy for safety. A more individualized approach is required, and the obvious one is a simple record of the heart rate at which untoward symptoms or signs develop. Working on this principle, a second nomogram has been devised (B) which permits the choice of a suitable starting level of exercise for the patient with symptoms, and his subsequent safe progress through the various stages of the tables. Decision on the starting level of the tables requires rather more trial and error than in the uncomplicated case.

Assuming that symptoms develop during a stress test, either carried out in the doctor's office or at home, then note is made of the pulse rate at which these occurred. I refer to this as the maximum heart rate, symptom limited, or max. H.R.[SL]. Using this figure, together with the resting heart rate (obtained as previously) then the training heart rate can be read from Nomogram B. A word of warning: If the difference between your resting heart rate and your max. H.R.[SL] is 40 beats per minute or less, then you should exercise only under the strict supervision of a physician. As you can see from the nomogram, the spread between training and progressing heart rates would be small in your case, requiring careful, accurate monitoring — too delicate a job for the average reader of this book. However, if this proviso does not apply to you, a trial one-mile walk is then taken, at a pace which is considered brisk, but not so fast as to bring on chest pain, skipped beats, or undue breathlessness. The pulse rate is taken in the 10 seconds immediately following the walk, and is compared with the desired training heart rate. Depending on the result, the speed is adjusted to the nearest appropriate level in Phase 1, always erring on the side of safety: that is, keeping the intensity of exercise below the level at which symptoms of cardiac ischemia develop. It may take one or two sessions to select the desired pace, but with patience and care, it is surprising how accurate one can be.

The following example will illustrate the method. Assume you have a resting heart rate of 72 beats per minute. While being tested, you develop evidence of ischemia, say chest pain, at a heart rate of 124 beats per minute. This means that you have a max. H.R.[SL] of 124. From the nomogram, this will give you a training heart rate[SL] of 110 beats per minute. You now go for a trial one-mile walk, choosing a level course, and keeping the pace slow enough to avoid chest pain or undue breathlessness. At the end of the

NOMOGRAM B
To Be Used for Calculating Your Training Heart Rate and Your
Progressing Heart Rate.

Maximum Heart Rate (Symptom Limited)
(beats per minute)

TRAINING HEART RATE
(beats per minute)

PROGRESSING HEART RATE
(beats per minute)

RESTING HEART RATE
(beats per minute)

For those who have not been able to complete a stress test because of the development of adverse symptoms or who have symptoms of coronary heart disease such as anginal pain, palpitations or breathlessness, etc. (see pages 119-23).

A line joining your resting heart rate and the heart rate at which your symptoms appear, your maximum heart rate (symptom limited), will intersect the centre columns at your training heart rate and progressing heart rate. Resting heart rates above 72 beats per minute should be charted at 72.

If the difference between your resting heart rate and your maximum heart rate (symptom limited) is less than 40 beats per minute, you should not attempt the training program in this book, except under medical supervision.

To obtain your heart rate (pulse rate) and resting heart rate see pages 139, 141-2.

measured mile, you discover that you have taken 20 minutes, and your immediate post-exercise heart rate is 108 beats per minute. This, then, is your starting level (Level 1, Phase 1 for an under 45-year-old) and over the next six weeks, you progress to two miles and then to three miles keeping the same pace of 20 minutes per mile. Using the same nomogram you can also tell what your progressing heart rate should be (in this example, 100 beats per minute). After each workout, you chart your pulse rate, and when this consistently fails to achieve 100 beats per minute for ten consecutive sessions, and provided you have none of the adverse symptoms mentioned above, then you progress to Level 2, Phase 1.

Not infrequently, a patient who initially shows evidence of myocardial ischemia during a test will, as he gets fitter, move into the category of an uncomplicated exerciser. This may take time, but nevertheless, for this reason, I feel that complicated cases should be exercise-tested every three months or so in order to have an objective measurement of improvement. When they can complete an uncomplicated test, then they can be progressed in accordance with Nomogram A. Complicated cases require much closer physician supervision than uncomplicated ones, and ideally should be enrolled in a formal post-coronary exercise rehabilitation class. In this way, they can be watched during supervised exercise sessions and monitored frequently during the workout.

In the early stages, the individual with symptoms during exercise will progress at a slower rate than his symptomless colleagues. This is to be expected, and should not be allowed to cause discouragement or depression. Above all, any temptation to progress faster than the tables indicate should be vigorously resisted. You cannot bully a damaged heart. This is one game where breaking the rules may mean more than the loss of a few yards or a touchdown; it may mean "game over" for the only player involved —yourself! So, have patience, and remember that if it took twenty years to get out of shape, you can't really expect to regain your fitness in a few months.

CHAPTER EIGHT

Some Do's and Don'ts

ATTAINMENT OF FITNESS

There are a few basic facts about physical fitness which should be borne in mind. First, each of us has an optimal level of endurance fitness which is appropriate to our age, sex and genetic background. Once we reach that level, more intensive training will result in only marginal gains. By the law of diminishing returns, the improvement will be minimal in comparison to the time and effort invested. Mark you, if one is a world champion, the extra effort may be worth it, for even fractional advances may make all the difference between victory and defeat. However, for most of us, such slender gains are of little cardiovascular advantage.

Let me give you an example of what I mean. An international long distance runner, with a maximum oxygen uptake of 70 ml/kg/min. is averaging, say 70 miles a week in training. By increasing this to 90 miles a week, he might conceivably improve his oxygen uptake by a few millilitres (although it is more likely to help him by increasing the ease or degree of mechanical efficiency with which he runs, thus allowing him to go further and faster on the same amount of oxygen); this slight improvement may be sufficient to reduce his time by 20 to 30 seconds — which is probably all that separates the top ten men in the world in his event.

For us lesser mortals, the requirements are not so exacting. The training tables have been devised to progress you to a level which is suitable for your age and general tolerance. They are based on maximum oxygen consumption levels attained by patients on the post-coronary exercise program, and should, therefore, be well within the capabilities of the vast majority of readers.

Of course, there are always exceptions to the rule. For example, some will be unable to progress to the end of Phase 3 in the tables. They may stick at an earlier level because of adverse symptoms, failure to achieve the progressing heart rate, or fatigue after the workout. Does this mean that they are wasting their time training? Definitely not. They have attained what is the right duration and intensity of workout for them, at least for the time being, and can rest assured that if they continue to work out at this level, they will maintain their maximum potential.

A case in point is Charles W., an industrial chemist, who was one of the first patients on the program. He sustained a severe heart attack at the age of 56. For the first week or so after the attack, his condition was so serious that he was not expected to survive. Complications included multiple cardiac arrests, and almost complete failure of the heart to function as a pump. For days, he was kept alive only by the heroic efforts of the coronary care team. When he arrived at the Centre his exercise test revealed a very limited physical tolerance, poor fitness level, and many abnormalities on the dynamic electrocardiogram. Not surprisingly, Charles found it impossible to progress to the end stage of the training tables. As a matter of fact, he never did succeed in getting beyond the walking stage. Yet, despite that, he obtained great benefit from the program.

Did it help? He thought so, and I would most certainly agree. Forced into an early retirement by the attack, he worked out regularly, rarely missing a day. As his fitness increased, so his general tolerance improved, until eventually he was able to contemplate work again. However, with a new lease on life, he decided that rather than return to his old job, he would offer his services to Canadian Executive Service Overseas (CESO), an organization of Canadian executives who assist in the establishment of vital industries in the underdeveloped nations. As a result, he travelled extensively in South America, the Caribbean, and the Far East. His exercise diaries arrived from all parts of the world, and he carried out his prescription walk in airports, around padangs, on board ship, in hotel corridors and, in fact, anywhere he could find a suitable space. When he ultimately died at the age of 70, it was from a non-cardiac cause. Whether or not the exercise program prolonged his life has to be a matter of opinion. What is not in dispute is that his regular walking regime vastly improved the quality of his last fourteen years.

There is a misapprehension about the development of fitness which I think it is important to dispel. Most people believe that a training program, carried out regularly, results in a gradual day-by-day improvement in your physical state. In actual fact, I have found that this is not the case. If you are expecting progress in this manner, then you are in for a big disappointment. What usually happens is that you plug away for weeks, or even months, without any apparent change, and then suddenly one day, you find the workout quite easy. At the same time, you will notice that your post-workout pulse rate has dropped a few beats or more. Or you will discover that you have completed the distance a few minutes faster than ever before. At first you will doubt the watch itself, but when you repeat the performance the following day, you will realize that you have suddenly and almost miraculously attained a new level of fitness.

What has happened? One of the major effects of training is to open up new blood capillaries in the skeletal muscle tissue so as to be able to transport more oxygen to the working cells. These new capillaries, so small that they can be seen only under a microscope, do not form gradually. They "open up," almost like a budding flower seen under time-lapse photography, and in response to the stimulus of repeated and prolonged training sessions. The duration of their formative period obviously varies from individual to individual, and is dependent upon the type and nature of the training program. The thing to remember is that the plateau is an essential part of the process. Don't get discouraged because your condition appears to be static. In actual fact, the preliminary work of capillarization is continuing apace; the next day may see a great leap forward.

HOW TO JOG

Recreational jogging for fun and fitness is reputed to have started in New Zealand. It was introduced by the world-famous track coach, Arthur Lydiard, who believed in marathon-type training for all his competitive runners, even his half-milers and milers. Since his protégés included such world champions as Peter Snell, is it small wonder that his training methods were imitated by coaches all over the world?

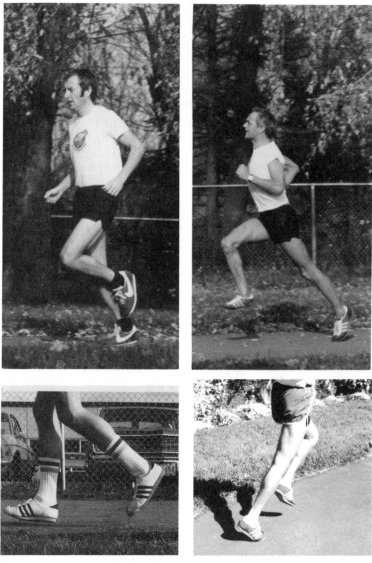

The right way (*left*) and the wrong way to jog. Note that the subject on the left is relaxed, the arms are carried at hip height and the body is upright. The close-up photo at the lower right shows good action for the youthful sprinter, but the close-up on the left shows the desirable style for the distance jogger, with a relaxed, flat-footed landing.

Winter training run; summer marathon run.

Apart from his interest in competitive track and field, however, Lydiard has always believed that physical fitness is the key to a happy and healthy life, and that slow long distance running is the best way to achieve such fitness. When Bill Bowerman, the highly succesful university track coach from Oregon, visited New Zealand, he was amazed to find that jogging was the national pastime. Young and old, male and female, all were caught up in the business of running for miles through the countryside at a slow steady pace, often in groups, joking and talking with one another along the way. Lydiard persuaded Bowerman to join his group for a jogging session. For Bowerman, it was his moment of truth. Within a matter of miles, he was having difficulty keeping up with runners in their 60s and 70s; to make matters worse, he later discovered that one of the "oldsters" who accompanied him for most of the way had deliberately held back in order to provide the visiting American coach with company! When Bowerman returned to the United States, he immediately launched a movement to introduce recreational jogging. Today, his home town of Eugene refers to itself as "The Jogging Capital of the World," with thousands of the inhabitants jogging regularly.

The next major development was the introduction by Dr. Kenneth Cooper, at that time in the United States Air Force, of endurance-type running as the main component in the service's fitness program. He later went on to introduce the same program to the population at large, through the medium of his book *Aerobics*.

Now we have the approach outlined in this book — the use of medically prescribed jogging and marathon-type training for the benefit of patients with heart disease.

Despite this impressive history, the technique of jogging still remains a mystery to many. It differs from running only in its speed of progression. In our particular context, jogging means running at a pace of 10 minutes per mile or slower. The action is simple; take short steps, about 2 to 4 feet in length, and always land flat-footed. The body should be erect, the shoulders and neck relaxed, and the head held naturally (if you fix your eyes on an imaginary spot about 30 yards ahead, this will give the correct head inclination). The elbows should be bent not quite to a right angle, so that the hands move backwards and forwards about the level of the hips; the more you bend your elbows, the faster your arms will swing back and forth, and this in turn will lead to an unconscious pick-up in the rapidity of your leg action and an undesirable increase in speed. The short stride and the flat-foot landing will ensure that your centre of gravity remains over the landing foot, thus preventing too much of a forward body lean, which is all very well for the sprinter or competitive middle distance runner, but plays no part in recreational jogging.

Middle-aged joggers should not try to emulate the running style of their teens. Running up on the toes, or practising an exaggerated heel roll, may have looked very impressive, but don't try it now — not unless you wish to develop a whole host of injuries which go by the impressive names of Achilles tendonitis, shin-splints, stress fractures, plantar fasciitis, tenosynovitis; need I list more?

EQUIPMENT

You will need a *stop watch* for counting your pulse and also timing your workout. A deluxe model is very nice, and if you can persuade your family to give you one for Christmas or Chanukkah, so much the better. However, the majority of people in my class manage quite well with a watch which costs around $55, has a 30-minute dial, and is marked off in 1/5ths of a second. Pressing the centre winding-knob starts the timing mechanism, a second press stops it, and a third press returns it to the zero position. Incidentally, there is not much point in having an accurate stop watch if you haven't accurately measured the distance you are walking or jogging. If you are using the local school track, then don't assume that each lap is a quarter of a mile. As a matter of fact, a great many school tracks have been constructed in accordance with the space available, and may need five circuits to complete a mile. If you are working out on the road, you will get an accurate enough reading from a car odometer; I have rarely found these to be misleading — unless, of course the hot rodder in the family has fitted your sedan with outsize tires!

Shoes are the most important item you will purchase, and you should not attempt to economize here. Just think of the number of times your feet will strike the ground when you are jogging five hours a week, week in, week out. Your feet require to be protected from the pounding they will receive, and it is precisely for this reason that special shoes have been designed for the long distance runner. While each manufacturer has individual variations, the following features tend to be common to all. They are relatively light, a pair often weighing less than two pounds. The sole is flexible but thick enough to absorb shock. It is frequently laminated, with layers of sponge rubber for shock absorption and high density rubber for stability. An arch support is usually built in, and the inner aspects of the tongue specially padded to protect the instep from the pressure of the laces. The upper is made of nylon, and the portion around the heel (the counter) is reinforced so as to grip the heel firmly and prevent it from wobbling from side to side as you run. Since the heel takes most of our body weight when we run, a special rubber heel wedge is often a feature and, to protect the Achilles tendon, or heel cord, the back of the shoe extends upwards in a soft padded tongue which adds additional support and prevents chafing.

Needless to say, no one shoe is ideal, and the individual will have to find the particular brand of running shoe which suits him best. At the time of writing, the major manufacturers in the field are Brooks, New Balance, Nike, Adidas and Puma. All of these manufacturers make a variety of shoes for runners. When you purchase, be sure to ask for a good "training" shoe. The so-called "racing flat" sacrifices some support for lightness, and while this is of value in an actual road race, this type of shoe is unsuitable for regular training.

A *sweat suit* is valuable, but not essential. A pair of slacks and a sweater will do just as well. It's purely a question of how natty you want to appear. Unless you live on the west coast, except for the summer months much of your training will be done in some form of garb which covers your legs and upper body. Therefore, a commercial sweat suit is probably the most convenient. My personal preference is for one which is made from a mixture of nylon and cotton, since this absorbs the sweat much better than a pure nylon suit. *Running shorts and T-shirt* are essential, but hardly represent a strain on the budget. While some runners like to run without *socks*, the majority prefer a light cotton pair in order to prevent blisters.

So you see, you don't require a mass of paraphernalia to embark on your training program, which means that if you are the sort of person who derives your greatest enjoyment from spending $300 or $400 on equipment for your latest whim, you should seek some more fashionable and likely less beneficial form of activity. You will never be able to blame jogging for that bank overdraft!

OVER-TRAINING

Training is achieved by overloading the body to the point where it has to work just a little harder to accomplish a given task. Measured doses of stress are applied, regularly and over a prolonged period, so that eventually resistance to that stress develops. The art of scientific training is to apply just enough overload, or stress, to achieve the desired result but not so much that the organism is overstrained and breaks down. Over-training, or staleness as it is usually referred to by track coaches, is characterized by chronic fatigue, irritability, susceptibility to minor infections such as colds and boils, insomnia, loss of appetite, lack of concentration, and decline in inclination and ability to train. The competitive athlete who is suffering from staleness may force himself to continue training but his performance steadily declines despite all his efforts. The ultimate answer is to rest for one or two weeks, and give the body time to recuperate. This is dealt with more fully in Chapter 12 under the heading "Build-up *versus* Breakdown."

While such an exaggerated state of affairs is unlikely to occur in the post-coronary jogger, nevertheless it is even more important in his case that he recognize the signs and symptoms of over-training, since his condition demands that there be a finer margin of error in the training process. Be alert, therefore, for such signs as excessive muscle soreness, an increase in your resting pulse rate, undue tiredness persisting to the next training session, premature ventricular beats or palpitations, increasing angina, marked breathlessness, or light-headedness during exercise. These four last symptoms are evidence of myocardial ischemia, and their consistent presence during exercise suggests that the coronary blood flow is not keeping pace with the other training responses. Their presence contra-indicates progression to the next training level. Indeed, if they appear for the first time or become more frequent in response to an exercise prescription, you should reduce your prescription to the next lowest level.

Having said this, I should also add the rider that almost all post-coronary patients experience exercise-induced angina or irregularity of heart action at some time or other in their program. How much to permit becomes a matter of fine judgment based on experience, and if you are not enrolled in a regular cardiac exercise class, then you should consult your physician on this matter.

Before blaming the prescription entirely for an increase in symptoms, you should consider whether or not you are under unusual business stress or are working prolonged hours. The typical post-coronary exerciser is usually enthusiastic and conscientious, and he often tries to maintain the prescribed level of exercise even during busy spells at his job. The result is that when he is at work he worries that he won't have time to carry out his exercise prescription, while during his workout he is worrying that the time spent in training could have been spent at work. I have learned to beware of various occupations at certain times of the year: for instance, accountants towards the end of the financial year, and departmental store workers during the Christmas season. At these times of stress, an exercise prescription which under normal circumstances is carried out easily and without symptoms may give rise to angina at the end of a long and worrisome day. The obvious solution is to cut back the exercise prescription until the work pattern returns to normal.

What if the high stress of employment looks like becoming permanent? The answer again may be to reduce the level of training. But, in the long run, it may be better to take a serious look at the job itself and your attitude towards it. Are you giving to your job more than your employer expects? Are you trying to carry out a job for which you lack the necessary aptitude? An honest answer to these questions may be very self-revealing.

Perhaps you should also re-examine your sleep habits. Chronic lack of sleep seems to be a feature of modern urban living. The long journey home from the office to the suburbs usually means a late evening meal, often followed by watching television until the early hours of the morning (have you noticed how late all the best shows start?). The occasional late night is inevitable, but don't make a habit of it and expect to reap the benefits of training. And don't assume the running program is making you feel overly tired when you haven't bothered to adjust your sleep pattern so as to allow for your additional energy expenditure.

From time to time, one of our joggers who has developed a relatively high level of fitness may experience premature ventricular beats on exertion. These are probably due to the high vagal tone which accompanies a training bradycardia, and usually clear up completely after seven to ten days' rest from training. In such cases, irregular beats do not have serious significance, and I find they occur even in fit long distance runners who are free from heart disease. However, this does not apply to the post-coronary exerciser who develops ectopic beats in response to activity in the early stages of training, and before he has had the opportunity to become truly fit. In these circumstances, they should be taken more seriously.

In the initial stages of the exercise program, it is almost inevitable that you will develop painful ankles and knees, Achilles tendonitis or inflammation of your heel cord, sore feet, and other relatively minor muscle tendon and ligamentous injuries that follow walking and jogging after years of inactivity. While not serious, they are a nuisance and can have an adverse effect on your motivation. A careful warm-up as described below can help but, once again, if the problem persists throughout a complete workout, or is felt between workouts, then a complete rest is indicated. Usually a week is sufficient, but if the trouble recurs on returning to exercise at the end of that time, then you should see your physician who will probably prescribe a course of physiotherapy. Close adherence to the tables, as well as the technique of jogging previously described, will reduce such injuries to a minimum. Remember also that dehydration from jogging in very hot weather can contribute to minor muscle tears, so drink plenty of fluids as advised. Our program's incidence of injuries over the years has been negligible, despite the fact that we are dealing entirely with the middle-aged sedentary individual who hasn't exercised for years.

A pleasant feeling of physical relaxation and tiredness should follow a suitable workout. In many cases, there is an immediate post-exercise sense of exhilaration (for this reason, some people prefer to workout in the morning or early evening rather than just prior to going to bed). Excessive fatigue may be defined as tiredness which is still present after a good night's sleep. It is usually accompanied by muscle soreness and pain and is a sure indicator of over-training. It may not be apparent after one or two exercise sessions, but the building-up from three or four sessions on consecutive days will make it obvious.

Usually after a workout, the pulse returns to its resting level within two hours; this may take a little longer on a hot and humid day. However, a fast heart rate (tachycardia) that persists for four hours or longer suggests that the workout has been too intense.

If you find that you are dreading your next workout, then this is a sure sign of over-training. A fit individual usually looks forward to the workout either as a relief from work-a-day tensions or out of sheer animal spirits. In the early stages of the program, you may not be quite this enthusiastic, but you shouldn't actively dislike the thought of training. If you do, then the exercise prescription is too ambitious and should be reduced.

Excessive irritability is not a symptom to treat lightly. In our experience, it may even herald another heart attack. Your wife may be the first to notice it, and it may be so marked that she takes the trouble to mention it to your family doctor. She may comment that you are ''becoming impossible to live with again,'' thereby implying that you are beginning to act similarly to the way you did before your initial heart attack. In a situation like this, it is essential that you look at your overall work and domestic situation in order to find and, if possible, minimize the cause of stress. In any event, your level of exercise should be cut drastically until the problem is corrected. If you are compulsive, you may resent this; but I am insistent with my patients that the exercise be reduced until at least I and the cardiologist have had a chance to assess the overall situation.

For those who are hooked on exercise, and are jogging five or six miles in an hour, the recognition of over-training may be difficult. The explanation for this may lie in Dr. Hans Selye's famous theory of stress. The application of mild and healthful stress produces both a feeling of elation and euphoria which may last for some hours, and also a change in the body's mechanism which makes it more resistant to that particular form of stress. However, if the stress, or training stimulus, is continued to excessive levels, then specific resistance develops at the cost of generalized resistance; in other words, the highly trained runner becomes extremely resistant to the fatigue of running, but less and less resistant to concurrent infections or mental stress. This may well be the explanation for the high susceptibility of world-class athletes to food poisoning, dysentery, and even such diseases as poliomyelitis. In any event, while the loss of generalized resistance may be obvious to the trained observer such as the physician or the coach, it is often hidden from the athlete by the short-lived sense of well-being which follows each training session. Thus, he may be losing weight, becoming more irritable, and developing many of the other symptoms described above; but each time he works out he feels great for two or three hours and so falls into the trap of repeating the training sessions in the hope that his overall condition will improve.

IF YOU SUFFER FROM ANGINA

If you suffer chest pain on exertion, then you should slow your pace until it goes away. If this does not work, then stop, and wait for it to disappear. As soon as this happens, start to walk again at a pace slow enough to prevent it recurring. Some individuals can "walk through" their angina, but I caution against this in the early stages of the program until you have become thoroughly familiar with your exercise response.

Use of Nitroglycerin

On occasions you may have to take a tablet of glyceryl trinitrate or some similar medication during the workout in order to remove the pain. An alternative is to take the medication ten minutes or so before your training session. I am frequently asked if this in some way reduces the effectiveness of the training. The answer is no. The fact that it enables you to complete your exercise session is, in itself, proof of its value. As you become more fit, you will find that the angina occurs less and less frequently, until eventually you are able to carry out a full workout without the necessity of medication. While on the subject of glyceryl trinitrate tablets, I should correct a common misapprehension. Your heart does not become accustomed to them, neither does their frequent use in any way aggravate your condition; in point of fact, they should be taken as required. It is surprising how many patients are reluctant to seek relief from nitroglycerin because of some imagined ill effect.

Warm-ups

Angina often occurs during the early part of the workout, and can frequently be obviated by practising a warm-up. This means spending five to ten minutes walking at a pace slower than the prescribed intensity, or performing a series of light flexibility calisthenics until your body breaks out into a light sweat. As soon as the sweat appears, you are then warmed up and may commence your prescription. This is very important for angina sufferers, and frequently works just as well as a nitroglycerin tablet. If your prescription is still at a low level, then you can enhance your warm-up at even slower speeds by wearing a sweater under your track suit in order to accelerate the stage of perspiration.

Exercise after Meals

Exercise should never be carried out within two hours of eating a heavy meal. This is particularly important for angina sufferers, since the digestion of food requires an extra supply of blood to the intestines, thus depleting the coronary circulation. In a situation where the coronary arteries are already narrowed, the loss of even a small reservoir of blood in this area can give rise to myocardial ischemia.

If you are an early morning runner and don't like running on an empty stomach then by all means have a roll, cup of coffee, or glass of orange juice before sallying forth; but don't try to trundle through the streets topped up with bacon and eggs, or corned beef hash.

A Flat Course

Hill running may be great training for competitive athletes, but it should be avoided by those with heart disease. It will certainly aggravate a tendency to angina, since the energy expended in running up a slope is a great deal more than that required to cover the same distance at the same pace on the flat. Consequently, all of the distances listed in the tables are assumed to be on a flat course. A slight gradient is permissible provided it is relatively short and is compensated for by an equal length of downhill course. Ideally, however, all of your workouts should be on the flat. If hills are unavoidable, then reduce your speed accordingly.

Cold Weather

There is no doubt that the body's reaction to cold puts a stress on the cardiovascular system. When body temperature falls the blood vessels in the skin constrict, shunting the warm blood away from the surface. This reduces further heat loss through conduction, convection, and radiation. It also ensures that the vital organs are maintained at their optimum operating temperature. The cost of this sudden narrowing of a major portion of blood vessel system is a precipitate rise in the pressure against which the heart is pumping—in other words, a rise in blood pressure. The additional load on the heart brought about by the increase in Double Product (BP × HR) may be sufficient to induce angina in an individual with narrowed coronary arteries.

How is it that tens of thousands of people, from the young to the elderly, can jog, cross-country ski, and skate, with considerable exhilaration and pleasure, despite finger-numbing temperatures? The answer lies in the fact that the body heat generated by physical activity balances the heat that is lost to the surroundings, skin temperature is maintained between 30°C and 35°C (86°F-90°F), and the state of comfortable equilibrium is reached. Cold-induced constriction of cutaneous blood vessels does not occur, and there is no increase in cardiac workload. However, of the two variables (heat loss and heat production), the ability to generate adequate body heat from exercise may be the most difficult for the person with coronary artery disease. If angina prevents vigorous physical effort, then heat loss may exceed heat production, and the chain of events just described is set in motion.

In practice, however, cold weather angina is not all that common in coronary artery disease patients. Wearing three or four layers of suitable light clothing (see the section on ''Cold Weather Jogging'' in Chapter 11) increases heat-retaining properties without adding to energy expenditure. For instance, an additional energy expenditure of only five or six calories per minute (for example, walking one mile in 15 minutes), can be accomplished in temperatures as low as −10°C (15°F) when you are suitably garbed. In those for whom even this level of exertion is impossible initially, then outdoor exercise is limited to higher temperatures until training results in a drop in resting and exercise heart rate, thus reducing Double Product, increasing anginal threshold, and eventually permitting a high level of outdoor activity in colder temperatures.

In patients who are capable of higher effort levels, but who suffer angina within a minute or so of beginning their exercise in the cold, the mechanism responsible is probably reflex coronary vasoconstriction. During exercise, mouth breathing becomes easier as respiratory rate increases. The warming effect of the blood vessels in the mucous membrane of the nose is bypassed, and cold air stimulates the nerve endings at the back of the throat. This in turn leads to spasm of the coronary arteries. Careful indoor warm-up exercise and the use of a woollen scarf or muffler covering the mouth is advised. In 1968 the Centre devised a simple plastic disposable oxygen mask that is attached to 12 inches of flexible tubing extending beneath the subject's T-shirt to about the level of the chest bone (see Appendix). At the cost of about $5, this easily produced apparatus is highly effective in preventing early-onset cold-induced angina. (It is, incidentally, equally effective for patients with emphysema.)

Interval Training

Assuming that your angina is so severe that you find it impossible to walk or jog continuously for the time prescribed, don't despair; there is another method you can use for training which I have found to be very effective. This is known as interval training; in its modified form, it consists of brisk walking for 15 to 30 seconds at a pace just below that which brings on the chest discomfort. Walk casually for a further minute, and then repeat the brisk walk for another 15 to 30 seconds. In this way, cover a mile, always staying below the level of effort which brings on the pain. You will eventually find that you can extend the distance to two or three miles in this way, with only infrequent episodes of discomfort.

Skipped Beats

These have been referred to earlier under "Exercise Testing" (Chapter 5) and "Cardiac Contra-indications to Exercise" (Chapter 7). Since they are so common, they are dealt with again in this section. You should know the other terms by which they are referred to: e.g., extrasystoles, premature ectopic beats (p.v.b.'s), premature ventricular contractions (p.v.c.'s), dysrhythmias. To be precise, skipped beats are actually extra heart beats which occur quickly on the heels of a normal beat, and are thus early, or premature, in the cardiac cycle. The correct description for them should, therefore, include the term "premature." Why ectopic? Each normal beat is initiated by the heart's natural pacemaker, an area of specialized tissue located in the right atrium known as the S.A. node. From here a signal passes across both right and left atria and then down both ventricles to reach all parts of the heart, at which point it contracts and empties itself of blood. A premature contraction occurs when a group of cells elsewhere in the heart decides to act as a temporary pacemaker. Since these cells are located away from the S.A. node, the origin of their signal is ectopic (Greek for displaced). The result is a beat which is not only premature, but, because the heart has not had enough time to fill completely, is also weak — frequently too weak to expand the peripheral vessels and cause a pulse wave. Therefore, the additional beat is usually not felt at the pulse. What is noticed is the long pause, or skip, which seems to occur before the next normal beat.

The development of an ectopic temporary pacemaker may be due to excessive intake of caffeine (tea, coffee, coca-cola), smoking, excessive alcohol (usually spirits), stressful circumstances, fatigue, or, in the case of coronary artery disease, shortage of blood supply to the heart muscle. Most people experience isolated skipped beats from time to time, but when they become frequent (every second, third, or fourth beat, or every minute), are aggravated by physical exertion, and are found in the presence of known coronary artery disease, then they should be reported to the physician before regular exercise training is undertaken. Various techniques for obtaining ambulatory electrocardiogram tracings are now available, and these can often pinpoint the precise source and help to establish the severity of the ectopic beats. A decision can then be taken as to whether they need to be suppressed by medication. The commonest and oldest substance used for this purpose is quinidine, originally obtained from cinchona bark. Other preparations are propranolol (Inderal), procainamide (Pronestyl), and disopyramide (Norpace). The decision as to which medication, or combination of medications, to use must rest with the individual physician. In the case of Centre patients who have been placed on medication following the detection of excessive skipped beats during an exercise test, or an exercise session, it is customary to carry out repeat ambulatory electrocardiogram monitoring to ensure that the ectopic beats have been suppressed, or reduced, before they are allowed to return to the training regime.

WARMING-DOWN

"Warming-down" is equally as important as warming-up for the heart patient. It is dangerous to stop exercising suddenly, because blood tends to pool in the legs, with the result that there is insufficient return to the heart. This causes a precipitate drop in the pumping force, and the coronary circulation is adversely affected. So, spend 5 or 10 minutes winding down after your exercise session, moving around and gradually letting your body return to its resting level. Many so-called "exercise deaths" occur after the exercise session is over and when the individual has returned to the locker room. There is now considerable experimental evidence to suggest that lack of adequate warm-down is a contributing factor in these cases.

While on this topic, a caution should be sounded against having hot showers immediately after a workout. This can be potentially dangerous, since the heat of the shower dilates the blood vessels in the skin, reducing the flow through the coronary circulation. This, following on an exercise session, may prove too much for the individual with coronary artery disease. So I advise all patients to wait 10 or 15 minutes after exercising before taking a lukewarm shower.

SMOKING

We have seen earlier that cigarette smoking seems to be associated with a high incidence of sudden death, and my personal experience confirms this. Although the number of fatal recurrences in our exercise group over the past seven years has been very low, the majority of these have been heavy smokers.

Smoking and exercise do not mix. The plain facts of the matter are that the smoke you inhale from your cigarette, cigar or pipe contains small amounts of carbon monoxide. Not only is this a poison, it is a very selective poison. It displaces oxygen from the hemoglobin molecule in your red cells, and so immediately reduces the effectiveness of your oxygen transport system. Furthermore, traces of the drug nicotine in tobacco smoke, by releasing the stress hormone norepinephrine into the blood stream, cause the blood pressure and heart rate to increase and the small blood vessels in the skin to constrict, thus making the heart muscle work harder than it needs to.

So if you smoke, you are defeating the whole purpose of endurance training. No matter how efficient your heart may become in pumping blood around the body, no matter how effectively your muscles learn to extract oxygen from the blood, it is all pointless if the blood is unable to carry its full quota of oxygen. Some authorities go so far as to say that for the smoker to undertake an endurance training program is a complete waste of time. While I would not subscribe completely to that statement, I do feel that the smoker has to devote a good deal more time in training to achieve the same effect. Three of his workouts are probably equivalent to one of the non-smoker's in terms of fitness payoff.

Before leaving this subject, I should draw your attention to the obvious fact that carbon monoxide is carbon monoxide, whether you inhale it from your own cigarette or somebody else's. Non-smokers who breathe the smoky atmosphere of night clubs, or share an enclosed space such as a car with a smoker, probably have high blood levels of carbon monoxide. The moral? If you stop smoking, try to persuade your relatives and friends to do likewise.

MEDICATION

Certain medications which are used in the treatment of coronary artery disease cause a drop in the heart rate, both at rest and during exercise. Currently, the most commonly used are those belonging to the group known as beta-blockers. They act by blocking the nervous stimulus to acceleration, and so reduce the work of the heart. For this reason, they may be very valuable in the treatment of anginal pain and high blood pressure. The most commonly prescribed of these substances go under the trade names of Inderal (propranolol), Lopresor or Betaloc (metoprolol), Corgard (nadolol), Blocadren (timolol), Visken (pindolol).

While small doses of Inderal may not affect heart rate, larger doses invariably do so, and this has to be allowed for in the training program. Individuals who are taking Inderal may have resting heart rates in the 50s, with a concomitant reduction at all levels of exertion right up to maximum. Attempts to achieve heart rates, either during exercise testing or workouts, based on age-related tables may be fraught with disaster. For this reason, I place all patients taking Inderal or a similar substance in the complicated category, and use Nomogram B for establishing both training heart rate and progressing heart rate. Over the years this has worked very well, and we have demonstrated repeatedly that patients who are taking beta-blockers can obtain a significant training effect. Of course, as they develop a training bradycardia their resting and working heart rates drop, and this reduction may be increased by the effect of the medication. Rather than have the resting heart rate become too slow, we customarily wait until it reaches the 40s, and then ask the patient's cardiologist to consider reducing the dosage by about one-third. This usually results in a return of the resting rate to the mid or high 50s. As training continues the rate eventually returns to the 40s, and again, the dosage is reduced by the same amount. Eventually the medication may be stopped completely, or, because there is now some evidence that small doses of a beta-blocker may reduce the incidence of a recurrent heart attack, possibly continued for a year or so.

Another problem that I have found in attempting to train patients who are taking Inderal is the difficulty of predicting the onset of fatigue; the individual suddenly becomes tired during a workout and then has to stop within a matter of 30 seconds or a minute. As one patient put it, "I find I poop out very quickly and without much warning."

Inderal in large doses may hinder the full utilization by skeletal muscle of its major fuels, fat and starch, and in this way cause early muscle fatigue. Of course, this is a small price to pay for its cardiac benefits, but where the fatigue is excessive, improvement may be obtained by switching to one of the other beta-blockers, particularly Lopresor or Betaloc.

Inderal is cleared fairly rapidly from the body, but this is a drug which should not be stopped suddenly. Recent reports indicate that a gradual reduction in dosage is advisable if untoward effects are to be avoided. Incidentally, this is a point to bear in mind if you are one of those foolhardy individuals (of whom I have come across more than a few) who, without consulting their physician, stop their medication when they are "feeling good."

Another commonly used medication which affects the heart rate is Digitalis. This has been used by physicians for many years, being derived originally from the leaf of the common purple foxglove; its main purpose is to strengthen the heart's action. It differs from the beta-blockers, however, in that while it may reduce the resting heart rate, in the dosages usually taken it does not appear to have much effect on the working or maximum pulse level. For this reason, it is less of a problem in a fitness program, although allowance must be made for the fact that it can produce a resting bradycardia, and this should not be confused with the effects of training. Digitalis accumulates in the body, and it may take as long as two weeks after its use is discontinued for its effect on the heart rate to disappear — an important factor if the physician stops the drug temporarily for the purpose of checking progress by means of an exercise test. Digitalis can also cause a false depression of the ST segment of the electrocardiogram during an exercise test.

Recently, a new class of heart drugs called "calcium channel blockers" has been approved in the treatment of heart disease. They act by slowing the rate with which calcium moves backwards and forwards into the cell via the special passages called calcium channels. Slowing the passage of calcium reduces the force with which cells work. The effect on the heart is to lessen the vigour and rapidity of its contraction, thus lightening its workload and so relieving angina. The arteries of the body, including the coronary arteries, respond to the calcium blockers by relaxing, thereby relieving spasm, allowing a greater supply of blood and oxygen to tissue, and reducing blood pressure. The three calcium blockers currently in use are Isoptin (verapamil), Adalat (nifedipine), and Cardizem (diltiazem). Each have slightly different actions, and your physician will choose whichever is most suitable in your case. Insofar as exercise training is concerned, I have found that, like beta-blockers, patients on these medications do very well. Indeed, by relieving symptoms, they often permit an otherwise immobilized patient to commence the program. With regard to effect on resting and exercise heart rates, nifedipine augments these, whereas verapamil and diltiazem slow them.

ISOMETRIC EXERCISES

Not so long ago, this type of physical activity became very popular as a method of building muscle size and strength. Its proponents reported major gains in these parameters by merely devoting a few minutes a day to isometric muscle contractions. The validity of these claims is not our immediate concern. On the other hand, the role of this type of exertion in the training program of the heart patient is very pertinent. The plain fact of the matter is that isometric exercises are entirely contra-indicated for this group. They are not conducive to endurance fitness, and, even more important, they may have a harmful effect on the damaged heart.

Let me be more specific. A maximum isometric muscle contraction is one in which the muscle contracts with full, or almost full force but without shortening. For example, the normal action of the biceps muscle in your upper arm when it contracts is to bend your elbow. If maximal contraction is carried out while at the same time flexion of the elbow joint is prevented, then the biceps muscle will not bunch up in the usual manner of "making a muscle"; you have achieved an isometric contraction of your biceps. Examples of isometric effort in everyday life are straining to raise a jammed window, or trying to lift a suitcase which is too heavy for you, or attempting to push an automobile which is stuck in the snow. This type of muscle action, as opposed to the "isotonic" movement in which the joint is allowed to move and the muscle to shorten, causes a precipitant rise in the diastolic blood pressure and a marked increase in the pressures within the chambers of the heart. If the heart wall is scarred from a previous heart attack, and if the coronary blood circulation is impaired as a result of atherosclerosis, then the results of such pressure increases can be

dangerous. Lifting of heavy weights is, for this reason, prohibited as a training endeavour or a recreational sport. Straining to lift
heavier and heavier loads may well build the body beautiful, but
the isometric element involved makes it an avocation suitable only
for those with the healthiest of cardiovascular systems.

A sad case reported by Dr. Bruce of Seattle may underline my
point even more emphatically. A patient of his on a post-coronary
exercise program seemed to be doing quite well, but then sustained a second and fatal heart attack while water skiing. The likely
cause of death, in the opinion of Dr. Bruce and his colleague Dr.
Pyffer, was the deleterious change in cardiac pressures brought
about by the intense isometric action of gripping the tow bar.

Another example of the adverse cardiovascular effects of an isometric effort is found in Lord Moran's book on Sir Winston Churchill:

> Washington, December 27. "I am glad you have come,"
> the P.M. began. He was in bed and looked worried. "It was
> hot last night, and I got up to open the window. It was very
> stiff. I had to use considerable force and I noticed all at once I
> was short of breath. I had a dull pain over my heart. It went
> down my left arm. It did not last very long, but it has never
> happened before. What is it? Is my heart all right? I thought
> of sending for you, but it passed off."

Sir Winston was obviously an astute observer of clinical symptoms. He was describing typical angina pectoris as a result of excessive load on his heart and coronary vasculature. He was lucky
not to have had a heart attack; in which event, the course of world
history might have been radically altered by an isometric muscle
contraction.

Certain types of power calisthenics contain an isometric-like
component and are to be avoided. Among the most popular of
these are "push ups" and "chinning the bar," proficiency in both
of which seems to be a measure of fitness, if not masculinity, in
the North American male. An additional problem with these, and
indeed all isometric exercises, is that the uninitiated tend to hold
their breath while carrying them out. While this may seem to
enhance performance in terms of power of lift or number of
repetitions, it introduces another element of danger for the person with heart problems. A not uncommon sight in any gymnasium is an exerciser slowly going blue in the face as he attempts to

strain himself to the limit. This is due to the fact that in holding his breath, he has closed off his windpipe, and in the course of his exercise is forcing the air in his lungs against the closed valve. This state of affairs is referred to in physiological circles as the ''Valsalva manoeuvre.'' Its effect, like that of the isometric muscle contraction, is to throw a heavy burden on a heart already severely taxed by the particular exercise which is being carried out. Hence power calisthenics, or any physical activity which encourages the Valsalva manoeuvre, is off limits for the individual at risk.

While on this subject, and particularly for those of us who live in colder climes, mention should be made of that bane of the householder's life, shovelling snow. The incidence of fatal heart attack and sudden cardiac death in any large city inevitably mounts in the three or four days after a heavy snowstorm. This is almost entirely due to snow-shovelling, which has particularly adverse effects on the elderly and those with coronary artery disease. Research studies have shown that the activity has all the components necessary to put the cardiovascular system in jeopardy. It is not only a very intensive form of exercise, equivalent to running a mile at anywhere between 7 and 12 minutes (depending on if you are moving heavy wet or dry light snow); it is also usually performed under unfavourable conditions of extreme cold. Add to that the most dangerous element of all—that it requires repeated isometric arm muscle contractions, customarily accompanied by the Valsalva manoeuvre, and you have set the stage for potential disaster. If you have to move snow, do it as follows. Dress for the cold in the manner advised under the section on ''Cold Weather Jogging'' in Chapter 11, and always warm up for four or five minutes before starting. Push the snow with a scoop rather than lifting it with a shovel; this allows your legs to do the work isotonically rather than your arms isometrically. Take a rest every three minutes or so and don't let yourself get out of breath. If you suffer from angina, or have severe coronary artery disease, give someone else the chore, and supervise them through the window!

Does this mean that you must go in constant fear of holding your breath or inadvertently carrying out an isometric muscle contraction? Of course not. As a matter of fact, the more endurance fitness you develop, the stronger your heart will get and the more it will be able to resist such stresses and strains. My point is that you should be aware of the dangers of these types of exertions, should not practise them on a regular basis, and certainly should not include them as part of your training program.

THE USE OF SAUNAS AND STEAM BATHS

Many people derive a sense of physical and mental well-being from the regular use of a steam bath. In recent years, the North American continent has seen a great rise in the popularity of the sauna, with the result that a significant number of high-rise apartments and even private dwellings now contain this facility. Consequently, I am frequently asked by the post-coronary patient if exposure to such extremes of heat is permissible on safety grounds. My interpretation of the limited number of studies which have been carried out on the effect of exposure to the heat of the sauna or steam bath on those with cardiovascular disease suggests a cautious approach.

Post-coronary patients have been found to develop electrocardiographic evidence of myocardial ischemia while in the sauna; these changes took the form of ST segment depression and frequent ectopic beats. They did not occur to anything like the same extent when these same subjects were exercised to an increased heart rate level equivalent to that attained in the bath. The reason for this seems to be that excessive heat, like emotional stress, releases into the blood stream a type of hormone which may have adverse affects on the myocardium. Potentially dangerous falls in blood pressure have been reported (especially when the subject is in the sitting position) with resultant decrease in coronary blood flow.

As a result of these potential hazards, one investigator has suggested that the middle-aged subject, and especially the sufferer from coronary artery disease, seek the cooler type of bath (temperature range 60°F. to 70°F.), or limit his stay in higher temperatures to five minutes; adopt the customary Finnish posture of lying down rather than our more usual one of sitting up, thus improving coronary blood flow; does not use the steam bath to "sweat out" symptoms which might well be the early portents of coronary artery disease (for example, "muscular" chest pain, excessive fatigue, "bursitis" in the shoulder); and, above all, does not, out of a false sense of pride, attempt to "tough it out with the fellows" if he feels himself getting dizzy, breathless, or developing an unpleasant thumping of his heart.

STICKING WITH THE PRESCRIPTION

Do not be overly ambitious. The coronary-prone individual is apt to over-estimate his capabilities and push himself to the limit. Not infrequently, he works on the principle that if something is good for you, more of it is even better. Apply this dictum to a medication, and you may pay with your life.

Exercise training in the presence of heart disease is no less critical a prescription. I am constantly having to warn individuals about trying to go too quickly. The lengths to which people will go to avoid this advice is a never-ending source of amazement to me. Intelligence and education have nothing whatsoever to do with it; the most unlikely subject, often one who should know better, will attempt to break through the training tables and achieve a personal best every time he works out. Witness the remark of a well-known cardiologist who has himself had by-pass surgery for coronary artery disease, attends the program regularly, and is in every other way a model patient. His exercise diaries showed an increasing escalation of his three-mile pace, and when asked for the reason replied: "I thought the whole point of training was to push yourself at each session." While this may be justified in training Olympic athletes (although Oregon's Bill Bowerman alternated heavy and light training sessions with his highly successful track men), it hardly makes sense for the middle-aged heart patient. Adherence to the tables and the method of progression will assure safety, as well as a desirable training effect.

A BENEFICIAL ADDICTION

Anyone who exercises regularly will tell you that they experience a feeling of exhilaration after each session — or, to put it in the modern vernacular, a "high." By the same token a layoff, even for a few days, will often result in a "downer," with symptoms of depression, anxiety or irritability. The more regular and intensive the training program the more marked the reaction to layoffs.

This urge to continue training is often so powerful that from time to time it will override common sense and lead the individual to persist in running throughout a period of heavy business or social commitments, or despite musculoskeletal injuries or attacks of flu which would obviously respond better to rest than physical activity. Small wonder that the sedentary onlooker refers so scathingly to the "fitness nut."

For many years I have recognized this compulsion to train in young athletes, and now I find it to be just as evident in the middle-aged jogger. It has all the hallmarks of a true addiction. But, you say, isn't that a bad thing? Not really. Provided you are aware of the compulsion and can leaven enthusiasm with common sense, then addiction to physical activity can be desirable.

How can this be explained? Well, a pair of medical researchers, Dr. Malcolm Carruthers and Dr. Peter Taggart, both of London, England, have put forward a fascinating explanation based on their own experimental work. They explain that stress situations such as rock climbing, parachute jumping, public speaking, acting, racing driving, et cetera are accompanied by emotional stress, the main components of which are anxiety, aggression and even aversion. These reactions cause the adrenal glands (two small bean-sized organs which lie above the kidneys), to release into the blood stream the stress hormones epinephrine and norepinephrine. Both substances, in high concentration, lead to a rise in blood pressure, an increase in blood sugar, and an elevation of blood cholesterol.

None of these changes are particularly desirable in the unfit sedentary individual, especially if he has heart disease. However, epinephrine and norepinephrine have a side effect which makes them attractive to the human body; they stimulate the pleasure centres in that primitive part of the brain known as the hypo-thalamus, by liberating a substance known as beta-endorphin. This is released from brain cells when the body is subjected to physical or mental stress. Its effect is to give rise to a mood of satisfaction and pleasure. Which explains why the racing driver, the rock climber, or the actor all derive enjoyment from constant-ly recreating tense and anxious situations for themselves. Vigor-ous physical activity, such as jogging, releases the same substances and therefore results in the same desire to recreate the pleasur-able stimulation. However — and this is the crucial point — vigor-ous sustained exercise does not bring about the same consistent rise in blood sugar or blood cholesterol which is associated with the more sedentary thrills. This is because it causes the body to burn sugar and fat as fuels. Here, then, is one beneficial addiction in which you can indulge yourself with safety!

CONCURRENT INFECTIONS

You are now aware that a number of viral-type infections can involve the heart muscle. The effect may be transitory, lasting only a matter of days or weeks. It may pass unnoticed by the patient, and leave no permanent damage. However, strenuous physical activity should be avoided during this time. Although severe viral myocarditis is relatively rare, mild forms of the condition may exist much more frequently than we suspect. Since a visit to the cardiologist is hardly justified every time you develop a fever, we work on the rule that it is better to be safe than sorry, and advise against carrying out the exercise prescription if you are suffering from any flu-like illness. To be further on the safe side, you should not work out until a full seven days have elapsed after your temperature has returned to normal.

Some time ago, a patient on our post-coronary exercise program collapsed while running on a community indoor track. Facilities for resuscitation were not available, and he was dead on arrival at hospital. An autopsy was not carried out, but it is probably safe to assume that he had sustained a further heart attack. His case was unique in that he was the first patient to suffer a myocardial infarction, fatal or non-fatal, during exercise, since the program had started in 1968.

Naturally enough, I enquired carefully into the circumstances of his death, hoping to learn something which would be of benefit to the rest of the group. The salient features which emerged were as follows. In his 40s, he had always been hard-working and ambitious, with a high sense of responsibility. For six months or so prior to his death, he had been working on a special project in his job. This required him to put in many hours of overtime. Despite this, he had made no concession to his training program, putting in five workouts a week in spite of the fact that he must have been feeling overly tired. He then developed flu. He didn't seem to be able to shake this, and it dragged on for two or three weeks. Again, he refused to cut back on his running, despite advice to the contrary by his colleagues on the exercise program who, like him, had been frequently admonished on this point. Finally, it emerged that he had been exceeding his exercise prescription, and running at a pace a good deal faster than he was required to.

None of these facts appeared on his exercise log. There is no proof that any or all of these factors contributed in any way to this individual's death. It may well be that his second and fatal attack would have occurred in any event, and irrespective of whether he was running, sitting at his desk, or watching television. And yet, one cannot help but wonder whether, had he adhered to the precautions outlined in this chapter, the outcome might have been different. The point to bear in mind is that all of the above advice is based on practical experience in the training of many post-coronary patients. The rules have been formulated in response to their reactions, both adverse and favourable, to the exercise regime.

HOW MUCH DO YOU WEIGH?

While obesity is less suspect than was previously thought as a risk factor in heart disease, it should still be considered an additional hazard for the post-coronary patient. Excess fatty tissue means excess work for the heart. Not only that, but overweight is consistently associated with a higher mortality from diabetes, hypertension, strokes, chest infections, digestive problems, kidney disease, and accidents. With a heart problem already, who needs the rest?

Body weight doesn't necessarily give a true measure of the amount of fatty tissue a person possesses. A heavy-boned or well-muscled individual may well be heavier than his slight-built counterpart, and yet not be obese. For practical purposes, however, and in our present-day affluent society, excess weight invariably means excess fat. There are a number of methods of estimating your percentage of body fat. One of the most accurate is underwater weighing, a laboratory procedure which has little practical application for the man on the street. However, you can obtain a reasonable estimate of your fat layer by pinching up the skin and fat over your abdomen an inch or so below your navel and parallel to the skin creases. Ideally, the distance between your finger and thumb should be no more than half an inch. The fat fold over the back of the upper arm, half way between the tip of your shoulder and the tip of your elbow is more convenient to measure; this should be no more than 1 inch (1½ inches in females). In the laboratory, these assessments are carried out using special skin calipers and taking the average of eight skin folds, but such refinements are unnecessary for most purposes. Another way of estimating your obesity factor is to use the Ponderal Index. Divide your height in inches by the cube root of your weight (in lbs.). Here are some cube roots, to save you frantically searching for your calculator:

100 - 4.64	125 - 5.00	150 - 5.31	175 - 5.59
105 - 4.72	130 - 5.07	155 - 5.37	180 - 5.65
110 - 4.79	135 - 5.13	160 - 5.43	185 - 5.70
115 - 4.86	140 - 5.19	165 - 5.49	190 - 5.75
120 - 4.93	145 - 5.25	170 - 5.54	195 - 5.80

For example, if you are 5'8'' tall and weigh 160 lbs., then you obtain your Ponderal Index by dividing the cube root of 160, (i.e., 5.43) into 68, or your height in inches, to give 12.5. The lower the index, the higher your amount of body fat. If it comes to less than 12.2, then your percentage body fat is over 30 per cent and you should start reducing.

It is customary in our society to assume that as one gets older, one "puts on a little weight." Mothers and wives, through generations of teaching, are made to feel that their sons and husbands should have a well-fed and plump appearance. The middle-aged Englishman of the eighteenth century was considered both handsome and dignified only if he were portly — all very well when leanness was a mark of poverty and malnutrition, but hardly applicable to our twentieth-century well-fed Western world. There is no earthly reason why anyone should weigh more at 45 than he did at 21. Competitive long distance runners, hardly an unhealthy breed, frequently have a body fat of less than 10 per cent. Ideal weights are hard to define. One rough calculation is to double your height in inches and add 10 per cent of the sum. A much more scientific approach has been taken by the American Society of Actuaries who studied the mortality rates of half a million insured individuals over the period from 1935 to 1954. The inference to be drawn from their data was that if you are of medium build, then the closer your weight is to the table on page 314, the more likely you are to achieve a normal lifespan.

If you do need to reduce, you should use a combination of dietary restriction and exercise. I do not intend to deal with the subject of diet, since this book is primarily concerned with exercise training. However, I have included some comments under a later section on Long Distance Running on page 192 which I think are pertinent.

A rough guide to the amount of calories we should be eating a day is obtained by the following formula: take your ideal weight in kilograms (plus or minus 5 per cent depending on your having a heavy or light frame), allow one calorie per kilogram per hour for a 24-hour period, and then add between 30 per cent if you are very sedentary, up to 60 per cent if you are very active; e.g.,

70 kg × Cal × 24 = basal   = 1680
if very sedentary, + 30 per cent basal =   504
        Total   = 2184
if very active, + 60 per cent basal   = 1008
        Total   = 2688

The ideal weight tables at the back of this book, together with a simple table of food calorie values, should allow you to approximate your daily intake.

ALCOHOL INTAKE AND EXERCISE

There is much uncertainty in the minds of the public about the effects of alcohol on the heart. Many can remember when the physician prescribed a daily ration of brandy or whisky for the post-coronary patient on the premise that it was a cardiac stimulant and dilated the coronary vessels. There is little to condone that practice today. On the contrary, recent evidence indicates that alcohol depresses heart function by decreasing the contractile force, or pump efficiency, of the myocardium, especially when it is the seat of ischemic changes or scarring from coronary artery disease. The amount of alcohol needed to cause this adverse effect in heart patients is quite small: in one study, just two ounces of Canadian whisky. There is also agreement among the experts that the heart muscle cells may suffer permanent damage from prolonged and excessive alcohol consumption, leading to the condition of alcoholic cardiomyopathy. Another practical consideration is the one of body weight; alcoholic beverages are high in caloric value, so you can scarcely expect to lose weight on a diet of cottage cheese, lettuce and beer!

For all of the above reasons, you should consider carefully whether or not to consume alcohol. If you have serious cardiac problems, you'd be better off abstaining. Chances are, however, that if you are capable of exercising, you're capable of drinking, but in moderation — no more than a shot of liquor daily (1½ - 2 ounces) or two bottles of beer, or a glass of wine.

Just as you shouldn't drink and drive, so you should never drink before jogging, especially if you suffer from heart disease. Not only is your heart less likely to be able to cope with the additional stress, but your judgment of pace and distance is probably impaired, as is your ability to count your pulse and interpret such warning signs as angina or light-headedness. If you must drink, then do so in moderation, and *after* your workout.

PHYSICAL CONDITIONS

Don't underestimate the effect of running into a head-wind. It has been shown that an athlete weighing 134 lb. and running at a 6-minute mile pace on a still day expends approximately 6 per cent more oxygen in the face of a light, 10 m.p.h. wind; to put it another way, he will have to put out the effort of a sub-5-minute mile pace! A 40 m.p.h. wind jacks the oxygen cost up by over 40 per cent. When you are talking oxygen increments of that order, you may be getting into a situation which is beyond your maximum oxygen consumption. Of course, I realize that you wouldn't deliberately set out to jog into steady gale force winds, but you can sometimes misjudge the wind force when the conditions are gusty. The trick is to back off if you notice yourself getting unusually breathless and tired on a windy day. Allowing for the wind resistance, the slower time will be giving you the same training effect anyway.

The best surface to run on is a smooth one. The hardness or softness doesn't really matter; your shoes should take care of that factor. An uneven surface increases the effort of running considerably, driving up your oxygen consumption and heart rate accordingly, and sometimes giving rise to anginal pain which would otherwise not occur. Some athletes feel that it is easier to run on a grass surface, and will seek one out if they are trying to nurse a leg injury. In my experience, this only makes matters worse, since beneath the deceptive green covering, the underlying ground is often rutted and uneven, making each stride a hazard and increasing the stress on tendons and ligaments. If possible, then, do your training on the road or on a track with a good surface.

PARTICIPATION IN OTHER SPORTING ACTIVITIES

When can I play tennis? What about golf? Is badminton okay? How about swimming? These and other similar questions are asked constantly by post-coronary patients who are on the exercise program. We try to answer each one individually, taking into account the patient's state of training, age, severity of heart attack, and presence or absence of symptoms. If you are working out in accordance with the training tables in this book, then you can use your achievement of the various levels as a rough guide to your ability to participate safely in a number of recreational physical activities (see table on pages 308-09).

While some of these recreational physical activities may be more enjoyable than jogging, they are harder to quantify in terms of energy expenditure and cardiac work. If you are good at a game, then you will perform it with greater skill, or to put it physiologically, with a higher degree of mechanical efficiency. Thus your oxygen consumption will be lower throughout the game than if you were a less proficient player. A poor swimmer will expend more effort threshing across the pool than his skilled counterpart will in an apparently lazy workout covering two or three miles. The squash player with twenty years' experience will finish a game hardly perspiring, while his sweating novice opponent may have just had the match of his life.

Actually, this is a problem with skill games, as a recent physician-patient of mine discovered to his cost. He had played squash for over twenty-five years and was so good that his daily workouts at the Y over the past five or six years had given him little if any training effect. The result was that when he was fitness tested, he scored no better than the average sedentary male of the same age.

Other variables in recreational sports include difficulty in pacing oneself, the effect of emotion and excitement, as well as extraneous factors peculiar to the game itself — as for example, the isometric component involved in gripping the golf club or the ski-tow bar, or the late nights (and possibly the hip-flask conviviality) associated with club curling.

CHAPTER NINE

Fads, Facts and Fallacies

Over the years I have developed the habit of holding 15- or 20-minute informal chats before each exercise session, answering patients' questions and discussing the implications of recent studies and experiments on heart disease, fitness and related subjects.

The following are some of the topics most commonly brought up in these sessions. I hope they will clarify a few of your own problems, or even correct some of the half-truths, fallacies and prejudices with which the exercising heart patient is surrounded.

SEXUAL ACTIVITY AFTER MYOCARDIAL INFARCTION

In a recent survey of 160 of our post-coronary patients, it was found that precisely half reported a reduction of sexual activity since their heart attacks. The main reason given was a fall-off in desire. A smaller number said that they were frightened of suffering another heart attack during intercourse, and a few actually reported adverse symptoms such as palpitations or angina pectoris during the sexual act.

The individual who becomes apathetic towards sex after his attack frequently shows high levels of depression and anxiety. He has lost some confidence in his masculinity and doubts his ability to function again in his role as head of the family. His reluctance to seek full satisfaction in sexual relations is perfectly understandable under these circumstances. As his confidence returns (and this often occurs with increasing physical fitness), the situation usually rights itself.

But what of the individual who is frightened of sexual intercourse because of its possible ill effects on his heart? Is there any
justification for his fears? Should he adopt special precautions during the sex act, and if so, what should they be? How long after his
heart attack should he wait before resuming a normal marital
relationship?

The answers to these questions may have been provided by
your cardiologist, but I find that many of the patients referred for
rehabilitation have not been so lucky. Beyond being told that they
should ''wait about a month'' before resuming sex, they have
been given little guidance in this area. The reason is not hard to
find. There has been minimal research carried out into the effects
of coitus on the damaged heart, and medical literature contains
little on the subject.

The sex act results in cardiovascular responses very similar to
those induced by exercise. There is a rise in heart rate and blood
pressure, as well as an increase in rate of breathing. However, in
terms of cardiac work, the cost of intercourse is modest, with
increases in heart rate about the same as that observed in climbing a few flights of stairs or walking briskly around the block. As
a matter of fact, much higher heart rates may occur during angry
discussions at work! ECG monitoring of fourteen subjects during
the sexual act showed that a small number developed changes
compatible with cardiac ischemia (ST segment depression and
ectopic beats), but these particular individuals experienced similar adverse signs during their usual occupational activities; in other
words, coitus did not have a disproportionately higher stress effect.

The vast majority of post-coronary patients can safely indulge
in marital sexual activity without fear of excessive cardiovascular
strain. Here we refer to middle-aged individuals who have been
married for a number of years. There are grounds for believing
that intercourse with a younger or less familiar partner may lead
to more profound physiological changes, with much higher increments of heart rate and blood pressure and so greater cardiac stress.
Extra-marital intercourse may well provide these ingredients, and
since it may also be accompanied by a bout of excessive food and
alcohol intake, might well be dangerous. It is probably in these
circumstances that the occasional coital death occurs — a death
dramatic enough to become more colourful in the retelling, and
so needlessly frighten the more conservative, ''non-swinging''
members of society!

Are there then any precautions to be taken after a heart attack? Sufficient time should be allowed for the infarction scar to form before indulging in intercourse. This means at least six weeks after the attack, and probably eight weeks to be on the safe side. If you suffer from angina during coitus, then try taking glyceryl trinitrate before commencing the act. Symptoms such as angina or ectopic beats may be relieved by changing your position. In the male-dominant position, much of your body weight has to be supported on your arms; this amounts to isometric exercise, and as previously noted, will lead to a disproportionate increase in blood pressure and cardiac workload. The effect is enhanced if the duration of the act is prolonged. Therefore, if you are bothered by symptoms, you might find it advantageous to try the side-by-side position or the female-dominant.

A proportion of my patients said that while they themselves were not apprehensive about having sex, their wives were unduly anxious. I have corroborated this on many occasions, both by questionnaire and frank discussion of the matter with wives. A fearful partner can put the husband at a disadvantage, and even increase his own doubts and uncertainties. In a situation like this, a knowledgeable family physician can be of great help.

To sum up, then, you are ready for sexual intercourse as soon as you can go for a brisk walk, or climb two flights of stairs without difficulty; this usually means about eight weeks after your heart attack. The chances of intra-marital coitus damaging your heart are remote and the sense of well-being associated with a normal marital relationship far outweigh the mythical dangers. If you suffer symptoms, then try taking glyceryl trinitrate or changing your position. Finally if you find the frequency with which you desire sex is diminished, then for goodness sake, don't panic. That may only make matters worse. Remember that improved physical fitness and the passage of time often works wonders.

DEPRESSION FOLLOWING MYOCARDIAL INFARCTION

Our own studies, as well as the work of others, have shown that a significant number of heart attack survivors are extremely depressed as a result of their attacks. Actually, one-third of the group we analyzed demonstrated this finding. Psychological testing and interview showed that, in addition to being depressed, they also have extreme tendencies toward hysteria and hypochondriasis—the so-called ''neurotic triad.'' This state of affairs was only evident after careful evaluation; it was not obvious to the onlooker. As a matter of fact, neither the patient's wife nor his physician had even suspected it. When confronted with the evidence of the psychological assessment, the unhappy individual invariably admitted his melancholy. The tragic thing is the frequency with which he felt that he was unique. A typical remark was, ''I envy the other guys. They seem to have accepted the fact that they've had a heart attack, and they never seem to worry about it. So what can I do? I'm scared stiff I'll have another one, but I can't admit it to anyone. So I play along, kibbitzing with the rest, and pretending that life is a big joke.''

Despite this facade, the depressed heart patient is very much lacking in confidence. He demonstrates less initiative at work, and is reluctant to make important decisions. He procrastinates, hoping that time will solve his problems. At home, he leaves more and more responsibility to his wife. Often this is in complete contrast to his pre-attack personality. This change was so marked in one patient that his wife, before leaving for a holiday, wrote him a note in which she abjured him to pull himself together, and revert to the strong-minded man she had married who had consistently called the shots for both of them. The trouble is that this is easier said than done. It takes time, a lot of patience and understanding, and sometimes the skill and advice of a professional.

Whether the depression is entirely due to the heart attack, or whether it is part of the patient's personality which has merely been brought to light by the illness is a moot point. There are some who believe that the depression is endogenous, and may indeed be a factor in actually causing the attack. If this is so, then psychotherapy may be advantageous not only in relieving the depression, but possibly in helping to prevent another heart attack. On the other hand, if the condition is entirely exogenous, then it should disappear with time and as general health improves.

In either case, there is little doubt that great benefit can be derived from an exercise rehabilitation program. Fitness improves the quality of life, and brings with it enhanced self-confidence and improvement in morale. Our depressed patients have gained considerably from the exercise program. However, we have learned to take a slightly different approach with our depressed as opposed to our non-depressed patients. The latter have little sense of insecurity; psychological testing reveals that they are abundant in self-confidence. Ambitious, driving, and over-competitive, they deny adverse symptoms and are obsessive in adherence to their exercise workouts. They are constantly matching their performances with those of others and setting themselves harder and harder goals. They are inclined to exceed their exercise prescription and have to be observed carefully in order to see that they do not do too much, or ignore the indications for a reduction in training intensity.

A depressed person is just the opposite. He tends to be overly protective, frightened of exerting himself too much, doubtful of the program's value, pessimistic about his own chances of improvement, and inclined to do less than the prescription calls for. He allows any number of trivial happenings to deflect him from his exercise session, frequently complains of leg muscle stiffness, or vague discomfort in the chest, and constantly seems to be searching for an excuse to drop out. He needs encouragement, reassurance, and a high degree of persuasion to see that he keeps on exercising at a suitable level. He is helped by observing the success of other post-coronary joggers who are obviously doing so well, and if he can just stay with it long enough to start feeling the benefits of fitness, he is well on the road to recovery.

Do you recognize yourself as belonging to either of these two groups? Whichever group you identify with, there is plenty to read, digest, and benefit from in these pages.

DIETARY SUPPLEMENTS

This is indeed a tangled web, spun by researchers, evangelists and ignoramuses alike. Nevertheless, the subject warrants consideration and so, without fear or favour or more ado, here are some thoughts for your consideration.

Vitamin E

Few subjects arouse more passion in medical circles than that dealing with the possible therapeutic value of this substance. The proponents of Vitamin E therapy angrily denounce their antagonists as being short-sighted, and accuse them of deliberately ignoring the evidence of innumerable case histories in which large doses of Vitamin E have been of value in heart disease, leg ulcers, skin infections and a whole host of other conditions. The opposition, however (and that probably includes the bulk of the medical profession), counters with the argument that there is a paucity of controlled clinical trials demonstrating that Vitamin E therapy is of any value, that deficiency states occur only rarely, and that Vitamin E is obtained in sufficient quantities from a normal diet without requiring to be supplemented by further intake. The battle has raged since Evans and Bishop of California discovered the substance, also known as tocopheral, in 1922. Present in large amounts in wheat germ and green leaves, its absence from the diet of laboratory rats was shown to cause sterility and a peculiar condition in which the muscles become swollen and weak.

In this brief section, it would be impossible to discuss all the pros and cons of Vitamin E therapy, and in any event, we are interested only in its real or apparent effects on heart disease.

The current rationale for the use of Vitamin E in the treatment of atherosclerosis is based on the theory that the present epidemic of coronary artery disease is largely due to a deficiency in this vitamin, resulting from our modern diet. The milling and purification of flour and other foodstuffs has led to the elimination of Vitamin E, it is argued, so that we now need to supplement this factor artificially. Among its reputedly beneficial effects are a reduction in the tendency for blood to clot, a dilation of peripheral blood vessels, and a reduction in the oxygen requirements of the tissue cells. Unfortunately, none of these properties has been consistently demonstrated by laboratory trials. In point of fact, the theory that coronary artery disease is due to inadequate amounts of Vitamin E, or indeed any other substance, in modern foodstuffs is still very much that — a theory.

When faced with the question whether or not it is advisable to take for therapeutic purposes a substance which has not as yet received the universal blessing of the medical profession, I am forced to fall back on two questions: Is it safe? And, is it expensive? Certainly, no toxic effects from the use of large doses of Vitamin E have ever been recorded in human beings. There have been occasional reports of side effects in rats, including increased deposition of cholesterol in the large blood vessels. I am told by a good physician friend of mine who prescribes Vitamin E for many conditions, that it should be used with caution in patients with high blood pressure, at least in the initial stages of treatment; and that it is contra-indicated in patients with certain types of valvular disease of the heart.

High intake of Vitamin E has been linked with a drop in the body's Vitamin K content. Vitamin K helps blood to clot, and so it is just conceivable that tocopheral, in destroying Vitamin K, may reduce the likelihood of thrombosis occurring within the coronary arteries. A more immediate implication of this finding, however, is that patients who have been placed on anticoagulant medication ("blood thinner"), after their heart attacks, might well be cautious about taking non-prescribed mega doses of Vitamin E for fear that the cumulative effect will result in excessive bleeding.

With the above proviso, I think we can conclude that Vitamin E is safe; but it is not cheap. However, if you have to cut down your smoking in order to be able to afford a year's supply of Vitamin E capsules, then it is money well spent.

Before leaving this contentious subject, I should make the point that I do not advise any of the patients on my exercise program to take Vitamin E. From questioning them, I know that a small minority do. On the other hand, just for the record, none of the individuals who have taken part in the marathon runs described elsewhere in this book have used Vitamin E as part of their training program.

Vitamin C

This substance is essential for the manufacture of collagen, the base substance which acts as a cement for much of the tissue and organs of our bodies. It occurs naturally in citrus fruit such as lemons and limes. James Lind, a physician in the British navy in the eighteenth century, empirically deduced that its absence led to the condition of scurvy. In the days of sail, long sea voyages meant that the crew would go many months without fresh fruit or vegetables. The result was that they frequently became ill with a disease which was characterized by fatigue, bruising of the skin, and a tendency to bleed easily from the gums and mucous membranes. These are the classical symptoms of scurvy, a disease which was the scourge of the British navy for hundreds of years before it was found that the addition of fresh fruit, such as limes, to the diet had a preventative effect. It was this insistence on limes in the British sailor's food store which led to his countrymen being referred to as "Limeys." It was not until 1932 that the specific protective agent in the lime was isolated in the form of Vitamin C; two years later it was first synthesized.

Recently, there has been renewed interest in Vitamin C for a number of reasons. The world-famous scientist and Nobel Prize winner, Dr. Linus Pauling, has advocated the therapeutic use of large doses of Vitamin C to help the body's defence mechanisms against infection. Once again, this subject is obscured by controversy. Time and time again, you will come across the arguments for and against the use of so-called mega-vitamin therapy. Orthodox medical teaching has established minimal daily requirements for all of the vitamins known to man. It has also identified a number of clear-cut conditions which result if these minimal daily requirements are not met. Scurvy, beri-beri (lack of Vitamin B), rickets (Vitamin D), night blindness (Vitamin A), are all examples of gross deficiency in vitamins. The mega-vitamin advocates, however, maintain that disease entities exist which are less dramatic and obvious in appearance, and are caused by a chronic partial shortage of dietary vitamins. This, they feel, is due to modern methods of food refinement and the addition of artificial food preservatives which tend to destroy the natural vitamin in the food. They aim to correct these conditions by supplementing the diet with large doses of the vitamin in question.

Their arguments are still tenuous, and valid scientific data to prove their point are still lacking. Nevertheless, to be fair, while large numbers of misguided, ill-trained enthusiasts and outright cranks are advocating all sorts of vitamin therapy for a host of conditions, both real and imagined, an increasing number of reputable physicians and scientists are devoting their attention to a careful study of even the most apparently outrageous claims. The opinion of an individual such as Dr. Linus Pauling cannot be ignored. Others, such as Professors Terry Anderson and Harding LeRiche, both of the Department of Preventive Medicine and Biostatistics, University of Toronto, are proceeding with carefully controlled and fascinating studies into the value of mega-vitamin therapy as well as the possible harmful effects of modern diet.

To return to Vitamin C. It is not too surprising to find that some researchers have claimed coronary artery disease to be a Vitamin C deficiency state. Their argument is that adequate quantities of this substance in the body will protect against atherosclerosis, possibly by reducing blood cholesterol levels. Again, there is no proof that this is so. However, there are certain facts about Vitamin C which are worthy of note. High levels of physical stress will result in a depletion of the body's stores of Vitamin C. Thus, an exhausting long distance run such as a marathon race, or two or three nights without sleep, will deplete our Vitamin C reserves. Now it is an interesting fact that our bodies cannot manufacture Vitamin C; we must obtain it from the environment, either in natural or synthetic form. Consequently, it is reasonable to argue that individuals who are under high physical stress will require increased doses of the vitamin. Another point to bear in mind is that smoking and alcohol both destroy Vitamin C.

With these facts in mind, it does seem reasonable to take Vitamin C as a supplement when you are under physical stress. In our context, this would include heavy training. The man who is jogging three or more miles five days a week would be included in that category. I recommend to my patients who are running five to six miles an hour, five times a week, that they take 500 mg. daily. If they are running longer distances, then I recommend higher dosages. I consider such a level of training to be stressful, and I have found that the incidence of muscle and tendon injuries in my joggers has been minimal. It is difficult to prove that this is the result of their Vitamin C intake without undertaking a large and expensive clinical trial, but I think that the proven role of Vitamin C in the formation of healthy connective tissue makes my assumption a reasonable one.

What about the cost and the safety factors? Of all the vitamins, surely Vitamin C must be the cheapest, so that does not constitute a problem. On the matter of safety, there are one or two provisos. The body can only store so much ascorbic acid in the tissues, and any excess is excreted in the urine. This tends to make the urine acid, and some authorities have stated that this could lead to the formation of certain types of kidney stones. While this is a remote hazard, it can be reduced by maintaining an adequate fluid intake. Further, stone formation seems to me to be likely only when the intake of the vitamin is truly massive.

The influence of high dosage is probably also a factor in a more cogent objection, namely that the body becomes accustomed to high Vitamin C levels, and if the high dosage is suddenly withdrawn, then a mild type of scurvy may occur. Again, this seems unlikely with dosages in the order of a half a gram to a gram; even so, I recommend that the long distance jogger reduce his intake gradually over a week or two if for some reason training is reduced.

"Bulk" Diets

Dr. Dennis P. Burkitt has suggested that a number of diseases which are characteristic of modern Western civilization may be due to a lack of bulk in our diets. In addition to appendicitis, cancer of the large bowel, ulcerative colitis, and various venous disorders, he also includes diseases associated with cholesterol metabolism. Of the latter, coronary heart disease and gall stones are undoubtedly the commonest.

The basis of his argument is that the past hundred years has seen a steady fall in the fibre content of our foodstuff, especially flour. The daily fibre intake from bread is now reduced to about a tenth of the level it was in the early part of the nineteenth century; packaged cereals, also poor in fibre, have replaced the high-fibre breakfast of porridge or oats. The effect of this lack of roughage in food is to reduce the weight and bulk of the fecal stools, and to increase the time of its passage through the intestine. Primitive peoples who still eat high residue diets pass large bulky stools, which pass through the intestinal tract in 35 hours or so, as opposed to 70 hours in those on a Western diet. In these individuals, diseases of the intestine are rare, as are such conditions as varicose veins, deep vein thrombosis, and hemorrhoids.

Of even greater importance, the presence of a high fibre content in the feces seems in some way to be connected with low serum cholesterol levels and the relative absence of ischemic heart disease. The mechanism for this is uncertain. Burkitt himself is careful to point out that a high residue diet may be only one factor in the causation of these various conditions, but his opinion is worthy of respect. How do you increase the fibre content of your diet? Merely by adding half a cupful of unprocessed bran to your diet daily. You can take it in the morning mixed with your usual breakfast cereal, or can mix it with soup and have it with lunch. It's cheap, and it can do you no harm.

Is Sugar Deadly?

Doctor J. Yudkin, Professor of Nutrition and Dietetics at the University of London, attributes the rise in atherosclerosis to an increase in the consumption of refined sugar. He points out that refined sugar, whether from cane or beet, is a relatively recent addition to our diet, only appearing in great quantities on our tables within the last hundred years. Already, however, the per capita consumption of this substance in the United States and Britain is an amazing one hundred pounds annually, if you count the sugar content of cookies, cakes, white bread, soft drinks, jams and other spreads, breakfast cereal, and so on.

According to Doctor Yudkin, experiments show that a high sugar intake is harmful for a number of reasons. First, it represents an inordinate intake of so-called ''empty calories.'' Since it is an unnat-

ural foodstuff the calories it provides are unaccompanied by vitamins or any of the other nutrients found in natural sugar sources
such as fruit. Furthermore, in sugar-sensitive individuals it leads
to a derangement of the body's ability to adjust its own blood
sugar level, and this in turn can predispose to a variety of ills, of
which atherosclerosis is but one. Finally, it is partially addictive
in that the more you take the more you want.

The atherosclerotic effect of sugar is brought about by increasing
blood cholesterol levels and enhancing blood stickiness. For more
details you can read Doctor Yudkin's book, *Sweet and Dangerous*,
which explains his theory in lay terms.

Doctor Ancel Keys of Minneapolis, who blames a high content
of animal fat in our diet as the chief cause for heart disease, has
taken issue with Doctor Yudkin's hypothesis, pointing out that
the relationship between high sugar intake and heart disease
breaks down in the cases of the South American countries and
also Sweden, areas with high sugar consumption and relatively
low incidence of heart disease. Furthermore, Doctor Keys' own
experiments have failed to show an elevation of blood cholesterol
levels as a result of diets containing as much as 40 per cent sugar.
Needless to say, Professor Yudkin has rebuttals for both arguments, and there is no doubt that his theory is an intriguing one.
On balance, however, I would have to say that at this time it has
relatively few adherents.

The Hard and Soft Water Controversy

A number of epidemiological studies have noted that there is a
higher incidence of deaths from heart disease in those areas where
the water is soft. Hard water flows over rocks rich in the mineral
dolomite, and so contains larger amounts of magnesium and
calcium. A low level of either or both of these substances in the
tissues may, it is argued, affect the rhythm of the heart and, if this
organ is already the seat of a disease such as coronary atherosclerosis, predispose to cardiac arrest.

Dr. Andrew Shaper, a research worker for the United Kingdom
Medical Research Council, in an article published in 1974 in the
Journal of the American Medical Association, describes how the death
rate from cardiovascular disease in Monroe County, Florida, was
found to have dropped considerably after the water supply had
been changed from a soft to a hard water source. Residents of the
hard water areas, both in America and the United Kingdom, have
been variously reported to have lower blood pressures, lower heart

rates, and lower blood cholesterol levels than their soft-water fellow citizens.

Whether it is the calcium or magnesium in the water, or both, which exerts a specific protective influence against death from circulatory disease is, in our present state of knowledge, impossible to say. Researchers from England and Finland have found that areas in which the soil is rich in both these minerals have a low heart disease rate.

Professor Terry Anderson of the University of Toronto has verified that the populations of soft water areas have a lower magnesium content in their muscle tissue (including their heart muscle) than residents of hard water areas. Since the hearts of persons who have succumbed to a heart attack are also found to have abnormally low concentrations of magnesium, he feels that his findings are compatible with the belief that waterborne magnesium exerts a protective effect. He also proffers the fascinating hypothesis that the basic problem is due to the critically low levels of magnesium in the highly refined Western diet, with the hard water inhabitants receiving just enough to avoid a heart muscle deficiency state.

Despite what might appear to be impressive evidence, most workers in the field are quick to point out that the whole matter is still very much open to question. Certainly there is insufficient data to warrant altering the water supply of the nation, or of advocating that physicians prescribe oral calcium or magnesium for their heart patients.

AIR TRAVEL

Nowadays, whether for business or vacation, most of us have to fly at some time or another. Can flying pose any special threat for the individual with coronary artery disease? Generally speaking, the answer is no. However, certain considerations have to be taken into account.

Jet planes usually cruise at altitudes of between 30,000 and 40,000 feet (9,144 to 12,192 metres). At these heights, the atmosphere is so rarified that, were it not for the pressurized cabin, passengers and crew would rapidly expire due to lack of oxygen. Pressurization ensures that the cabin altitude remains between 5,000 and 7,000 feet (1,524 to 2,134 metres). While it is possible to pressurize the cabin to sea level when flying at heights in excess of 25,000 feet (7,620 metres), it is not economical to do so; and, indeed, for most travellers it is not necessary. In effect, the majority of trips are made at cabin altitudes between that equivalent to Denver, Colorado (5,000 feet), and slightly less than Mexico City (7,523 feet). This is not a problem, since our blood's ability to absorb and transport oxygen isn't materially hindered until we are exposed to altitudes of 10,000 feet and above.

However, individuals with chest disease, such as chronic bronchitis or emphysema, may have difficulty getting sufficient oxygen at lower atmospheric pressures than 10,000 feet. In which case, they may require supplementary oxygen during the flight. Obviously, any chest patient who is breathless at rest, or on minimal exertion, will only fly after very careful medical assessment. As for those with coronary artery disease, the ability to climb two flights of stairs easily or walk 100 yards briskly without breathlessness should ensure a problem-free flight.

How long after a heart attack should one wait before flying? Published reports indicate that less problems occur in those whose heart attack has occurred two to six months before the flight, than in those who fly less than eight weeks after their attack. Those in whom the attack was accompanied by complications, or in whom there was a history of more than one previous attack, also have a higher occurrence of inflight problems. It would seem wise, then, to defer flying for at least two months. However, British Airways recommends that if the journey is essential, an uncomplicated case can fly as early as two weeks post-infarction.

Actually, in my experience, patients have suffered more episodes of angina on the ground than in the air, as a result of the strain and frustration of crowded airports, flight delays, customs and immigration inspections, and lengthy waits at baggage conveyors.

Apart from the matter of cabin altitude, there are other aspects of air travel which are probably more important. Alcohol and cigarette smoke intensify the ill effects of low blood oxygen, and so are best avoided, or at least reduced, during long flights. Since the atmosphere in the cabin is dry and rarefied, dehydration can be a problem. Remember, then, to drink plenty of non-alcoholic fluid. Another point to note is that gas expands at altitude. That includes the gas in your stomach. Therefore, on a long flight wear loose clothing, and don't consume too many carbonated drinks, or you'll bloat up like a balloon. Take a walk up and down the cabin every half hour or so to keep the circulation flowing and to avoid blood "pooling" in the lower limbs. If this is not possible, straighten your knees and ankles and clench the thigh and calf muscles from time to time. Finally, and most important, always carry a three days' supply of your medication on your person or in your cabin luggage. If you pack it in checked luggage, you will sooner or later face the problem of lost bags and, at best, the inconvenience of having to find a local physician to prescribe replacements.

LONG DISTANCE RUNNING

The theme of this book is the value of endurance training in post-coronary rehabilitation. More specifically, the beneficial effects of LSD or long slow distance. Why is it necessary to work out for an hour at a time? After all, hasn't a popular book on fitness extolled at length the benefits which accrue from a mere 30 minutes of exercise weekly (a gospel with a built-in appeal for a population conditioned to looking for the instant solution to everything)? Why should you have as your goal the ability to run five or six miles? The answer is simple; instant fitness, if such a thing exists, is about as durable as instant art, or instant music, or instant scholarship. Unpopular and unpalatable as it is, the fact remains that no one becomes proficient at anything by practising a mere 10 minutes a day. If you intend to achieve a worthwhile state of cardiorespiratory fitness, then you have to impose some degree of overload, either in terms of intensity or duration, on your cardiovascular system. Since your heart has some degree of damage, the intensity component has to be limited. Duration, on the other hand, has a much wider margin of safety.

Slow jogging for up to an hour has a number of benefits to offer. It is an excellent way to relieve tension and anxiety. Problems have a way of solving themselves during the workout, largely because they are seen in perspective. Jogging permits only a superficial, holistic type of thought; minutiae and trivia recede into the background, leaving only the important high points for consideration. You no longer miss the wood for the trees. There is also the ego-building factor. The first time you complete five or six miles, no matter at what speed, you know you have set yourself apart from the majority of your fellow men. You are no longer "the guy who had the heart attack."

The psychological benefits of long distance recreational jogging should not be underestimated. In fact, we now have reports from psychiatrists who recognize its value in the treatment of mental illness. Dr. Kostrubala, a psychiatrist practising in Los Angeles, has formed a long distance jogging group for his patients, and carries out group therapy during training sessions. He reports considerable improvement in his patients as they become fitter. This has been the experience of many depressed, tense and anxious individuals after starting a distance jogging program — so much so that if they miss a few training sessions, they often notice the build-up of tension again.

The physiological gains are also immense. After half an hour of steady exercise, you begin to fall back on your stores of body fat as fuel. Fatty acids are burned, and the body relies less and less on its sugar stores. In addition to the metabolic advantages in terms of blood lipid levels, the actual caloric expenditure is considerable. A 160 lb. man running for an hour at a steady 10-minute mile pace will burn 600 calories. This, repeated five times weekly, means that he will burn 12,000 calories a month — which equals 3 lbs. of fat. The surprising fact is that caloric expenditure is more dependent upon the distance you cover and your body weight than upon the speed of your run. For example, a fit young athlete may run five miles in 30 minutes, while you may take 50 minutes for the same task. You are burning less calories per minute (10 calories as opposed to 18 calories, to be precise), but since you are running for a longer time, you both finish up even. The heavier you are, the more energy you need to keep your bulk on the move, and so the more calories you spend.

You never see an obese long distance runner. I believe that he burns his body fat more efficiently than the sedentary person and this is borne out by experimental work. Not only that, but I find he automatically tends to eat less starchy and thus less fattening foods. He shuns sweet desserts. He avoids rich cuts of steak, usually heavily marbled with fat. Animal fat is easy to store, but hard to burn; vegetable fat is much more readily used, and maybe this is why the long distance runner tends to prefer it. Many long distance runners tend to adopt the same dietary habits. Is it by accident or design? One cannot help but wonder if the body naturally chooses the foodstuffs most suitable for its needs. And maybe it is not coincidental that the runner's diet happens also to be the one most suitable for prevention of atherosclerosis.

Before leaving the subject of body weight, mention should be made of the work of Mayer, who ascribes the relationship between appetite and weight to the activity of an appetite centre in that primitive portion of the brain known as the hypothalamus. He believes that in sedentary individuals, this control centre becomes inactive with the result that the nice balance between appetite and body weight is lost. Fat stores increase, but appetite remains high. Obesity encourages less activity, less activity leads to even less energy expenditure, and so even greater fat storing. In this way, the vicious circle continues. Finally the fat person may indeed come to eat less than his slim colleague, but he still continues to get fat.

Cinephotography has shown that obese subjects in a girls' camp were consistently more sluggish in all physical activities. For example, during field games they moved around as little as possible, and during swimming practice they rested much more frequently than their slim, active friends. A physical activity program reactivates the control centre in the brain, restores the balance between food intake and energy expenditure, and ensures the success of a sensible, moderate reducing diet.

Many of us require a goal to aim for, and recreational joggers are no exception. For those of us who spend a major portion of our spare time plodding through the streets and parks, the ultimate distance is 26¼ miles — the marathon race. Merely to have completed such an exhausting trial, at no matter how slow a speed, is a triumph in itself. The aim is not to race against anyone. We leave that for the fleet-footed athletes who disappear from sight at the sound of the starting gun, never to be seen again by those of us who make up the rearguard. Our needs are few; merely to be privileged to leave with the pack at the starting signal, and lucky enough to be able to cross the deserted finishline on our feet — three, four, five or even six hours later. With such simple wants, how can we be denied?

Let us be certain of one thing, however; like most things in life, the travelling is often more rewarding than the arriving. By that I mean that it is the training needed to ensure successful completion of the marathon that confers the benefit. There is no magic in the race itself from a health point of view. Thus, I cannot agree with my good friend, Dr. Tom Bassler, the Los Angeles pathologist, who believes that anyone who completes a marathon race in under 4½ hours is immune from a heart attack for the next five years. (He excludes smokers.)

The so-called "Bassler imperative" seems to be not only an exaggerated claim, but also a totally unnecessary one. We have discussed the undoubted physiological benefits to the heart which accrue from endurance training. We have looked at the evidence

The author with Mr. Magdi Yacoub, cardiovascular surgeon, discussing the training project for heart transplant patients, Harefield Hospital, London, England.

Author and staff at team meeting.

in favour of exercise as a preventive measure in coronary heart disease. We have considered the sense of exhilaration and well-being which accompanies the trained state. To make any greater claims is to destroy the force of our arguments to date. This I will concede; the lifestyle associated with marathon-type training is hardly likely to contain too many heart attack risk factors. On the other hand, completion of a marathon run is no guarantee of immortality.

One of our patients who, some three years earlier, had finished a marathon run in five hours, died in his sleep. Autopsy failed to show any evidence of recent coronary thrombosis or myocardial infarction; it must be assumed that he had suffered a cardiac arrest. He was a smoker, and in the five or six months immediately prior to his death, had increased his cigarette consumption considerably. Running does not permit you to flout all of the other risk factors — especially when you have already had one or two previous heart attacks and know that the dice are already loaded against you.

For those who are interested in marathon running, I have discussed the matter in some detail and included suitable training tables in Chapter 12.

More and more doctors are appreciating the value of jogging, although I must say that their numbers are still minuscule when viewed in terms of the profession as a whole. Nevertheless, there is now an active group of physicians and allied healthy professionals who have formed the American Medical Joggers Association. Under their neurologist president, Dr. Ron Lawrence, they have championed the cause of jogging for health. They encourage their members to take part in long distance road races, including marathons, and schedule their medical meetings around such events as the Boston Marathon, the Mission Bay Marathon, the Honolulu Marathon and the London Marathon. The papers given by the members are invariably stimulating, and ample time is allowed for frank and free-wheeling discussion. The tone of these meetings is friendly and frank, without the scientific constraints which are customary in many medical conventions and which, at times, have a rather stultifying effect on verbal interplay. It is strange to attend a medical meeting where practically all of the members go for a jog after the day's proceedings, and wind up the whole affair by entering a marathon race. The post-marathon dinner is a euphoric affair, with each member discussing step by step his experiences during the race held earlier in the day. Equally unusual, there is a noticeable absence of smoke and liquor to accompany the proceedings! The members of the association now exceed 5,000, with a significant proportion of them Canadians. They include the Honolulu cardiologist, Jack Scaff, who is a keen jogger himself, and who introduced the Cardiovascular Division into the First Honolulu Marathon in 1973, having been stimulated by the example of the Toronto men in Boston nine months earlier. Dr. Tom Bassler, referred to earlier, is also a member, as is the author.

Another medical group which has long recognized the value of exercise in cardiovascular disease is the American College of Sports Medicine. This group is considerably larger than AMJA, and consists of physicians, physiologists and physical educators who are interested in the scientific and medical aspects of sports. The association journal, *The Physician and Sportsmedicine*, frequently contains articles on exercise therapy, and the annual meeting invariably has a section dealing exclusively with exercise and coronary heart disease. Membership in this association is growing rapidly, and this signifies the burgeoning interest in the subject. The emphasis here is more scientific than that of AMJA, with heavy stress on experimental work, both laboratory and clinical.

For the reader who has never been involved in an exercise program before, and who on reading this book intends to start exercising, I hope the above will provide the necessary motivation. If nothing else, it should at least indicate to him that he is anything but on his own. There are thousands of us out there in the street, so come on out and join us! A wave of the hand, and a short "Hi" as we pass in the night, and you've been initiated.

HEART SURGERY AND RELATED TOPICS

Coronary Artery Bypass Graft

In May 1967, Dr. Rene Favaloro carried out the first coronary artery bypass graft (CABG) procedure on a patient suffering from severe coronary atherosclerosis. Since then, the operation has become an increasingly viable alternative form of therapy for those patients in whom medical treatment is ineffective. In fact, it is no exaggeration to say that it has now become a commonplace procedure in all of the major medical centres of the Western world.

Although technically quite complex, the operation is simple in concept. Using a length of vein taken from the patient's thigh (or

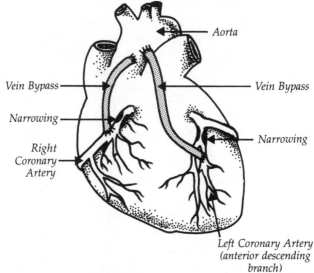

Aorta

Vein Bypass

Vein Bypass

Narrowing

Narrowing

Right
Coronary
Artery

Left Coronary Artery
(anterior descending
branch)

Figure 21   Bypass Surgery–Narrowings in right and left coronary arteries are bypassed, using two lengths of vein from the patient's leg. Blood now flows from the aorta, around the narrowed segments, and on through the healthy artery beyond them.

a segment of artery taken from the chest wall), the surgeon bypasses the atherosclerotic narrowing in the coronary artery by stitching (i.e., grafting) one end of the vein into the base of the aorta and the other end into the portion of coronary artery beyond the narrowing (Figure 21). The ideal situation for grafting is where you have a localized narrowing, as opposed to an elongated, or series of ''beaded '' obstructions. Preferably the narrowing should be high up, and a wide healthy artery should exist below the narrowed area. Furthermore, the heart muscle supplied by the coronary artery should be relatively healthy; it would not make sense to provide an increased blood supply to tissue that is already too badly damaged by disease to benefit from it.

Given these conditions, any number of grafts can be done at the same time, depending on the skill of the surgeon. Over the years, as technique has improved, the operative risk involved in the procedure has diminished until today it is considered to be of the same order of magnitude as, say, a gall bladder operation.

Are there any complications? The two most common are a perioperative myocardial infarction (a heart attack occurring during surgery), and a blocking of the graft. The former is not necessarily of any consequence, and is often only detected from routine post-operative electrocardiograms. Graft blockage occurs in about 10 per cent of cases, and, if it happens at all, almost invariably does so within six to twelve months of surgery.

Who should be considered for bypass graft surgery? This is obviously a matter of fine judgment, the decision to recommend an operation usually being a joint one involving cardiologist and cardiovascular surgeon. In general, however, surgery is usually reserved for those who are suffering from severe incapacitating angina which is not responding to adequate medical treatment. Needless to say, the severity and extent of the atherosclerotic lesions have to be taken into account, and this is determined by a diagnostic procedure known as coronary angiography. Here a fine hollow catheter is threaded up a leg or arm artery so that its tip lies just at the origins of the left and right coronary arteries. A contrast fluid is then injected into the arteries through the catheter, and its passage down all of the branches of the coronary vascular tree is visualized and recorded on a cine-x-ray. Any narrowing or blockage can thus be identified (Figure 22). Thereafter, more contrast substance is injected into the ventricles in order to outline the size of the heart in systole and diastole and thus see how well it contracts (ventriculography). After this the catheter is removed, a compression bandage is placed over the tiny puncture mark in the limb artery, and the patient can rest overnight and be discharged from hospital. There is little or no discomfort involved (indeed the method was developed by a Dr. Werner Forssmann who first carried out the procedure *on himself* in 1929 in order to gain more information from x-rays of the heart!) Risk is minimal, and everything is carried out with the patient sedated but awake. Obviously, one has to have an angiogram before being considered for surgery.

Broadly speaking, the benefits of coronary artery bypass graft surgery can be twofold: first, an alleviation or abolition of anginal symptoms; and secondly, an improved life expectancy, at least in certain cases. Which cases? Despite some areas of uncertainty here, there is a growing body of evidence to suggest that patients with atherosclerosis involving only one coronary artery, or mildly involving two, do equally well whether treated medically or surgically. On the other hand, patients in whom all three coronary arteries are seriously diseased, or who have marked narrowing of the beginning portion of the left main coronary artery (just before it divides to form the circumflex and left anterior descending branches), would seem to have a better survival rate if treated surgically. That is, of course, always assuming that the other criteria of operability are present, and remembering that each case must be judged on its own merits.

Does it sound as if CABG surgery is the quick cure-all for coronary artery disease? Only the most naive would come to that conclusion. First of all there is a risk. Granted that the risk is an acceptable trade-off in certain situations, the fact remains that even in the hands of the most competent surgical team, things can go wrong. Then you should remember that there is no procedure which can be carried out on the human body that carries a warranty. The human mechanism is too complex for that. So no surgeon can give you a 100 per cent guarantee that the result will be exactly as you both want. All of which means that you do not rush into surgery until you and your medical advisers are satisfied that all avenues of medical therapy have been very thoroughly explored.

As bypass surgery has become more common, so the number of such cases referred to the Toronto Rehabilitation Centre's program has increased, until at the time of writing they constitute 20 to 25 per cent of the total. Surely there can be no better expression of the way in which exercise rehabilitation has been accepted to complement and supplement medical and surgical treament of heart disease.

I have always believed that if the full benefits of CABG surgery are to be realized, in terms of quality as well as quantity of life, then the post-surgical patient should be advised regarding exercise and lifestyle change. After all, while the graft averts the consequences of a potential blockage, it cannot of itself affect the rate of development or the consequences of any new atherosclerotic lesions. Unless the risk factors associated with the presence of the disease in the first place are effectively removed, then it is hardly surprising to find that the patient has to return in five years or so complaining of similar symptoms as before, only on this occasion emanating from an atherosclerotic narrowing in what was previously a healthy artery, or even narrowing in the graft itself. Indeed, there are increasing reports in the medical literature of a type of accelerated atheromatus plaque growth occurring in the graft of those patients who do not reduce their risk

Figure 22 Angiogram–X-ray of coronary arteries (angiogram)
showing narrowing (arrow) in upper portion of the anterior
descending branch of the left coronary artery.

factors. All the more reason, then, that the CABG patient, now
free from angina, should take advantage of a rehabilitation training program to obtain true functional benefit.

Percutaneous Transluminal Coronary Angioplasty

Since 1977, there has been an alternative procedure to bypass surgery for certain potential surgical candidates. In that year, Dr.
Andreas Gruntzig of Zurich, performed the first Percutaneous
Transluminal Coronary Angioplasty (PTCA). The method consists
of inserting a thin catheter, with a distensible balloon at its tip,
into the coronary artery until it reaches the narrowed area. The
balloon is then inflated, so as to flatten the atherosclerotic plaque
and thus restore normal blood flow (Figure 23). Compared with
surgery, PTCA is a relatively minor procedure, not unlike a routine coronary angiogram. There is no surgical scar, the patient is
only in hospital for a few nights, and can resume normal activities in two or three days. Most major medical centres now per-

1   Atherosclerotic plaque in
    coronary artery

2   Dilating catheter is
    passed beyond narrowed
    segment of artery

3   Balloon inflated,
    flattening plaque

4   Catheter withdrawn, with
    reduction in size of plaque

**Figure 23   Percutaneous Transluminal Coronary Angioplasty
(PTCA)**

form the procedure, and although it is not entirely free from risk,
the mortality rate is lower than that for CABG surgery. Best results
are obtained when the blockage is localized to the upper (proximal)
part of the coronary artery, is fairly soft and recent without too
much calcium deposit, and is not more than five millimetres or so
in length. Ideally, only one coronary should be diseased, although
with increasing experience physicians are now dilating two or three
vessels. As with surgery, the major indication for PTCA is severe
angina of effort, not amenable to routine medical treatment and
drugs. Problems encountered may include difficulty in passing
the catheter past the blockage, and damage to the wall of the coronary artery as the balloon is inflated. Because of these possible
complications, patients must be prepared for immediate emergency CABG surgery.

It is too early to say what the long-term results will be, since the
procedure has not been in common use for long. Nevertheless,
patients followed for up to three years show a high percentage of
success. It is doubtful, however, that PTCA will be a substitute for
bypass surgery. By present standards, I would hazard a guess

that about 20 per cent of potential bypass graft patients will be offered PTCA as an alternative.

Heart Transplants

Before leaving the topic of cardiac surgery, I should mention the exciting new developments in the area of heart transplantation. After some false and shaky starts in the 1970s (due largely to overly optimistic predictions and subsequent bad publicity), the 1980s saw the establishment of a firm foundation for future widespread success. The discovery of new medications to overcome the major problem of rejection has not only enabled the patient with his new heart to be out of hospital and back to work in a matter of weeks (as opposed to months in the past), but it has also improved the five-year survival rate to well in excess of 70 per cent.

At the moment, the number of centres in the world where heart transplants are being carried out is limited, but I have no doubt that this will change in the near future. Obviously this is not the answer to the epidemic of coronary artery disease. Only prevention will solve that problem. However, the heart transplant procedure will save many valuable young lives in the meantime.

One of the leading centres in the world for heart transplant surgery is Harefield Hospital in London, England. The surgeon, Mr. Magdi Yacoub, is a firm advocate of post-surgical exercise rehabilitation, and in 1984, he and I set up a joint research project between Harefield and the Toronto Rehabilitation Centre. This has involved the exercise testing and training of English transplant patients by senior members of the Centre's staff who spend five days or so in Harefield every three months working with the new patients and reassessing previous ones. In the intervals between these visits, communication is maintained by mailed exercise logs, in similar manner to the system adopted for patients on the home program.

Amazing as it seems, patients are put on the training program as early as eight weeks after the transplant. Some are at the jogging stage by twenty weeks! A far cry from the situation a few years back, when all were kept at rest and almost in total isolation for two months. It would be unrealistic to suggest that we know all there is to know about the effects of training on the transplanted denervated heart, but the indications to date are that our efforts will be rewarded by at least as gratifying results as we have seen in post-heart-attack and post-bypass patients.

CHAPTER TEN

The Woman
in the Picture

IN THE FOREGROUND

I have referred earlier to the peculiar fact that the current epidemic of fatal heart attacks, which commenced in the 1920s, shows a very high ratio of male to female deaths. Prior to 1920, that ratio was approximately one to one — that is, equal mortality in both sexes. Subsequently, however, the death rate in males increased disproportionately, particularly in the age group under 50, until today fatal heart attack and sudden cardiac death is about ten times higher in men than in women. Interestingly, when we look at the other manifestation of coronary artery disease, angina pectoris, the sex difference almost disappears. The reason for these findings still remains unknown.

In recent years, as women have achieved increasing equality in our society, we have braced ourselves in anticipation of an epidemic of female heart attack deaths. So far, this has not occurred. Possibly the failure of women to catch up with men in this area merely reflects the degree to which they have fallen short of complete equality. If this is so, then the 1990s may see the hard-driving, hard-working, highly stressed, sedentary career woman claim equal time with men in the coronary care unit.

On the other hand, heart attacks are not the sole prerogative of the male. Approximately 10 to 15 per cent of patients referred to the Toronto program are female. The majority are in their post-menopausal years, which suggests that female hormone exerts some protection from myocardial infarction. Further support for the hormone protective theory lies in the evidence which has accumulated since the 1960s linking the birth control pill, which acts as an artificial regulator of female hormone levels, with certain types of cardiovascular disease, such as vein thrombosis, stroke, and heart attack. These oral contraceptives usually contain two hormones, progesterone and estrogen. The risk seems to be greatest when the amount of estrogen is high, and this has led to the development of pills containing only micro-dosages of that particular hormone. Older women are particularly in jeopardy, and those over the age of 35 should discuss alternative methods of contraception with their physician.

As for the pre-menopausal group, the risk factors seem to be similar but not identical to their male counterpart. A number of studies have shown that cigarette smoking is particularly dangerous. Examination of all the available data reveals that the young woman who smokes a pack of cigarettes a day has as much as ten times greater risk of having a heart attack as her non-smoking female friend of the same age. More than a pack and a half, and the risk is twenty times greater. Here, then, is one risk factor which is totally under the control of the individual and can be eliminated at will. In view of the gruesome evidence, it is surely in one's best interests to do so.

Another potent risk factor for women is diabetes. Female diabetics, particularly those requiring medications to control their blood sugar, have the same incidence of coronary artery disease as males — i.e., ten to fifteen times greater than non-diabetic females. In our present state of knowledge there is no cure for diabetes; but once detected, it can be held in control and many of its unpleasant consequences avoided. An annual check-up should always include urine and blood analysis, particularly in those women with a family history of heart disease, and the diagnosed diabetic should adhere strictly to the dietary and medication regime prescribed by her physician. With regard to family history, particular significance has been attached to the occurrence of a heart attack or stroke, before the age of 60, in a mother or a sister.

Obesity, in the absence of other risk factors, seems to be of little significance in the pattern of female heart disease. Similarly, the status of elevated blood cholesterol is much less clear-cut than in men. One reason is the very high levels of HDL cholesterol found in young pre-menopausal women. This may in itself protect against the development of atherosclerosis. It should also be noted that after the menopause not only does the level of total cholesterol tend to rise, but this elevation applies particularly to the LDL cholesterol fraction.

As with males, untreated high blood pressure acts as an independent risk factor for coronary atherosclerosis, and can augment risk as much as six-fold. Again, the answer lies in detection and, since total cure is rarely possible, strict adherence to a medically prescribed regime which may include weight control, regular exercise, and anti-hypertensive medication.

Insofar as the role of physical activity in the primary prevention of heart disease in women is concerned, there have been no major studies published to date. You will recall that the earlier reports involving all-male populations dealt with those engaged in heavy manual labour. Only relatively recently has the effect of leisure-time physical activity been considered. Today, as more women take up jogging, cross-country skiing, cycling, aerobic dancing, and other cardiovascular conditioning activities on a regular basis, the opportunity for further research will increase accordingly. In the meantime, our current knowledge of the psychological and physiological effects of training in the female leads us to believe that the protective effect of exercise applies equally to both sexes. Women joggers have been shown to have higher HDL cholesterol and lower triglyceride levels than sedentary women. Women police cadets in Los Angeles demonstrated the same improvement in cardiac performance after a period of jogging training as did male cadets. Women patients referred to the Toronto program have fared equally well as men in terms of symptom reduction, improved morale and mood, increased maximum oxygen consumption, and reduced incidence of recurrent heart attack.

Today, of course, the female athlete is no longer considered a rare phenomenon. In fact, in many sports, the women's events are as exciting as the men's. Women race all distances up to 3,000 metres on the track, often at a faster pace than the male Olympic champion of twenty or thirty years ago. More and more women are entering marathon runs, and the 1984 Olympics saw the introduction of the women's marathon. Dr. Van Acken, the famous German coach and physiologist, maintains that a woman's metabolism is better adapted to feats of endurance than a man's, and he forecasts that women one day will outperform men in distance running. Men may continue to dominate those activities requiring pure muscle power and speed, but the day might well come when a suitably trained woman will capture the world's long distance running, swimming, or cross-country title.

All of the foregoing explains why the women referred to the Toronto program are treated exactly the same as the men. They should use the training tables exactly as described, with the same age division and precautions. For the women reading this book, there is no earthly reason why you shouldn't progress to the 4-mile distance and even to the marathon if you are prepared to devote the time. I recall when the T.R.C. Joggers were out on a training run a few years back, we first met a middle-aged lady jogger proceeding leisurely along the same park track. Our next encounter was when we watched her finish a determined and gallant last in her first full marathon race. Today, at 64, Judith Kazdan has twenty-five completed marathons to her credit. She runs mostly on her own in training, occasionally with her husband.

IN THE BACKGROUND

Strictly speaking, I should use the term spouse here, but as I have explained, the vast majority of heart attack patients are male, and so woman and spouse are very likely synonymous. In any event, whether you be male or female spouse, let me emphasize right now that this section is probably one of the most important in the entire book. Why so? Because the message this book is trying to impart involves a change in lifestyle which, in a partnership, means a change for both parties. I will go further. Only with the full and complete cooperation and understanding of the spouse can the heart attack patient hope to successfully adhere to this or any other cardiac rehabilitation program. I can quote literally hundreds of cases to prove my point. And yet, I am all too aware of the difficulties involved.

From our own experience, we know that the problems start immediately with the onset of the heart attack. Nearly half of the wives we interviewed reported being "numbed," or in a state of shock on hearing the news. Like their husband, they echo the phrase, "This can't be happening to him." This sense of unreality is quickly shattered, however, by the day-to-day problems which arise. There are the daily visits to the hospital which, for the young wife, may be complicated by having to look after the children, while at the same time keeping up a brave face. Working wives are fearful of losing their jobs, and can only hope that they have a sympathetic and understanding employer. Even after the husband's discharge from hospital, symptoms of anxiety and depression are common. Complaints of fatigue are frequent. Many wives develop the symptoms of ill-health themselves, requiring visits to their doctor. There are so many unanswered questions, and all too frequently so little proffered advice.

For the first few weeks after discharge the patient is dependent, and even childlike in attitude. The older wife may even encourage this, substituting for the grown-up family which has maybe only recently left home. But how far do you go? As one wife said, "I am scared stiff that I will lose my temper, raise my voice, criticize or do anything that will make him ill again."

The questions are legion. How much can he lift? How much can he do about the house? To what extent can you insist on him not smoking, or keeping his weight down? Is it safe to have sex? How long will it be before he can accept responsibility, or stop acting like a spoiled child? Is it any wonder that some marriages are brought to breaking point by the frustration and irritability that often occur during the stage of convalescence following the heart attack. And yet, this need not necessarily be the case. If both partners can recognize and discuss the possible areas of strife, then they can introduce a greater warmth and affection into their relationship than ever before. Again, to quote the wife of one my patients, "I don't think either of us knew how much we had until we nearly lost it."

That's all very well, you say, but how do I go about dealing with my particular problem? First of all, read the rest of this book carefully. It will give you a good idea as to how much exercise your husband should be doing. It will also indicate the risk factors he should be avoiding. A feature of the Toronto program is an evening with the spouses of newly referred patients. This provides an occasion to meet with the staff, and allows me the opportunity to explain the nature of heart disease, its possible causes, and the role that exercise plays in primary and secondary prevention. After the talk, the questions start. With audiences of about one hundred assembled, you can imagine that the queries are many and varied. I try to answer each question as honestly and as carefully as I can, pointing out that in matters of judgment, as opposed to fact, my response has to be based on my personal opinion, which in turn is based on my experience with my own and other programs. The vast majority of my audience are, of course, women, and their sole purpose in attending the meeting is to learn how to help their husbands. They are encouraged to ask questions which have been bothering them, and which they have never had the opportunity to ask previously. Since the patients are not present at the meeting, the spouses can be as frank as they wish in expressing their fears, doubts, and concerns.

Some of the questions dealt with are too individual to be answered in general terms, others have been dealt with elsewhere in this book. However, the following paragraphs are based on the questions most often asked by the concerned partner, and hopefully will be of help.

Overcoming Despondency

It is now accepted that rehabilitation should start as soon as the patient gets out of the coronary care unit and returns to the general ward. The hour-to-hour battle to save his life is over, and the time for healing has begun. For the moment, the patient is glad just to be alive, but as the days pass, that feeling of relief is replaced by one of despondency. The mind is plagued by doubts and uncertainties, all revolving around the ability to be able to do all of the things which were part and parcel of everyday life before the attack. As one patient said to me, ''I wanted to get out of the hospital, and yet I was scared to go home. Activities which I had always taken for granted now became a first; the first time you walk up the stairs, you wonder if it's safe, and you breathe a sigh of relief when you get to the top of the flight and nothing happens. The first day you mow the grass, or clean out the basement, or go back to work, it's the same feeling — will you make it? It's as if you're trying to pick up the pieces of your life again, and never being sure if they'll fit together properly this time.''

Of course, a good post-coronary rehabilitation program helps to overcome much of this fear. No program, however, can help as much as a well-informed wife. What, you say, can I do? First of all, take a positive approach right from the first hospital visit. Don't avoid discussing the future. The vast majority of heart attack patients return to their previous jobs. If your husband's is the exceptional case, it still does no harm to discuss alternatives. To make small talk and steer away from a topic as important as future work plans is a great mistake; to the depressed patient, it can only mean one thing—there is no future to discuss. Even if he doesn't feel inclined to pursue the subject in great detail, he will thank you later for displaying such confidence.

When the day comes for your husband to return home, don't make the mistake of one of my patient's wives who automatically picked up his suitcase and carried it to the car. That one action, well-intentioned as it was, put the seal on all his fears. Four years later, he still sees it as his most humiliating moment. Better to have let him offer to carry it himself (after all, how much personal belongings can you accumulate during a two-week stay in the coronary ward?); or if lifting has been entirely prohibited by the physician, make some remark to the effect that you are obeying doctor's orders, which means lifting is out, for the time being. The main thing is to avoid being over-solicitous. Exercise sensible precautions, but don't fuss. No doubt there is an increased element of risk in certain physical activities, but then driving an automobile isn't exactly 100 per cent safe these days, and no one can live his life completely immune from risk. Besides, until recently, the tendency, has been to exaggerate the dangers of physical effort for the heart attack patient. We now know that many of the things that he will want to do are perfectly safe.

In the first few months after the attack, there is often a reluctance to make decisions. This is perfectly natural, and is just another manifestation of the depressed mood. Eventually, the situation rights itself. Just be patient, and whatever you do, don't get into the habit of making all the decisions in the home. If you do, you may well find yourself stuck with the role of decision-maker permanently. Every so often, give your partner the opportunity to regain the initiative.

How to React to Symptoms

Symptom-claiming is not unusual in the early days following the attack. It is an expression of insecurity, and represents a need for reassurance. It may last a matter of months only, but it can be a real trial for the wife who never becomes quite inured to a succession of frightening complaints of chest pain, numbness in hands, dizziness, and so on. Often the symptom complex is similar to the one which heralded the initial attack, and it is difficult not to push the panic button and call the physician on every occasion. However, each wife knows her own husband, and very often will have an instinctive feeling for the true state of affairs; as likely as not, it will be safe for her to follow that instinct and give him the reassurance he is seeking. If, on the other hand, she is not all that sure of herself, she will usually learn from the first few false alarms.

Is it not better to be sure than sorry? Within reason, yes. However, a man cannot spend half his life running in and out of the doctor's office or the hospital emergency department. If he is to live a normal life, he must learn to exercise judgment and maturity in assessing the significance of various symptoms. To get into the habit of requiring an electrocardiogram every time he gets an ache or a pain is to follow the path to cardiac neurosis — in my experience, one of the most difficult of all conditions to cure. The ironic thing, of course, is that the electrocardiogram is by no means infallible. If this preoccupation with symptoms persists beyond a six-month period or so, and shows no signs of responding to simple reassurance on your part, then it should be mentioned to the family physician or the cardiologist. Psychiatric treatment may be indicated to relieve the condition before the pattern becomes set.

Once again, it should be borne in mind that reluctance to make decisions or to take responsibility, as well as exaggeration of symptoms, are merely expressions of depression, a not uncommon reaction to a heart attack in a certain personality type. Depression recedes with time, although since the trait is probably inborn, it never disappears entirely and may reoccur in response to some other misfortune. Frank depression, accompanied by a mournful, long expression, is rare. The depressed individual is more likely to cover up his real feelings, and feign a cheery, jocular mood. In many cases, his act is good enough to deceive even those closest to him, including his wife. However, the underlying mood cannot help but express itself in the more subtle ways already described.

There are certain symptoms which should be taken seriously, since they may herald a recurrence. Complaint of severe pain in the chest, left arm or jaw and which is accompanied by pallor, sweating and alteration in pulse rate is classical; it will be underestimated by only the most ineffectual or callous observer. Such a picture demands urgent medical attention, and precious time should not be wasted "waiting to see if it will go away."

An analysis of the patients referred to the Toronto Rehabilitation Centre showed that a high proportion of them had six hours or more warning of their attack. The manner in which the attack started varied (see Figure 24), but pain in the chest or arm was the commonest. Since the survival rate is highest in those who receive medical care quickly, the recognition of warning signs is of para-

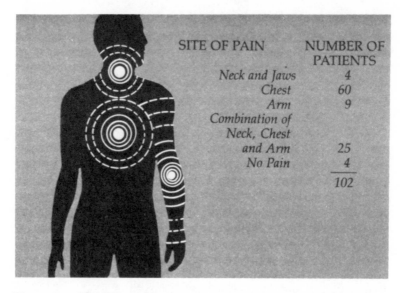

SITE OF PAIN	NUMBER OF PATIENTS
Neck and Jaws	4
Chest	60
Arm	9
Combination of Neck, Chest and Arm	25
No Pain	4
	102

Figure 24   The Sites of Pain in Heart Attack as Reported by 102 Patients Referred to the Centre's Post-coronary Exercise Program

mount importance. The problem is compounded by the tendency for some men to deny that the symptoms they are experiencing are those of a heart attack. Blame is usually laid at the door of the gastro-intestinal tract. Beware the severe attack of "indigestion" which lasts more than half an hour, does not respond to simple antacid medication, and is made worse by lying flat.

There are other indications of impending trouble which, although less dramatic than chest pain, should nevertheless be heeded. In some ways, they may be more important, since they may antedate the attack itself and so allow more time for preventive action. Foremost among these intangible and often vague signs is excessive fatigue. Tiredness which is not relieved by a good night's rest should be considered suspect in the recent post-coronary patient, and search should be made for the cause. A heavy workload or an overcrowded social itinerary is usually the culprit, and steps should be taken immediately to adopt a more sensible and relaxed routine. Dr. Nixon, cardiologist at the Charing Cross Hospital in London, places great emphasis on irascible mood as an ill-omen, and I agree entirely with him. Frequently, the wife is the first to recognize the onset of a cantankerous, irritable manner which was so typical of the first attack. Both fatigue and irritability may be the result of a return to the old, driving, overcrowded lifestyle, with its business and financial worries, impossible work schedule, and absence of physical activity and recreation. In short, a repetition of the very set of circumstances which probably triggered the initial acute attack.

Sexual Activity

We have dealt with this subject previously, but let us return to it again briefly, looking at it from the spouse's viewpoint. Many post-coronary patients, both male and female, quickly regain their interest in sex after the acute stage of the attack is over and they have returned home to their routine daily activities. The chances are that their level of interest will be the same as previously. However, for couples who have not received explicit instructions before hospital discharge, there may be uncertainty and fear regarding the safety of intercourse. Actually, such fears are largely groundless. It has been said that if you can walk up two flights of stairs, you are physically fit enough to have sex. Unless the heart has been extensively damaged, there is no more danger after the heart attack than there was before it. So don't enter the situation in obvious fear and trepidation. Nothing is more destined to put your partner off, and increase feelings of depression, insecurity, and worthlessness.

There are individuals who do experience genuine symptoms during intercourse, either angina of effort, or palpitations (skipped beats), or extreme breathlessness. In my experience a good exercise program, which improves cardiovascular fitness, will almost invariably eliminate these problems. Some doctors recommend the use of a medication such as glyceryl trinitrate immediately before sex in order to prevent angina. Others suggest a change in position. The point to emphasize is that the persistence of symptoms during sexual activity should be discussed openly and frankly with your physician.

There are certain medications which, in some patients, may reduce sexual urge. One cannot be specific here, since the individual variations are wide, and also because it is frequently very difficult to distinguish between a true chemical side effect and a host of other less tangible causes. However, there have been reports of reduction in libido following the taking of various drugs used to lower blood pressure, certain beta-blockers, as well as some blood-fat lowering agents, tranquillizers, and anti-depressants. If one of these medications is suspected of reducing sex desire, the matter should be discussed with the prescribing physician. On no account allow your spouse to stop a medication on the grounds of suspicion. After all, it has been prescribed for a reason, and in the case of a blood pressure medication, is usually required to be taken indefinitely. It is often relatively easy for the physician to substitute another substance which is equally effective but does not carry the same side effects. While we are on the subject, incidentally, let me remind you that the two commonest drugs which have been shown to reduce sexual appetite are non-prescription — alcohol and cigarettes!

Preventing Another Attack

Recognition of dangerous symptoms is one thing; preventing them from appearing is a far more worthwhile goal. What positive steps should you take to help your partner keep from having a further attack? It can be expressed in a phrase: "Assist him in his efforts to change his lifestyle." His previous way of life contained the seeds of his attack. He has been given a chance, maybe his last, to alter the situation. This means a suitable diet which is low in cholesterol and animal fats, a physical fitness program, a veto on cigarette smoking, and moderation in both work and play.

Sounds easy? Well, maybe. It's no use applauding these aims and then getting irritable because this new lifestyle precludes some of your favourite social engagements and habits. After all, if he has to jog in the morning, he may not exactly relish a late party the night before — even if it is with that delightful Jones couple you feel you "owe" it to. He may want to go to bed around 10:00 p.m. or so, without that 11:00 p.m. nightcap which he used to look forward to so much. He may object to your smoking, especially if he is suffering the tortures of the damned trying to give it up himself! He will be learning to say no to things which he really doesn't want to do (or knows he shouldn't do), instead of always saying yes to every request, trivial or otherwise.

As the wife of one patient put it, "Bill isn't the same anymore. He used to be so kind and thoughtful, and took me wherever I wanted to go. Now, he says he isn't going anywhere just because he has to. Last week, he refused to go to my cousin's wedding.

Sometimes when we have company and it gets late, he just excuses himself and goes to bed at 11:00 p.m.''

Bill has had two heart attacks, is now a dedicated jogger and is fitter than he has ever been in his life. My guess is that if he keeps on playing it so smart, he'll live out his normal lifespan.

You will need to accommodate to this new partner. The more accommodation needed, the more you can console yourself with the thought that the rehabilitation is proceeding successfully. You may have to arrange mealtimes so as to fit in with exercise sessions. Don't nag because you have to keep food hot while you wait for him to come back from his jog. If you can't jog with him, then take the trouble to acquaint yourself with the distance he has to go and the time it should take, and then plan accordingly.

If you feel that this is a chore, just think of Mrs. R. whose husband had a heart attack when he was 29 years old.

"Certainly Herman's running is time-consuming," she related at a recent meeting of the Ontario Heart Foundation. "In fact, our daughter was two years old before all three of us ever had Sunday dinner together; Herman was always out training with the cardiac marathoners. But that's a small price to pay to have him alive and healthy. Besides, we were only married two years before his attack, and the picture looked so bleak, that we decided that it would be irresponsible of us to start a family. However, he improved so much on the running program that we changed our minds."

Herman R. has run eighteen marathons in all, his fastest being in 3 hours, 10 minutes. In 1975, he was the first heart patient ever to officially enter the Boston Marathon, where he placed 1,500 out of a field of 2,500 and returned a time of 3 hours, 20 minutes. Three months after that, in August 1975, his second daughter was born.

If you are to play an intelligent role in the rehabilitation program, you should take the time to read this book carefully. Master the training tables, understand the method of progression, and become familiar with the signs of over-training. Learn how to use a stop watch, and check your husband's jogging times. Have him complete a daily workout diary, and check to see if he is going too fast or too slow. Discuss his progress with him and congratulate him on each upward step he makes in the tables. Encourage him when he plateaus, and keep his spirits up when he seems to stick for too long at one level.

In short, aim to be his mentor and his coach, remembering that no one can really consistently train themselves; from time to time, everyone needs the objectivity of an informed onlooker, one who will not only urge them on to greater heights, but one who will also apply the brakes when the signs call for it. As the "coach" of a cardiac athlete, you have additional responsibilities. Never forget that this particular jogger has a scar in his heart, and that excessive enthusiasm or competitiveness is uncalled for and even dangerous. The name of the game is health through fitness, not fitness for competition.

As your spouse's condition improves, there will be a simultaneous improvement in symptoms, including angina and tolerance for heavier physical work. Eventually, he will be carrying out physical tasks which are far beyond the level of his pre-attack capabilities. This may in itself cause problems. He may wish to discontinue the prescribed medication. Most of the time, this is all to the good, but try not to let him do this before he checks with his physician. I am constantly having to remind my patients of this.

Another side effect of increasing fitness is the desire to take up new and sometimes more strenuous leisure activities, such as camping, sailboating, backpacking, cross-country skiing. Often allied with this is an increased interest in the simpler pleasures; walking in the rain, a good novel, a fall outing on foot to catch the colours. If you are prepared for this changed outlook, you will hopefully adapt your lifestyle accordingly.

Can you adapt to this? I still recall with crystal clarity the bemused tone with which one of my earliest "successes" described his wife's reaction to his newly awakened yearnings. "You know what she said, Doc?" he intoned sadly. "I wish you hadn't changed. We were so happy when you were the way you used to be."

Before closing, let me touch on a delicate subject. If you have read the early chapters, you will have noted that the life expectancy of the individual who has had a heart attack is less than normal. Maybe the adoption of a new lifestyle will correct that; if we didn't think so, it would hardly be worth the effort. Nevertheless, the unpalatable fact of your partner's possible early death may be hard to live with. Yet this is a fact of life, which may help to put my whole argument into perspective. Don't dwell on the negative side. Accept the odds, then make up your mind to reduce them to a minimum. You cannot live your life by statistics, otherwise you would take no risks at all. Get on with the business of living, and may you both live happily ever after.

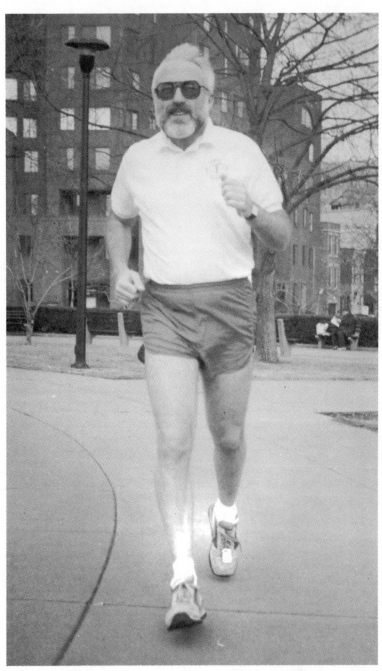

Dr. Ron Lawrence, President, American Medical Joggers Association.

Part Three

RUNNING AND YOUR HEALTH

Write the vision, and make it plain upon tables, that he may run
that readeth it.

Habakkuk 2:2

CHAPTER ELEVEN

Loping and Coping

In recent years, more and more individuals have become increasingly interested in the healthy active lifestyle, adopting many of the principles advocated in this book. People are becoming more concerned with the positive attainment of health, rather than merely the absence of disease. This may explain why in Canada and the United States the incidence of death from heart attack is slowly declining. Not that we can afford to be complacent about this. After all, coronary heart disease is still our number one killer. Nevertheless, if the trend continues, the twenty-first century might well see the end of the epidemic. If this forecast proves to be correct, then there is no doubt in my mind that prevention rather than cure has been responsible.

No one's life is problem-free, and the jogger is no exception. Time is precious, and the conscious decision to spend some of it on regular jogging sessions may meet resistance from unsympathetic family or friends. Excessive zeal may lead to injuries, minor in the overall scheme of things, but sufficient to put a temporary halt to your workouts, lead to a chorus of "I told you so," and make you miserable and mad with the world. The air around you may be so thick with gasoline fumes and industrial pollution that you wonder if you wouldn't be better off to buy a stationary bicycle. You are bombarded with contradictory advice about jogging shoes, dietary supplements and a whole host of "essentials" for the jogger. You pick up the paper one morning to find jogging is *the* road to health and fitness, only to read the next day that the middle-aged jogger is dicing with death.

The veteran jogger will have learned to roll with the punches, temper enthusiasm with common sense and use a mixture of guile, deafness of convenience and sheer indifference in order to keep family, job, friends and himself together — and still jog! He can probably teach you the tricks of the trade — if he has the time. Otherwise, you are going to have to learn the hard way. Hopefully some of the topics covered in this chapter will set you thinking in the right direction.

INJURIES

Let's face it, jogging is a safe sport. Compared with football, ice hockey, English rugger and the like, it's pretty tame. The ancient Irish game of hurling (reputedly the fastest field game in the world and without doubt the most dangerous-looking) makes jogging look about as perilous as threading a needle; no badly smashed bones, dislocated shoulders, eight-inch lacerations, fractured skulls, broken noses, tendons and ligaments shredded like crab meat. And yet, even the gentle game of golf can give rise to the painful condition of ''golfer's elbow.'' Swimmers can develop ''swimmer's ear,'' a rather painful exzema of the ear canal. Prolonged knitting can result in a tenosynovitis, or inflammation of the wrist and finger tendons. I cannot think of a single physical recreation, no matter how mild, that does not carry with it the possibility of injury. Nevertheless, you should be aware of some of the more common injuries which can occur so that you can recognize them in their early stages and take swift corrective action.

Cause of Injury

Jogging injuries are self-inflicted wounds. They are due to carelessness, vanity, unwarranted enthusiasm, over-estimation of one's capabilities, or just sheer stupidity. This may sound harsh, but time and time again when confronted with the forlorn victim pouring out his tale of woe and demanding instant relief so that he can quickly return to his hobby, I can usually elicit a history of excessive speed, duration or frequency of workouts — all without adequate build-up. Frenetic training on hills, not making due allowance for headwinds or rough ground, allowing one's shoes to wear so badly that they no longer provide adequate support or protection are all examples of the sort of thing I mean. Some

joggers are more susceptible to injury than others because of congenital structure weaknesses in their feet or knees, but these cases
are relatively rare, and even they can avoid problems if they use
care and moderation.

There is little excuse for the health jogger to hurt himself. Unlike
the competitive runner, there is no element of pressure or urgency in the workouts, no running against the stop watch, no need
to teach the body to ignore the intense discomfort of muscle-
screaming fatigue; this is the lot only of those whose talent and
temperament have destined them for one goal and one goal only,
to be first across the finish line. Such heroics are not for us. The
name of our game is cardiovascular fitness and health, and this
can be achieved quite adequately without the risk of bodily insult.
That is the first and most important principle you can learn.

Essentials of Treatment

Jogging injuries rarely occur dramatically. A sprinter or a jumper
who tears a muscle in full flight will often collapse like a shot rabbit,
clutching the injured leg wildly. Muscle tears in joggers are com-
paratively rare. Injuries are usually the result of chronic over-use.
The feet of a relatively short-striding jogger will hit the pavement
about 1,500 times for every mile covered. As the mileage goes up,
so does the possibility of injury. Pain is invariably the warning
sign. When it occurs during the run, it is a signal for you to slow
down and evaluate the situation. Where is the pain located? Is it
sharp or aching? Have you experienced it before? Does it feel similar to a previous injury? If slowing your pace removes all trace of
discomfort, then gradually pick up your speed again and note
what happens. If all is well, then chances are you have merely
experienced one of the countless and transitory inconsequential
musculo-skeletal aches and pains which are the lot of every sports-
man. A return of the pain at a quicker pace, however, is a clear
signal to back off and finish the workout at the pain-free level. If
the same thing happens on the next workout, then accept the
fact that you have an injury, relax, and skip the next two or three
training sessions.

Seems obvious? Well, maybe it does, but it is surprising how
many joggers adopt the opposite approach. Their motto is ''When
in doubt, run it out.'' With such a philosophy, a relatively minor
injury, which would respond quite well to a few days' rest, is
aggravated to the stage where it becomes chronic and requires

not only prolonged rest, but often professional treatment. The vast majority of joggers' problems can be detected by the alert jogger at a stage early enough to respond to rest. If rest doesn't work, then a cause for the difficulty must be found and appropriate remedial steps taken.

Let me give you a simple example. Today, as I write this chapter, I have just returned from a 10-mile jog with a group of my post-coronary marathoners. We had six inches of fresh snow last night. Despite this, the sky was blue, the sun was warm and our usual route through the park adjoining the Centre was a delight. On the other hand, this was the first snow of the winter, and our legs have not, as yet, toughened to the countless unaccustomed compensatory movements needed to keep one's balance. Our captain, Harry B. has had trouble in the past with his knees. After five miles, he noticed a slight discomfort in the left knee. Immediately, he slowed and then, after half a mile, walked back to the safety of the ploughed pavement where he finished his workout on an even surface. Had he continued to soldier on with the rest of us, there is a strong likelihood that he would have let himself in for a lengthy layoff and a time-consuming period of physical therapy treatments. As it is, I have no doubt that he will be jogging again tomorrow, free from complaint. After years of jogging, he knows that prevention is a good deal easier than cure.

Assuming that a period of rest has not been successful, then usually the next stage in treatment is one of a number of *physiotherapy* treatments, some of which can be employed by the jogger, others which need professional application and then usually only after the condition has been diagnosed medically. Cryotherapy, or the therapeutic application of cold, is often used in the initial stages of an acute injury to relieve pain and reduce swelling. It can also be used over a chronically inflamed tendon, such as in heel cord (Achilles) tendonitis. Cold is applied in the form of a commercial cold pack or, more usually, by massage with an ice cube. The ice is held in a towel and then applied directly to the skin over the painful area. Care should be taken to see that skin sensation is normal to start with, that you are not one of those individuals who is hyper-sensitive to cold (the skin becomes red, ''wealed,'' and swollen within minutes), and that the area has not been frostbitten at any time in the past. The ice is used in a circular or back-and-forth movement over the skin, which first feels cool, then burns, and then after about three minutes, begins to ache. Finally, the area becomes numb. Ice massage should not be used for longer than five minutes and can be repeated morning and evening, and after workouts.

Therapeutic heat often relieves discomfort and increases circulation to the affected part, thus accelerating the healing process. Superficial dry heat can be administered by use of a heating pad (caution: severe burns have occurred as a result of people falling asleep while the heating pad is still on), or an infra-red heat lamp (for maximum effect, the feeling should be one of comfortable warmth, *not* excessive heat; the lamp should be about 1½ to 2 feet away from the area being treated and the treatment time should be about 20 to 30 minutes). Examples of moist heat applicators are the so-called wet pack or hydrocolator. These are canvas packs which contain a heat-retaining substance; they are placed in boiling water, heated to a temperature of 160° F., wrapped carefully in a towel so that they do not burn the skin, and placed carefully over the painful area. If you have never used one before, it is advisable to have your physician or physiotherapist demonstrate their use first.

Contrast baths are excellent for foot and lower leg injuries. To carry this out properly, you will need two buckets, or plastic waste baskets. Half-fill one with water at a temperature between 55° (12°C) and 65° F. (18°C), the other with water at a temperature between 95° (35°C) and 100° F (37°C). Place the injured leg for 3 to 5 minutes in the hot water and then for 1 to 2 minutes in the cold; alternate for about 30 minutes and remember always to start with the hot and end with the hot. Small whirlpool baths are also useful for lower leg injuries, although one should recognize that dangling the leg in a whirlpool for 30 minutes or more can sometimes aggravate the condition by giving rise to gravity-induced swelling. Individuals who suffer from diabetes or restricted circulation to the lower limbs should not carry out any of these self-prescribed procedures without first seeking the advice of their physician.

A deeper form of heating can be achieved by the use of machines which generate high frequency electrical currents. The three commonest deep heating currents used today are short wave diathermy, microwave diathermy, and ultra-sound; all have to be used with great caution since there are situations and conditions in which they can cause unpleasant and sometimes quite serious side effects. Specialized training is required for their use, and they should be applied only by a suitably qualified professional. They can, however, be particularly valuable, either used singly or in combination, for treatment of deep-seated tendon or joint injuries.

Massage can be used to relieve pain, increase blood supply, reduce swelling, and both stretch and soften tendons and scar tissue. There are numerous techniques, the commonest being light or deep stroking, kneading, or deep friction. I find that the last is particularly valuable in the treatment of chronic Achilles tendonitis. Briefly, the foot on the affected side is held in the relaxed position with the toes pointing down so that the tendon is loose and mobile. Then, using the straight middle finger reinforced by the index finger on top of it, pressure is applied over the painful area of the tendon just above the heel bone and a side-to-side sawing motion is carried out for about 10 to 15 minutes. By then, the tendon will feel quite numb but free from discomfort. The treatment is repeated every second day for about a week or so. For the treatment to be effective, the painful area must be very accurately defined so that the treatment is given precisely. The movement of the massaging fingers must be across, or at right angles to the direction of the tendon itself, and great care must be taken to see that the massaging finger and the skin over the tendon move as one so that it is the fibres of the tendon itself which are being massaged and not the overlying skin. Failure to observe the final point will lead to reddening and damage to the skin itself. A physiotherapist familiar with the technique can readily teach you so that you can carry it out on your own.

Medication

The most common non-prescription medication likely to be used by the injured jogger is acetylsalicylic acid, more frequently referred to as ASA or aspirin. Aspirin is primarily an anti-inflammatory drug. Its pain-relieving property is not all that powerful, and yet the public tends to see it purely and simply as a pain reliever. In point of fact, aspirin is often the drug of choice to reduce a high temperature or take the redness and swelling out of inflamed joints. It is therefore a useful drug for the over-use syndrome frequently met with in joggers. The chronically inflamed knee or Achilles tendon will often respond well to a combination or rest, physiotherapy and aspirin.

The drug comes in two strengths, 300 mg. and 600 mg. and, under normal circumstances, the average individual can easily tolerate up to 1,200 mg. daily. Like all medications, however, there are side effects. The most prominent is irritation of the lining of the stomach. If you have an ulcer, beware of taking aspirin. You can get enteric-coated aspirin tablets which pass through the stomach and dissolve in the intestine, but even these are likely to aggravate a peptic ulcer. Remember that aspirin makes you sweat and may make you susceptible to dehydration if you are continuing to exercise in the very warm weather. It also destroys Vitamin C, so you might be wise to increase your intake of that vitamin when you are on aspirin therapy. Finally, it has a tendency to make your blood less sticky. If you are on blood thinners (so-called anticoagulants) you should consult your doctor before using aspirin. Barring these precautions, you will find that, from time to time, aspirin will give considerable relief for sore joints or tendons.

Other anti-inflammatory agents include phenylbutazone (Butazolidin), oxyphenbutazone (Tandearil), indomethacin (Indocid), ibuprofen (Motrin), naproxen-sodium (Naprosyn) and cortisone. All these medications are obtainable by prescription only, since they can have adverse side effects. Another prescription drug which is neither anti-inflammatory nor a pain-killer is sometimes prescribed in sports injuries. This is methocarbanol (Robaxin). Its action is to relieve the muscle spasm which is often secondary to a joint or deep tendon lesion. The spasm is really a protective mechanism, an attempt on the part of the body to reduce the mobility of a moving part. Muscle spasm is not always beneficial, however, sometimes giving rise to its own particular form of pain, or by persisting too long, preventing the joint from regaining its full range of movement after the underlying problem is cured.

Therapeutic Exercise

This plays a large role in the treatment and prevention of sports injuries. It is prescribed most frequently to improve mobility and/or strength. Range of motion exercise can be either *passive*, in which the therapist moves the relaxed muscle or joint without help of the patient, or *active*, in which the patient performs the work entirely unaided. The active type is the most frequently used in sports medicine. The commonest form of active range of motion exercises is *stretching*, the purpose of which is to restore or achieve normal range of movement or alignment in a joint.

Strengthening exercises can also be divided into two types. There are the *isometric* exercises, in which the muscle is contracted but the joint which it helps to move is held motionless. A further refinement of this is to force the contracting muscle to work against an added weight. An example of this is the so-called "static quadriceps hold," where the patient keeps the knee joint in the fully extended position by contracting the thigh muscles, while at the same time, the therapist applies appropriate weights to the foot. This manoeuvre is particularly valuable if you are dealing with a situation where you want to build up the strength of the anterior thigh muscle (quadriceps) while at the same time not aggravating a painful knee condition by bending and straightening the knee joint too much. *Isotonic* exercises build strength by having the muscle contract, but at the same time allowing the joint to move. This is usually carried out against the resistance of a weight and, since the weight is increased as the patient's tolerance permits, the procedure is known as *progressive resistance exercise*.

Over-use injuries, when not due to excessive zeal, are often the result of either inappropriate or badly worn *shoes*, or *gait defects*. For this reason, I usually ask the injured patient to jog or walk once around the track while I observe him. Badly worn shoes are a frequent cause of trouble. Heel wear tends to cancel the advantages of the heel raise. A worn sole exposes the front of the foot and the bases of the toes to excessive pounding. All materials deteriorate with time, and it should be no surprise that the nylon and rubber composite in the shoe lose some of their resilience and flexibility with the passing months, especially after being exposed to conditions ranging all the way from sun-baked pavement to snow-covered parkland. A 30-mile-a-week jogger, even if light-footed, is probably ready for new shoes every twelve months. When you do buy a new pair, don't forget to break them in properly. I usually take four to six weeks to do this, using them for only one workout the first week and then wearing them for an additional workout every five to seven days or so. No matter how well the new shoes fit, no matter how comfortable they feel, they are never quite the same as the old ones and will require minor adjustment of gait to accommodate to the differences in weight, balance and resilience.

While the subject of jogging shoes has been written about ad nauseum, it does no harm to mention some of the features we should be considering when choosing a new pair. Weight is important. If they are too heavy, they can give rise to a form of shin splints. Too light, and they start to come apart and wear excessively in a few months. The only way to be sure is to try them on, and remember that the heavier you are, the more sturdy the shoe you will require. The heel should be sufficiently raised, probably about three-quarters of an inch, and the outer layers of cushioning should be sufficient to break the shock of landing, but not too spongy, otherwise you will develop soreness in the lower calf. Once again, the amount of heel cushioning you require is dependent upon your body weight. The exaggerated heel flare which was so common a few years back proved to be valuable when running on soft ground or fresh snow, but was much more than the foot required when jogging on hard pavement. The result was excessive mobility in the knee joint, with resultant increase in knee injuries. So, avoid the excessive flare, and choose one which is more modest. The heel counter, or back of the shoe, should be made of a firm material and should fit the heel snugly enough to prevent side-to-side movement. A sloppy-fitting heel counter or one that is made of a soft flexible material puts excessive strain on the heel cord and is a common cause of Achilles tendonitis. A good shoe has a sole and shank which is flexible in the heel/toe direction but has a fair degree of torsional rigidity, thus allowing the foot to bend, but not to twist. The degree of inside padding in the shoe is a matter of personal preference, but the built-in arch support which is now standard in all jogging shoes should at least fit the natural contours of your own arch. Finally, make sure that the toe box is sufficiently spacious to accommodate your toes without cramping; the tip of the big toe or longest toe should be about one thumb's breadth from the end of the shoe; if you have high flexed toes, they should not rub against the top of the shoe. A marathon jogger's feet will swell during the 26-mile jog and if the shoes do not allow for this (not infrequently the swelling amounts to half a size), then expect to finish with blackened toe nails.

By watching the jogger in action, or even while he is walking, you can detect a number of defects which are characteristically associated with the more common over-use injuries. In the normal stride, the leg and foot pass through the *swing* phase (when the foot is in the air), and the *stance* phase (when the foot is in contact with the ground). The stance phase can be divided into three stages—heel-strike, mid-stance and toe-off. Our major interest is in the stance phase. The heel should strike the ground slightly to the outside of a vertical line drawn through the centre of the heel bone. Proof that the heel-strike is correct can be found by inspecting the jogger's shoes. The maximal point of heel wear should be about a half an inch to the outside of the mid-line. As the body's centre of gravity moves forward and over the heel, weight-bearing continues along the outer aspect of the foot to the base of the little toe. This is the stage of mid-stance. Finally, as the heel leaves the ground, more weight is taken in sequence by the heads of the fourth, third, second and first metatarsals — that is, the bases of the fourth, third, second and big toes. At the time of take-off, then, most of the body weight is over the base of the first and second toes, the area commonly known as the ball of the foot. If the gait is normal, inspection of the shoe will show the maximal area of wear in the sole to be the outside edge and the area just over the point where the first and second toes bend up during toe-off.

The precise mechanics of gait are, of course, a great deal more complex than I have described. For the detection of simple gait disorders such as are associated with the more common jogging injuries, however, a knowledge of the basics will suffice.

To being with, however, it is important to understand what is meant by the terms *pronation* and *supination*. Since there is a tendency at the moment to ascribe practically all jogging injuries to defects in gait or malalignment of the feet, these two terms have been working overtime. In essence, they both describe the position of the feet in two extremes of rotation around an imaginary axis which extends from the centre of the back of the heel through the full length of the foot and out through the tip of the second toe. Inward rotation of the foot around that line is termed pronation; outward rotation, supination. You can observe these positions on your own feet by carrying out the following manoeuvre. Stand with your feet about 18 inches apart, the toes pointing forward; without sliding your feet, rotate your upper body as far as it will go to the left. Your right foot is now in extreme pronation, with the inside border, or longitudinal arch, touching the floor and the heel bone canted outward. The left foot has assumed the position of extreme supination, with the outside border of the foot jammed against the floor, the longitudinal arch high and withdrawn from the floor, and the heel bone canted inward.

Pronation and supination should not be thought of as twin evils. As a matter of fact, the foot is in slight pronation during the heel-strike portion of the stance stage, and then becomes supinated through the stages of mid-stance and toe-off. So pronation and supination must occur if the gait is to be normal. When the foot is in the pronated position, it is mobile, with all the joints flexible and loose. In the supinated position, joint motion is more limited and the foot is rigid. It is this ability to flow easily from a supple to a rigid position that imparts to the normal foot its amazing versatility. Not only is it capable of supporting the entire body weight concentrated through its small surface area, but it can also act as a fulcrum over which that weight shifts safely and smoothly.

Excessive pronation is the cause of a number of injuries to the foot, the bones of the lower leg and the knee. The feet are frequently in the "ten-to-two" position, toeing outward in the standing position and also in walking and jogging. The heel strikes the ground on its outside edge rather than just half an inch or so lateral to the centre line, and the feet have a flat appearance. When viewed from behind in the standing position, the heel cords, instead of bisecting the heel, appear to be displaced inward. This is because the heel bone itself is tilted outward. A glance at the shoe shows much more wear to the outside of the heel than normal.

Excessive pronation may be due to abnormalities of the muscles or joints of the foot itself, so-called fixed pronation. Or it may be the result of malalignments elsewhere in the leg, in which case it is known as compensatory pronation. You can demonstrate the most common form of compensatory pronation by carrying out the following experiment. Stand with your feet about 6 inches apart, the toes pointing forward. Then, with the ankle completely relaxed so that the foot droops down and the knee held straight, raise one foot off the ground by a "shrugging" action of the hip. Now rotate the hip outward; the leg and foot will follow suit. A short step with this leg will result in the foot striking the floor in an exaggeratedly pronated action. This exercise shows that if you hold your hip externally rotated you will have a marked pronated gait and will suffer from all of the difficulties associated with it. What is the cause of the externally rotated hip? In the vast majority of cases, tightness or shortening of the hamstrings and external rotator muscles which straighten and externally rotate the hip joint. The cure for this type of compensatory pronation is to carry out stretching exercises for the shortened muscles. There was a time in my distant youth when army physical fitness instructors and the like taught that the correct way to stand and walk was with the toes pointing slightly outward. The hip joint, of course, had to follow suit and also rotates outward. After a number of years, the hip joint muscles which normally carry out this rotatory action become shortened, and so we now have a permanent case of compensatory pronated gait.

There are two causes of excessive pronation which one comes across from time to time. If you ask the jogger to stand up straight with knees touching and find that he can then not place his heels together, he is displaying evidence of knock-knee deformity. The effect of this on the feet will be to bring the inner borders closer to the floor, thus exaggerating pronation. A jogger who can stand straight with heels together but then has a wide space between his knees is suffering from bow legs. The bow-legged individual again has to pronate both feet excessively to get the inner borders of his feet to the floor.

Excessive supination of the feet is much rarer than excessive pronation, and is usually found in the individual with a high arch. The supinated foot is a locked and rigid structure which transmits the shock of heel-strike abruptly to the bones of the lower leg and knee. Small wonder that the deformity is associated with fatigue fractures of the foot and leg. Protection from this should be sought in shoes which have good interior padding and more than the average degree of resilience and softness in the sole and heel. Jogging over rough uneven surfaces should be avoided.

Whether the pronation or supination deformity is fixed or compensatory, its ill effects can often be counteracted by the use of modifications to the shoe. These can either be *external* or *internal*. The commonest type of external modification is the heel wedge, which is placed on the inside or outside edge of the heel, depending upon the deformity being treated. Basically, the wedge is intended to restore the heel bone from its tilted position to a more vertical one. Obviously if the heel moves inside the shoe, then the wedge is of little use. Other examples of external modifications are sole wedges, transverse bars at various points on the sole and "raises" of different heights. However, the internal shoe modification, or *orthotic*, is frequently used. We seem to have reached a stage where the jogger without an orthotic feels underprivileged. There are five basic types of internal shoe modification commonly prescribed and made by the orthotist. They are the longitudinal arch support, the metatarsal arch support, the internal heel wedge, the heel bar, and the internal heel lift or pad.

The longitudinal arch support is most useful in the treatment of excessive pronation. Such inserts can be either soft (made out of moleskin, orthopedic felt or piano felt), semi-rigid (made out of cork, leather, fibreglass and flexible plastics), or rigid (made out of rigid plastic and acrylic). These orthotic devices can be transferred from shoe to shoe, but the rigid, and sometimes the semi-rigid, types are made from a casted model of the foot and can be very expensive, costing anywhere from $200 to $300. The rigid ones take some getting used to, and many joggers have difficulty tolerating them unless they are extremely accurately fitted and made. Obviously, not all cases of pronated foot require a rigid orthotic device. In many cases, the semi-rigid type will do, and if you want to save money, you can always try the type of arch support obtainable in any drug store first; it usually costs less than $20. The grossly deformed foot which is the source of recurring injuries, however, will inevitably require custom-made orthoses.

Finally, let me again stress that jogging technique is all-important in avoiding injury or reawakening an old one. The pace should be comfortable, the body erect and the stride short. If you visualize your foot landing flat rather than with an exaggerated heel-first or toe-first strike, then not only will the foot behave normally, but your speed will be more controlled. A loose arm carriage with the elbows bent to about 30° or 40° short of a right angle (so that the hands are held at about hip level), relaxed shoulders and neck muscles, and the head erect — all contribute to a controlled jogging posture which is free of strain and tension and less prone to bodily hurt. At the time of writing, over 5,000 post-coronary patients have passed through the Toronto Rehabilitation Centre's exercise program. They have logged over a million hours of walking and jogging. The incidence of injury is extremely small, and I can think of very few patients who have been forced out of the program through an injury which was resistant to treatment. Yet the average age of the men is 51, the women 54. The program has its fair share of individuals with pronated feet, histories of back trouble, old football knee injuries, all the wear-and-tear problems to which joints are prone with the passing years. The low incidence of injury is due entirely to a combination of careful jogging technique, insistence upon suitable jogging shoes, and a training procedure which stresses slow build-up over a period of many months.

COMMON JOGGING INJURIES AND RELATED MEDICAL PROBLEMS

Runner's Knee

This is not a medical term, but has been coined in recent years to describe pain in the knee which afflicts some long distance runners. In a typical case, pain is experienced usually over the inside but sometimes over the outside of the knee joint. The pain comes on anywhere from three to ten miles into a jog, and can be severe. There is rarely any redness or swelling present, but pressure over the painful area will usually elicit discomfort. On occasion, the complaint will be of pain under the kneecap. In severe cases, the pain is brought on not only by running, but also by anything which causes the front thigh muscles to contract strongly — for example, doing a full squat or climbing stairs.

The knee joint is a complex structure and obviously the causes of pain can be many and varied. Most physicians, therefore, feel the term runner's knee can be a catch-all for a number of conditions involving any one of the various tissues and structures which contribute to the joint and its action. For our purposes we will restrict its use to knee pain brought about by faulty gait associated with exaggerated foot pronation. As we have seen, the pronated foot tends to ''toe out,'' with resultant outward rotation of the entire leg, including the hip joint. This puts the knee at a mechanical disadvantage. The hinge has to move obliquely to the body's line of progression instead of parallel with it. There is an abnormal pulling force to the inner side of the joint, resulting in strain and inflammation of the structures in that area. In addition a grating develops between the kneecap and thigh bone, causing its under-surface to become painfully roughened and eroded. This latter condition is known medically as *chondromalacia patellae*. Since the kneecap is attached to the upper end of the shin bone (or tibia) by a tendon (the patellar tendon), the grating can also involve this structure, inflaming it and giving rise to the condition of *patellar tendonitis*.

Satisfactory treatment almost invariably requires correction of the pronation deformity by means of an orthotic device. This doesn't have to be of the rigid custom-made type. Indeed, you should first try a temporary soft support which you can make yourself or, if you wish, buy a semi-rigid one from the drug store. It should lift and support the arch of the foot and also the inner side of the heel bone. If you find after two or three weeks that this is not helping, then you may have to consider the more expensive orthotic. If the hip tends to externally rotate, then stretching exercises for the hamstring and hip rotators should be instituted. Quadriceps strengthening exercises are essential, but because of the undersurface roughening of the patella, they should be of the isometric or static weight-loading type with the knee joint fully extended as described on page 227. If quadriceps exercises are not carried out and a jogger begins to favour the leg by restricting knee movement, noticeable wasting of the thigh muscles will occur within a matter of two or three weeks. An elastic knee support should never be worn; it tends to press the kneecap against the thigh bone. You can modify the support, however, by cutting out a hole through which the kneecap protrudes; this will relieve the pain, and can be used while jogging. In the early acute stages of the condition, ice therapy will help and later heat in the form of hot packs or short-wave diathermy can be tried. Aspirin will also help.

Don't expect a cure in a matter of days; it may take months. This is not to say that you won't be able to jog for months. You can keep going if you slow your pace, avoid hills, stay off roads which are highly cambered, avoid rough surfaces, and maintain a good jogging technique. Don't be afraid to back off your workouts for a day or two if the condition flares up, but start up again as soon as you notice signs of recovery. Don't become discouraged if progress seems to be slow. In some cases it can take as long as a year for the condition to resolve, and even then it has a tendency to recur from time to time.

Shin Splints

This again is an imprecise term which has no medical meaning, although it is very familiar to physicians who make a habit of treating injured track men or joggers. It merely means pain in the shin region. It can occur in two forms, depending on the location of the pain. An *anterior* shin splint refers to pain felt in the muscle of the front of the lower leg and along the outside border of the shin bone. The commonest causes are over-striding, the wearing of shoes which are too heavy, excessive downhill running, pronated foot deformity, and strength imbalance between the muscles of the calf and front of the leg.

In all these situations the front lower leg muscle (the anterior tibial muscle) is being made to work too hard. In the case of over-striding, the toes and forefoot are too high in the air at the moment of heel-strike, and so, in order to prevent uncontrolled foot-slap, the anterior tibial muscle has to work like a stay-rope, gradually paying out the tendons attached to the top of the foot and letting the sole meet the ground with a minimum of shock. Repeat this thousands of times in a run, and you can see why the muscle would start to complain of over-use. Heavy shoes require effort to keep the toes from stubbing against the ground during the swing-through phase of jogging — again, extra work for the anterior tibial muscle. Pronated feet are "loose" feet, and the excessive joint mobility has to be compensated for by additional muscular work. As for the muscle strength imbalance, most joggers have very powerful calf muscles which tend to overpower the anterior tibial muscles. Since the action of the calf muscles is to rotate the foot downward, and the action of the anterior tibial muscle is to pull the foot upward, it can be readily seen that weak anterior tibials are constantly fighting to resist the action of the calf muscles.

There is another symptom sometimes associated with anterior shin splints. Because the anterior tibial muscle shares a rather cramped compartment in the front of the leg with both a nerve and an artery, swelling of the muscle due to over-use sometimes compresses both these structures, particularly the nerve. This results in numbness and tingling in the foot and sometimes stubbing of the toe because of weakness in pulling the toes up during the swing phase.

In the acute stages of anterior shin splints, treatment consists of ice massage. Correction of over-striding, choosing shoes of suitable weight, the fitting of an orthotic device, and strengthening exercises for the anterior tibial muscle are all measures to be used if indicated. Once the cause of the condition has been established, then the treatment becomes obvious.

Posterior shin splints describes pain in the lower leg along the inside border of the shin bone. Again, the culprit is the pronated foot. To understand this, you have to realize that one of the major deep muscles of the calf, the tibialis posterior, is attached at its upper end to the back and inner border of the shin bone and then forms a tendon which hooks around the inside of the ankle to fan out and be attached to most of the bones which form the sole of the foot. The action of the muscle is to pull the foot into the supinated position. Therefore in the pronated foot, the tibialis posterior muscle is working constantly to correct the deformity. The greater degree of pronation during jogging, the greater the likelihood that the muscle will give trouble. First, the workload may be so great that tiny parts of the muscle attachment to the back and side of the shin bone tear away. In a bad case of posterior shin splints, you can feel tiny bumps if you run your finger along the inside border of the shin. These can be very tender and probably represent the areas where fibres of the muscle have pulled away from the bone. This is the commonest presentation of the condition. Another symptom of the overworked tibialis posterior is pain and swelling just behind and beneath the inner ankle bone, where the tendon is constantly sliding back and forth through a tunnel formed by bone and fibrous tissue. If this movement is excessive, then the tendon becomes inflamed, swollen and sore. The way to treat posterior shin splints is to correct the pronation deformity. In the acute stage, once again one can use ice massage to the painful area, and reduce the workouts to a level which do not cause pain.

I have heard it said that shin splints occur most frequently in inexperienced runners whose enthusiasm leads them to change too rapidly from slow running to speed training, or from soft to hard running surfaces. This may be so, but I haven't found that the novice has any monopoly on these errors, and, in fact, some of the most stubborn cases I have ever treated have been in world-class distance runners. In these individuals, excessive mileage may be an additional aggravating factor, but I am satisfied that in the chronic case, relief can only be achieved by successful treatment of the foot deformity.

Stress Fracture

These are fine, almost invisible, cracks in the bones of the foot or lower leg, and are due to excessive mileage, faulty jogging technique, foot or leg deformity, non-resilient shoes or a combination of any or all of these factors. In a way, they resemble the fatigue faults that develop in a metal that has been exposed to excessive stress. The symptom of the stress fracture is pain, usually severe enough to stop your jogging, present at night, and throbbing in character. Occasionally, there will be swelling also. Tapping the bone in the area of the stress fracture will aggravate the pain. X-rays are of little value, since the crack is so fine that it doesn't appear on the x-ray until it has started to heal and lay down a fine line of extra calcium which then shows up on the x-ray plate. The treatment is rest. On no account try to run through a stress fracture; otherwise, you will only delay healing. The healing period is about six weeks, and during that time, you should attempt to maintain your fitness level by switching to some non-weight-bearing exercise like swimming or cycling. There is no need for you to sit around and mope because you are missing your customary daily jog.

Most stress fractures occur in one of the long bones (metatarsals) of the foot, although they can also occur in the two long bones of the lower leg (the tibia and fibula). A stress fracture in the tibia should be treated more seriously than elsewhere because this bone bears a good deal of the body's weight and occasionally even excessive walking may extend the fine hairline crack into an out-and-out break. Otherwise, stress fractures heal very well. Indeed, the bone is a good deal stronger after healing than it was before. If you wish to avoid a recurrence of the condition, you have to be careful not to repeat the cause. Since the supinated foot is more susceptible because of its relative inability to absorb landing shock, insoles and well-padded shoes are a must.

Runner's Heel

The muscles of the sole of the foot are covered by the plantar fascia, a sheet of tough tissue which is attached to the front of the heel bone, passes forward under the longitudinal arch and then fans out to insert into the under-surfaces of the toe bones. Because of its fore and aft attachments, it acts as a sort of tie, joining the two ends of the bony arch of the foot. Since this arch flattens when the foot is taking body weight and resumes its curved shape when the foot is off the ground, the plantar fascia is being stretched and relaxed with every step. Excessive mileage, or unaccustomed sprinting (an action which requires powerful "toe-off") or just the old fault of too much too soon, can result in plantar fascitis, or inflammation of the structure. Miscroscopic tearing of fibres occur at the attachment of the heel bone and sometimes further forward, closer to the arch of the foot. The complaint is one of pain under the heel just where the heel pad joins the arch when walking or jogging, and pressure in this region, even when the foot is resting, reproduces the discomfort.

Runner's heel is particularly likely if you start to train too vigorously after a long lay-off. The weeks of inactivity tend to tighten and weaken the plantar fascia. Shoes that have poor arch supports or are too stiff, requiring a vigorous toe-off in order to bend them, will obviously throw an extra strain on the fascia. On occasion, the area where the fibres pull away from the front of the heel bone becomes infiltrated with calcium and forms a so-called spur, which is seen on an x-ray. Some surgeons advocate the removal of this spur, although in my experience this rarely helps. The general treatment is to look for and eliminate the cause; however, in the early, very painful phase, an internal heel raise with a cut-out which coincides with the painful area, together with an arch support, will help. Some physicians advise local cortisone injections, but while this does relieve some of the inflammation and soften the scar tissue, it may cause even more tearing to occur especially if the individual persists with his jogging. Cortisone should only be used as a last resort, and then only if you are prepared to lay off for a period of one week after the injection. Physical therapy treatments consist of ice massage, or application of ultra-sound.

Achilles Tendonitis

This is the inflammation of the heel cord and is a major headache for a significant number of runners. The reason is not hard to find. Even under normal everyday circumstances, the heel cord has to take an incredible strain. If you balance on one foot, and then stand on tip-toe, your heel cord is being subjected to a pulling force equivalent to twice your body weight. For the average jogger, that means some 250 to 300 lbs. on each heel cord with each step. If you start to sprint, which means landing and driving off the toes rather than the heel of the flat foot, then the strain is even greater. Actually, the healthy heel cord, or Achilles tendon, is capable of taking the strain of up to 5,000 to 6,000 lbs. per square inch before it snaps, and can bear about one third of this weight with perfect safety. Notice, however, that I said the *healthy* tendon. By the time we get into our mid-thirties, the blood supply to the tendons begins to get less, with the result that the safety level begins to drop. This is why in elderly individuals an apparently minor strain, such as stepping awkwardly off the curb, can result in rupture of the tendon. While a partial or even complete tear can occur in joggers, it is relatively rare. More likely are the repeated microscopic tears in the deep fibres of the tendon, resulting in a generalized inflammation. The commonest causes are tight heel cords (you should make a point of carrying out stretching exercises to alleviate this), a shoe with an inadequate heel lift or one which allows the heel to wobble from side to side, running up hills, excessive speed work, or running on the toes. If you have perfected the short stride, flat-foot landing, then you should rarely be troubled with Achilles tendonitis.

In the early stages of the condition, the jogger notices aching pain in the heel cords both during and after the run. He finds that when he gets up in the morning, he has to hobble across the room for the first few minutes before the tendons loosen up. As the condition develops, swelling and thickening is apparent. The treatment consists of reducing the intensity and duration of the workouts, adding a half-inch heel raise, and correcting any shoe faults. Ice massage can be carried out after each jogging session, and aspirin often helps. In severe cases, the physician may want to apply a plaster cast to prevent the tendon moving too much during ordinary walking. I have rarely found this necessary, and when it is, an attempt should be made to find an alternative form of exercise for the sufferer. Under no circumstances should cortisone injections be given into the tendon. This is only likely to soften the tissue up and lead to an extension of the tear, or even a fully fledged rupture. If the tendon does tear through, then surgical repair will be necessary. Ultra-sound using a technique in which it is given through water may help to reduce chronic inflammation. In the final analysis, however, improvement in jogging technique is the only answer.

Before leaving the subject of Achilles tendonitis, mention should be made of *calcaneal bursitis* or inflammation of the fluid sac which forms an interface between the back of the heel bone and the heel cord at its point of insertion. This is usually caused by ill-fitting shoes which press against the back of the heel and rub up and down with each step. The fluid sac becomes inflamed, reddened and painful. The differentiation between this condition and Achilles tendonitis is largely by location of discomfort. Pain from bursitis is lower down, often over the back of the heel bone itself, and is aggravated by thumb pressure in this area. The cure is removal of the offending pressure from the shoe. In the acute stage, ice, ultrasound, or even a hydrocortisone injection into the sac itself will bring quick relief.

An occasional cause of foot pain in the jogger is *Morton's metatarsalgia*, named after Dr. T. G. Morton, who first described it in

1876. This is due to the development of a spindle-shaped swelling, or neuroma, about three-quarters of an inch long, on the small nerve which lies between the third and fourth toes. Actually, it is a thickening of the nerve sheath, or covering, which has been irritated by constantly being nipped between the adjoining bones that form the base of the third and fourth toes. It is seen most frequently in an individual with the broad, or splayed, forefoot. It occasionally occurs between the second and third toes, or the fourth and fifth toes. The presenting symptom is sharp or burning pain in the ball of the foot, sometimes shooting into the affected toes. It is not constant, but occurs at varying intervals, and each attack has a sudden onset. Characteristically, relief is not obtained by sitting down and taking weight off the foot, but by taking off the shoes and squeezing or manipulating the forefoot. Diagnosis is usually made on the history, and by the fact that the pain can sometimes be aggravated or brought on by squeezing the bases of the toes together. Very occasionally, it is possible to detect a patch of numbness on the affected toes. X-rays are negative, since nerve tissue doesn't register on an x-ray plate. Treatment consists of altering the alignment of the toe bones by the use of an orthopedic felt insert which raises one of the two offending toe bones so it no longer squeezes the nerve. A shoe with a broad toe box is also advised. In addition, injections of cortisone and local anesthetic between the affected toes can often help. In the last resort, the neuroma can be removed by a relatively simple surgical procedure.

Ever since the New Jersey cardiologist Dr. George Sheehan referred to the subject of Morton's Toe in his *Runner's World* column, joggers have become excessively conscious of the length of their toes. Dr. Dudley J. Morton, in his book, *The Human Foot*, described a congenital abnormality consisting primarily of a shortened big toe or, more precisely, a shortened first metatarsal (the long bone which extends from the base of the big toe to the apex of the longitudinal arch). Because of this shortening, the big toe cannot take its fair share of bearing the body's weight, with the result that the second toe and the corresponding second metatarsal bone have to take an additional load. The result is a painful callous on the ball of the foot under the second toe and discomfort in the forefoot due to the excessive motion of the second metatarsal. X-rays will show the shortened first metatarsal, and also a thickening in width of the shaft of the second metatarsal, due entirely to its extra weight-bearing chores. This is the so-called atavistic foot, or Morton's Toe. How common is it? Not very, in its classical and complete form. Just because your second toe is a smidgeon longer than your big toe doesn't give you the right to blame Dudley Morton for all your foot woes. In short, I suspect the condition is probably grossly over-diagnosed.

The condition can be relieved by fashioning a metatarsal insert which, by providing a platform under the base of the big toe, shifts the maximum point of weight-bearing away from the second toe back to where it belongs. The painful callous under the second toe, if present, is pared down and should not recur.

Hematuria

This is the medical term for the passage of bloodstained urine. It can occur in long distance runners and joggers after a particularly hard workout. Needless to say, it is a frightening symptom, especially since, in a sedentary individual, it usually heralds disease of the kidney or lower urinary tract. However, careful investigation of a large number of marathon runners who were found to have the problem failed to reveal any evidence of the disease. What then is the cause of the bleeding? We have always assumed that it was due to a temporary failure of the kidney's filtering system, allowing red blood cells to leak into the urine along with other waste products being excreted. Since in the vast majority of cases the filtration failure was temporary, no structural damage ensued, and only very rarely was investigation of the kidney positive. But in 1977, a British surgeon, Dr. N. H. Blacklock, came up with an alternative explanation. By passing an instrument through the penis and into the bladder of runners with "10,000 metre hematuria," he observed that the back wall of the bladder showed considerable bruising and tiny bleeding points. He concluded that this was the origin of the bleeding and that the state of the posterior wall was due to repeated banging against the base of the bladder during running. The only way that this could happen would be if the bladder were flaccid, or empty. On questioning the runners, it was indeed found that invariably they had not taken any fluid before or during their runs. The moral, then, is never to undertake a long, hard jog without ensuring a partially full bladder by adequate intake of fluids. Finally, if blood-stained urine recurs, the jogger should seek medical advice regarding full investigation of the kidneys.

Not all red-stained urine contains blood. On occasions, the colour may be due to the breakdown of red cells, releasing the pigment from the blood protein hemoglobin into the urine. Why do the red cells break down? The theory is that as they pass through the fine blood vessels in the sole of the feet, the more fragile ones are literally pounded apart with the impact of each jogging step. Hemoglobin pigment is a harmless substance and its excretion does not damage the kidney. The remedy for the situation is to be found in good-quality jogging shoes which contain well-padded soles.

Another brownish-coloured substance which when present in the urine may mimic hematuria is myoglobin. This is a muscle protein, and its presence in the urine indicates some muscle destruction, the commonest causes of which are severe and exhausting bouts of exercise, or advanced dehydration amounting almost to heat stroke. Neither of these situations should occur, except in the most imprudent or fanatical jogger. Myoglobinuria is a dangerous business. The muscle breakdown substance does not pass easily through the kidney and can, in fact, block its filtration mechanism and lead to renal failure and death.

In general, then, blood-stained urine occurring occasionally in a long distance jogger is a benign condition which can be controlled by ensuring a partially full bladder. However, a sample of the urine should be examined by a physician to confirm that no other substances are present which might indicate true kidney disease. The bleeding usually clears up quite rapidly, within a couple of days. If it lasts longer, however, or recurs frequently, then the physician should assume it is due to some other abnormality until thorough investigations have proved the contrary.

Minor Discomforts and Irritations

It is the little things that get you. You finish your first marathon, you bask in the awe-struck deference of your sedentary fellow species, and that night you drift off to sleep in a mood of jubilant ecstasy — only to get out of bed the next morning, and find that you have developed an exquisitely painful pea-sized bluish swelling at the edge of your anus. Which reduces your triumphant healthy stride into the office into a sort of crab-like shuffle. You have developed a thrombosed *external hemorrhoid*. It is really nothing to do with the internal hemorrhoids that sedentary individuals frequently complain of; this is a clotting of blood in a small subcutaneous vein close to the opening of the anus, and it is caused by friction. Despite the acute pain, it usually settles down of its own accord within a few days. If not, then the out-patient treatment is evacuation of the hardened clot by making a small incision through the wall of the vein after injection of a local anesthetic. Prevention is easy. Just apply a liberal amount of vaseline between the buttocks before the marathon starts.

Muscle stiffness after a lengthy jog can be avoided. The longer you have been jogging, the less likely you are to be bothered by this problem. However, it can be a nuisance, and in the early stages of your jogging career, you may find that large doses of Vitamin C (500 to 1,000 mg daily) may help. If you can manage to jog just two or three miles the day after a long run, it helps to relieve muscle discomfort. The first few steps may be difficult, but take your time, don't be afraid to walk every so often, and you'll be surprised to find that at the end of the first few miles, you feel a good deal better.

Numbness of the toes, usually the third, fourth and fifth, bothers some joggers. It usually comes on after about five or six miles, and once started, is difficult to relieve except by slowing to a walk. You can avoid the problem by lacing your shoes quite loosely or, better still, not lacing the bottom two or three holes. Again, prevention is better than cure. I find that once the numbness commences on a run, even loosening your laces helps only partially. The high arched foot is particularly susceptible to this condition. When buying jogging shoes, it is better to choose ones in which the lace holes are continued down to the level of the toes; this allows you to ensure looseness at the lower levels.

Some joggers complain of *swollen, tingling fingers* after a lengthy workout. This may be due to two causes. Holding the elbows in the bent position for too long without straightening them restricts blood flow and so gives rise to a puffy swelling which, in turn, causes the nerves of the fingers to tingle. Middle-aged joggers who have wear and tear degenerative changes of their spine and run with hunched shoulders and tight neck muscles may compress the roots of the nerves which emerge between the neck vertebrae and pass down through the arms to the hands. This will also cause tingling and numbness. Learn, then, to run loosely, with relaxed shoulder and neck muscles, occasional straightening of the elbows and clenching and unclenching of the fingers.

Nipple irritation, soreness, and even frank bleeding will occur during a long jog in hot weather when the running shirt becomes soaked in sweat and rubs against the unprotected nipples. Vaseline is the runner's friend. It should be applied liberally to all potential areas of friction, especially the nipples, in the anal cleft and the insides of the thighs.

Regular joggers expose their skin to the sun for long periods of time. In the sunnier climates, this can lead to bad cases of *sunburn*, especially in light-skinned individuals. The best solution is to apply any one of the commercial sun screens which contain the substance Paba. You can use these in various strengths, depending on the susceptibility of your skin to sunshine. I have had good results with Pre-Sun, and Coppertone's Supershade, both screens containing 5 per cent Paba. (The former stains clothing slightly.) Some individuals are allergic to Paba, and so they should try a small amount first and then check for the development of a skin rash. Heavy sweating will tend to dilute the effect of the screen; reapply it every hour or so. Tanning oils do not give adequate protection and, in fact, in a very hot sun, merely "fry" the skin. Remember to wear a hat with a sufficiently wide brim to protect your face. White clothing tends to reflect the sun, but the light material of a running shirt will often let a high percentage of the sun's rays through. The more porous the material, the more likely this is to happen. Constant over-exposure to sun and wind will dry your skin out, and age it prematurely. Both in winter and summer, then, it makes sense to apply a protective cream or lotion. Skin cancer is on the increase, and is directly related to the number of hours of exposure to the sun. It is slow-growing, does not spread to other parts of the body, and can be cured by a simple surgical excision or exposure to radiotherapy, but better to avoid it in the first place. Classically, the skin cancer appears anywhere on the face above the level of the mouth, commences as a small pearl-like tumour with raised edges and dimpled centre, often with a scale-like covering from a slight discharge. It you knock this transparent crust off, it quickly forms again. Anything resembling this should be checked out by your dermatologist.

THE AIR WE BREATHE

If you live in a large city, you have to be prepared to pay a price for the vocational and avocational advantages of massive "togetherness." There, in a word, I may have alienated those readers whose whole aim in life is to find some quiet, sparsely populated retreat in which only the sound of the wind or sea or solitary bird call disturbs their contemplative life. So be it. I have always loved cities, and found their fascinating mix of inhabitants both personally and professionally stimulating. I am aware of the dire predictions about the imminent demise of the urban way of life; yet, like the hundreds of millions of city dwellers all over the world, I continue to live where I feel I can best fulfill my mental, emotional and material wants.

There are, of course, drawbacks to this type of living. Among other things, we have to contend with the pollution of our air by the waste products of our automobiles and our industrial plants. Lately, the jogger has had to contend with the charge that all of the benefits which he thought he was getting from his hobby are being neutralized by the increased inhalation of these harmful substances. All that huffing and puffing, say the local Jeremiahs, fill your lungs with so much poison that you would be better off sitting in your living room with all the doors and windows tightly closed, watching television and enjoying a six-pack. I think this argument may be somewhat exaggerated.

What are the common air pollutants? What effect do they have on us? The answer to the first question depends to some extent on the area in which you live. In Los Angeles, for instance, the pollutants are composed largely of compounds that arise from the chemical interaction between sunlight and the various combustible products of automobile fumes. In other cities, we may be dealing predominantly with carbon monoxide, sulphur dioxide, or a number of airborne chemicals in particulate form.

Carbon monoxide is a major component of cigarette smoke, and we have already described its cuckoo-like occupancy of the red cells of the blood, displacing the vital oxygen being carried to the body's cells. Inhaled even in minute quantities by the jogger, in theory, it could reduce the efficiency of his oxygen transport system and turn an easy workout into a relatively tough one. Inhalation of enough carbon monoxide to affect about 20 per cent of hemoglobin, the oxygen-carrying protein in the blood, will lead to headache behind and over the eyes, breathlessness, muscular weakness and dizziness. When about 40 per cent of the available hemoglobin is saturated with carbon monoxide, there is a feeling of nausea together with dimming and blurring of vision; judgment becomes impaired and the individual becomes belligerent.

Since the major source of carbon monoxide is from automobile exhaust fumes, the highest concentration will be along heavily travelled highways. Exhaust smoke disperses slowly, so if your regular jogging route is 40 to 60 feet or more away from the edge of a busy highway, you should be home free.

Ozone is a key component in the smog which results from the action of sunlight on fuel oil hydrocarbons and nitrogen dioxide. It has been found in aircraft cabins at altitudes above 30,000 feet, and also in association with various welding devices. In recent years, a good deal of work has been done on the effect of ozone on the human body, and while much is still to be learned, we do have some indications that in high concentrations (greater than 0.15 parts per million of air), it can have some toxic effect. Its major target is the respiratory organs, where it can cause breathlessness, chest pain and coughing. Experimental animals have been shown to develop edema of the lungs and pulmonary hemorrhage when exposed to very high concentrations of ozone. In addition to the respiratory symptoms, high ozone levels can cause headaches and reduce one's ability to concentrate. The heart rate may drop, and this can give rise to increases in blood carbon dioxide. At ozone levels in excess of 0.2 parts per million there may be a considerable decrease in central visual acuity and ability to see in the dark, together with an increase in peripheral vision. Some coaches have reported that when ozone levels are high, athletic performance is adversely affected.

A few cities now operate an ozone alert when the level reaches more than 0.15 parts per million, which warns susceptible individuals to reduce physical exertion. When the level becomes in excess of 0.2 parts per million, even healthy persons should limit their outdoor exercise. It is possible, however, to defeat the ozone problem if you remember one or two basic principles. In the first place, keep in mind that on a sunny, humid day the maximal ozone levels are between 11 a.m. and 6 p.m., and the lowest levels are in the early morning. Therefore, if you wish to be on the safe side, run early in the morning or late at night. Older individuals (and that means us) are more susceptible to the effects of ozone than young people. Don't forget that the hotter it gets, the more ozone is produced. For instance, a rise of 15°F. (9°C) from 75°F. (23°C) to 90°F. (32°C) doubles the amount of ozone which can be generated. Secondly, if you have a chest infection, you are obviously more susceptible. Interestingly, the ingestion of Vitamin C would appear to substantially reduce the effect of ozone on the lungs. Finally (and this must be a consolation to Los Angeleans), the more exposure you have to ozone, the more likely you are to develop a tolerance toward it. At least you are less likely to be overcome by the more acute and unpleasant symptoms. Whether the long-term effects are worse, only further research and time can tell. Again, a sensible jogger who understands the dangers and is prepared to alter his normal workout times to suit the conditions has little to fear.

There is no doubt that running in the city on a hot, humid, muggy day when the traffic is heavy and the industrial pall is hanging close to the ground can be uncomfortable and sometimes downright unpleasant. Nevertheless, if you follow some of these simple guidelines you should not come to any harm, and the benefits of jogging will far outweigh any minor and transitory discomforts brought about by breathing polluted air.

THE PERILS OF HEAT

Whenever I watch an old late-night movie about the exploits of the British army in India or the French Foreign Legion in the Sahara, I make a bet with myself that more soldiers or legionnaires died from dehydration than ever succumbed to a tribesman's bullet. In those days, the way to avoid sunstroke was to protect the head and back of the neck. The most essential article of tropical kit was the pith helmet; it practically became the symbol of Empire, the Raj, Kipling and all that. Unfortunately, picturesque as it may have been, the sun helmet did little to protect from the real killer, fluid lack from excessive sweating — in other words, dehydration. But can we, in our daily jog or our easy-going marathon attempt, become dehydrated? If so, can the results really be that serious? What precautions can we take to avoid them? To answer these questions, we should know how dehydration occurs.

Our body temperature results from heat generated by our working muscles and organs and heat absorbed from the surrounding atmosphere. As you sit reading this book, hopefully relaxed and calm, with easy breathing and slowly beating heart, you are generating about 75 calories of heat every hour. If you were to put the book down (not yet, please), stand up and go for a three-mile walk, you would have generated about 300 calories. Intense brief activity can burn about 800 to 900 calories an hour.

If the body had no means of dissipating its internal heat, then even under resting conditions, your temperature would rise about 2°F. (1°C) an hour; under moderate working conditions, the rise would be in the order of 9°F. (5°C) an hour. Like any other machine, the body has a temperature at which all the various parts function most efficiently, 98.6°F. (37°C). If the inside temperature of the body climbs above 108°F. (42°C) or falls below 84°F. (29°C), essential organs such as the heart, kidneys and liver, cease to work, and death is imminent. But since, as we have seen, even staying alive generates enough heat to kill us in a matter of hours, we must have a very efficient mechanism of dissipating this excess heat and holding the body temperature consistently close to the 98.6°F. (37°C) level. How does this system work?

Exercising requires oxygen, and this results in the shunting of as much as a gallon of blood through the blood vessels of the muscles every minute. Since these muscles are working, their internal temperature is raised, and this heats the blood which passes through them. This heated blood then returns to the heart where it is pumped around the body again. As it flows through the brain, it triggers off the "Benzinger Reflex," a mechanism by which the blood vessels to the skin are reflexly opened up and the sweat glands stimulated to work overtime. Warm blood can now dissipate its heat into the surrounding cooler air by the processes of convection, conduction and radiation. Notice I said *cooler* air — that is, air temperature lower than the skin temperature. What happens when the air temperature is high, approaching that of the skin? Under these circumstances, the body has to depend more and more on the evaporation of sweat to drop the body temperature. The mere act of sweating has no cooling effect per se; it is the vapourization, or evaporation of the sweat from the surface of the body which is all important.

A 1-calorie increase in body heat can be balanced by the evaporation of about 1.5 c.c. of sweat. But there is a limit to the rate at which one can sweat. In the average unconditioned individual, this amounts to about two to three pints per hour; in a trained, heat-acclimatized jogger, this figure may be increased to as much as five pints per hour.

Evaporation of sweat can be influenced by a number of conditions. If the air is humid, it is already saturated with moisture and cannot accept any more. So the sweat will not vapourize; it will merely drip down the face and body like water, in which form it cannot have a cooling effect. In conditions of very high humidity, therefore, sweating becomes less effective as a means of reducing body temperature.

On a windy day, the mechanism of evaporation has an advantage. The air next to the sweating skin, as soon as it becomes heavily laden with sweat moisture, is blown away, and its place is taken by air which is drier and more receptive to further vapourization.

Clothing is an important factor. It should allow free movement of air over the skin. Trapped pockets of air become saturated with vapourized sweat and prevent further evaporation from that area. Air is a very good insulator, and prevents body heat from escaping by conduction or radiation. Perfect examples of clothing which prevent adequate heat loss are the rubberized training suit, or the footballer's uniform, with its plastic helmet and padding, designed to protect against bodily contact injury but not against the ill effects of high heat conditions. Deaths from heat stroke due to the wearing of such apparel are, sad to say, recorded from time to time in the medical literature.

The fourth condition affecting sweat evaporation has to do with blood volume. Why is it that when you go for a long jog on a very hot day (usually the first hot day of the summer, when you are not as yet acclimatized to the heat), you tire so quickly? As we have seen, a portion of your circulating blood volume is shunted into your muscles during exercise; furthermore, because of the heat of the day, you are sweating heavily and losing water from your blood stream at a rate of five pints an hour. Unless you replace the sweat loss by drinking fluids, the net result will be a reduction in blood volume. But as long as you keep jogging, your muscles require oxygen and thus your heart is committed to pumping a steady supply of oxygen-laden blood to the scene of action. With the drop in the amount of blood available, however, there is a concomitant drop in the amount ejected with each heart beat — i.e., the stroke volume. The only way that the heart can now maintain its output of blood is by increasing the number of strokes per minute. In other words, the heart rate must go up if the heart is to maintain an adequate blood supply to the exercising muscles.

But, as we have seen in Chapter 5, each of us has a maximum heart rate; if we continue to jog at the same intensity, this maximum is eventually reached. When that happens, cardiac output cannot keep pace with demand. Actually, we can gain a very slight respite by constricting the blood vessels of the skin, a stratagem which can be detected by the sudden change which occurs in the jogger's complexion, from ruddy and sweating to ashen pale. This constriction of the skin's blood vessels shunts some blood back into the central pool, raising the central blood volume, and making more blood available, again, for the heart to pump. For a short period of time, stroke volume increases and cardiac output is maintained. Unfortunately, the price you have paid for this temporary postponement of the inevitable is a high one. By diverting blood away from the skin, you have deprived yourself of your major mechanism of heat loss. Thus the temperature inside your body rapidly begins to climb and the whole heat control compensatory system begins to break down. Unless you stop exercising, or unless you have been drinking ample quantities of fluid to keep your blood volume up, you have reached the stage of dehydration.

There are three clinical conditions associated with exercising in the hot weather, and although they may merge imperceptibly and insidiously into one another, it leads to a better understanding of the whole mechanism of dehydration if they are dealt with as separate entities.

Heat Cramps

Heat cramps occur in highly trained individuals who have been working out for some time in hot weather. In the case of the jogger, the cramps occur in the legs. They may come on toward the end of a run (the last four or five miles of a marathon) or after the jog, for example, in the shower or walking home. They can be extremely severe and may last for many minutes. Sometimes they involve the muscles of the abdomen and then may simulate a surgical condition, such as an acute appendicitis.

Such cramps are thought to be due to a chronic lack or loss of sodium. As I explained earlier, the highly conditioned athlete has a copious sweat production, much greater than the sedentary individual. While his sweat contains less sodium than normal (the body's attempt to conserve its supply), this can be outbalanced by the speed with which sweating occurs, so that eventually, he tends to lose sodium. He can replace the fluid by drinking water, but this does not replace sodium. Ingestion of a dilute salt solution (1 teaspoonful of salt to 2 pints of water) will relieve his cramps very rapidly.

The average jogger is not likely to be bothered by this. It is much more frequent in the individual who is training for long periods in the heat, such as the competitive marathon runner who is averaging 150 miles a week in a hot climate. Incidentally, your best sources of salt are catsup, bran, fish, nuts and meat. Do not use salt tablets; they are far too concentrated.

Heat Exhaustion

This is due to inadequate replacement of the water lost in sweat. The early signs are fatigue and weakness. I cannot emphasize enough that thirst is a very poor indicator that you need fluid. There are several reasons for this. It has been shown that the mere act of putting something in the mouth, a pebble, for instance, reduces the sensation of thirst for about 15 minutes. Also, laboratory experiments have shown that the introduction of a small amount of fluid through a tube directly into the stomach has the same effect — even though the water has not been absorbed through the stomach wall. So a jogger may take just a mouthful of cold water, swallow it, no longer feel thirsty, and carry on for another half an hour before he feels he needs to drink again. Yet the amount of fluid taken is totally inadequate, and dehydration is inevitable.

With water losses of up to 5 per cent of his body weight, the dehydrated jogger develops a flushed, hot skin, his judgment becomes poor, and he may become uncoordinated and irrational. I recall an athlete in Boston, screaming at his coach and a group of people who were providing fluid, that they had given him ''the wrong bottle.'' In fact, he was given the fluid that had been made up for him, but in his confused state, he didn't recognize it. It didn't taste right to him, and he became extremely belligerent. After the race, he couldn't remember the incident at all!

Other symptoms of heat exhaustion are light-headedness, a very rapid heart rate, and severe frontal headaches. Heat exhaustion can occur in varying degrees of severity, and may become chronic during a long spell of hot weather training, until noticed by a coach, a friend, or the jogger himself who is familiar with the effect of dehydration. Drinking adequate water before, during and after training jogs is just as important as during a marathon race. Heat exhaustion can also develop rapidly during a run and may progress to heat stroke, the third and most dangerous manifestation of dehydration.

Heat Stroke

Heat stroke is the popular term for hyperpyrexia, that is, body temperature in excess of 108°F. (42°C). Again, the cause is lack of water. Its onset can be insidious and rapid. The victim, after demonstrating evidence of extreme heat exhaustion, collapses into a coma, from which he may never recover. Death is frequently due to renal failure.

The effects of heat stroke on the body are widespread. In the posterior portion of the brain, the cerebellum, there is destruction of specialized cells. This is why survivors may be left with staggering gait, or speech disorders. Bleeding into the cortex of the brain is responsible for various mental disturbances. The kidneys can be irreparably damaged, making renal dialysis necessary. Hemorrhage into the heart muscle, and even heart attacks in spite of perfectly normal coronary arteries have been reported. The liver may be damaged, causing intense jaundice. Clotting of blood in the blood vessels may lead to damage in a whole host of organs. As you can see, an incredible number of deadly pathological changes all stem from simple failure to drink adequately during a hot weather run.

How to Avoid Dehydration

Anyone who exercises on a hot day, old or young, male or female, jogger or runner, is a potential dehydration victim. If you are a fun jogger, never forget that the number of calories burned (and therefore the amount of body heat generated) doesn't depend on the speed you jog, but rather on the distance you cover. For example, whether you jog three miles in 24 minutes or in 36 you will still burn approximately 300 calories. Actually, the slower the pace, the longer you are exposed to the sun, and so the greater the likelihood of dehydration. The heavier you are, the more calories you will burn as you jog and, therefore, the greater your need for fluid. The following rules apply equally to the middle-aged novice jogger and the highly trained athlete:

1. Allow time for heat acclimatization. The body learns to cope with heat if you give it enough time to adjust. The process takes about 7 to 10 days, and during this time, the workouts should be low key to commence with, gradually building up to your usual intensity and duration. When the temperature is above 85°F. (30°C) and the humidity above 30 per cent, the cardiac jogger should miss out the session altogether. (See page 307 for use of the Heat Safety Index.)

2. Always prehydrate 10 to 20 minutes or so before exercising on a warm day. Drink about half a pint of fluid, then another half a pint every 20 minutes or so while working out. Don't wait to feel thirsty before drinking. You should train yourself to prehydrate and hydrate, otherwise you won't be able to do it in competition. Carried out for the first time under the stressful conditions of an official marathon, your stomach will feel distended, you won't be able to absorb the fluid, and it will swill around inside you at every step.

3. The best fluid to use is water. It should be comfortably cold (best temperature for absorption is 40°F), and if you require a flavour you may add a little fruit juice according to taste. Minerals such as sodium and potassium aren't really essential; the body can replace them later. However, if you do add sodium, it should be in small amounts of 1 teaspoon of salt to a gallon of water.

What about potassium? During prolonged physical exertion, potassium leaks out of the muscles, resulting in relatively high levels in the blood. Even though some of this excess is excreted in the urine and sweat, it is rarely enough to drop blood potassium levels below normal. Therefore, there is no need to add potassium to the fluid which is taken during the run. It has been our experience that most proprietary hydration fluids contain too much potassium and, therefore, if given consistently during the marathon, result in excessively high potassium levels. After the run, however, potassium passes back into the muscles, dropping the blood concentration. Therefore, potassium should be used in the post-race drinks, in concentrations about half that normally found in sweat. Diluted orange juice is an excellent source.

Chronic potassium loss in sweat and urine can occur from exhaustive hot-weather training day after day, especially before heat acclimatization takes place. This is best prevented by eating a diet high in potassium-containing foods, e.g., whole grains, nuts, fruits such as bananas, oranges and prunes, tomato catsup. In general, the potassium-deficient athlete will have a craving for such foodstuffs, and will not have to be urged to eat them.

Some post-coronary joggers may be taking hydrochlorothiazide medication, a diuretic which is given to treat mild cases of high blood pressure. Diuretics encourage the kidneys to excrete sodium and, therefore, water. Potassium is lost in the urine at the same time, and the prescribing physician often suggests that a patient on such medication increase his consumption of potassium-containing foods or, alternatively, prescribes a potassium pill to take. Obviously, a patient taking diuretics (trade names, Diuril, Hydrodiuril, Esiberix) is most susceptible to low blood potassium levels in high heat training and should be aware of this. Too much or too little potassium in the blood can give rise to various abnormalities of cardiac rhythm, and in unexplained cases of palpitations or skipped beats appearing in a healthy jogger, analysis of a blood sample for potassium concentrations should be carried out.

Sugar, usually in the form of glucose, is often added to replacement fluid to provide energy. Actually, there is little to recommend this practice. Glucose solutions which exceed 2.5 per cent strength are too concentrated to be absorbed through the gut wall and therefore lie in the stomach, causing nausea and vomiting. Worse still, to dilute the glucose, water is actually drawn out of the blood stream and cells of the body into the intestine, thus aggravating the dehydration! If, on the other hand, you prepare a solution containing less than 2.5 per cent glucose, the amount of energy provided is probably too small to be of any value.

The best replacement fluid, then, is still cold water, plus a mild flavouring agent if desired.

4. Clothing should be light, porous and comfortable. Fishnet vests are most suitable, allowing easy circulation of air and free evaporation of sweat from the skin.

5. Cold water sponging helps, as will putting ice under your hat. If you sponge your legs, be careful not to wet your shoes and socks, otherwise you will run into problems with blisters.

6. Get into the habit of weighing yourself naked before and after each workout. If you have hydrated adequately, you should have lost no more than 3 per cent of your body weight; more than 5 per cent, and you have definitely dehydrated.

7. Finally, when the air temperature and humidity are both extremely high even copious quantities of water will not hold your body temperature down. Slowing your pace, or even walking, will reduce your body's rate of heat generation, but it you start to develop symptoms of excessive high body temperature (severe muscle and abdomen cramps, dizziness,

extreme irritability, a tendency to stumble), then smarten up and drop out of the run. Failure to do so may have very unpleasant consequences.

COLD WEATHER JOGGING

While indoor exercising has its advocates, I believe that walking and jogging out of doors is of most benefit. Apart from the sheer boredom and discomfort of indoor exercising (when did you last sweat your way round four miles of a "26-lap-to-the-mile" track?), the outdoor jogger achieves an exhilaration and sense of satisfaction which can only be obtained by physically coping with the natural elements. The feeling one gets from hacking four miles through the pouring rain or driving snow is no less rewarding than the pleasure of an early morning run through the park in the spring. Even allowing for your reluctance to accept this philosophy, there is another more cogent reason for advocating out-of-door exercising. If you are going to work out five days a week for the rest of your life, surely the most convenient way to do so is by stepping through your front door and using your own district as a training ground. You fit your exercising into your lifestyle, and you make it part of your daily living.

I have found that patients who resort to indoor stationary exercycles and the like rarely persist with their programs. Instead of arranging their day's activities around their one hour workout, they attempt to fit the exercise session into their already rather hectic lifestyle. They try to watch television while cycling, or rig up a stand so that they can read a book during the session. They fit the activity in just before supper, and if they arrive home late from work, they find it all too easy to miss out "just this once." Eventually the bicycle, or rowing machine, or other exercise gimmick, is relegated to the basement because it looks so forlorn, untidy and unused in the living room; and that's the end of that. As for the indoor fitness club, this certainly has its place, provided you don't have a half hour's drive each way, and provided its facilities include a jogging track big enough to allow you to cover four miles without injuring your ankles, knees or inner ear balance mechanism from pivoting around a minuscule circle.

There are, of course, some hazards associated with jogging in the cold. In addition to the possibility of cold-induced angina (see Chapter 8) we have the problem of snow-covered and icy surfaces, which impose greater energy expenditure and increase the likelihood of injury. Head winds increase chilling effect and air resistance. Rain or wet snow reduces the insulating properties of clothing and allows body heat to "wick out" to the atmosphere. Paradoxically, dehydration can be as much of a problem in the winter as it is in summer. Although body heat loss by conduction, convection, and radiation is more efficient in the cold, the evaporative process continues, making excessive fluid loss by sweating possible. Moreover, exposure to cold air strongly suppresses the sense of thirst, and drinking to replace fluid is often ignored.

Fortunately, the body heat generated by jogging is usually sufficient to offset loss of heat to the surrounding cold air. Where there is imbalance in favour of heat loss, this can be prevented by wearing suitable clothing.

The purpose of clothing in cold weather is to insulate the surface of the skin from the surrounding environment and prevent heat loss. Clothing traps air and modifies the skin's so-called microclimate. The fabric is less important in this regard than the weave. Layering garments and varying the closeness of the weave or knit allows considerable flexibility in achieving the desired level of heat retention. However, insulating properties may be changed drastically by the action of water or sweat. Tightly woven cotton with little interfibre air-trapping sticks to the body when wet, eliminates large air pockets, and reduces insulation. Wool, on the other hand, retains its insulating properties with its natural oils and greater air-trapping interstices even when wet. In recent years, man-made fibres have been woven and knit in various ways to develop systems of functional clothing for cold-weather activities of all types.

The layer next to the skin should be tightly woven ribbed material that provides some insulation while allowing for evaporation during excessive sweating. The middle layer (loosely woven wool or a fish net cotton and synthetic mix) should absorb some of this excess sweat but again allow for evaporation. The third layer (a tighter woven wool, wool/cotton combination, or synthetic fibre) should have some degree of stretch to permit variable insulation by opening and closing our pores in the material in response to body movement. A fourth layer is needed only in conditions of high wind and extreme cold. It should protect against wind, rain, and snow and yet be permeable to body heat. Man-made materials have performed these functions with considerable success.

If possible, all upper body garments should be zipped or buttoned in such a way that they can be loosened at the neck when the body overheats or closed up if chilling occurs. Dark or coloured outer garments tend to conserve body heat; they should be adorned with reflective strip material so as to be visible in the darkness.

The legs rarely require more than two layers. Track suit pants over panty hose will suffice on even the coldest days. Long underwear is fine, although it tends to restrict knee movement if it is not cut down. Socks should be a wool/cotton mixture or a ribbed and channelled, woven synthetic material. Hands, susceptible to cold because they are poorly muscled and used little in jogging, are best protected by wool mittens which trap more air than gloves. Since considerable body heat is lost through the head, a woollen hat that pulls down over the ears to prevent frostbite is necessary. The exposed parts of the face should be protected from chapping and cold sores by applying petroleum jelly. Shoes with waffle soles give greater purchase on ice, and slightly flared heels provide greatest stability on soft snow.

Air temperature is only one of the factors that should be taken into consideration when planning workouts in cold climates. Wind conditions, presence or absence of sunshine, and humidity levels all affect the body cooling rate. A 15-mile-an-hour wind can make a still-air temperature reading of 2°C feel like −9°C; thus a wind chill chart should always be consulted on a windy day (see Appendix, page 307).

Is the sun shining or is it overcast? Direct sunshine is worth an additional 7°C (12°F.). This can be critical. You may start your walk on a calm day with the sun shining brightly, and if you are using an out-and-back course, by the time you head for home you may find yourself battling a 10-mile-an-hour wind, with the sun long since disappeared behind the clouds. You are no longer adequately dressed, and things begin to become pretty miserable. You can, of course, pick up your pace to generate more body heat. But this may require a level of exertion beyond your capabilities, in which case you will fatigue, lose your body heat even more rapidly or, if you are a post-coronary patient, develop angina and have to slow down again.

Probably the greatest threat to maintaining equilibrium between heat production and heat loss is wet clothing. Whether the result of driving rain, melting snow, or drenching perspiration, the effect is the same. Evaporation from the wet material will drop your body temperature at an alarming rate. This is one of the most potent causes of hypothermia. With every one degree (1°) fall below normal, you go through the successive stages of slurred speech, uncoordination of hands and feet, unsteadiness, confusion, collapse, and finally coma. Hypothermia is hardly the lot of everyone who goes for a jog on a cold day and gets his clothes wet, but you should take precautions to see that you never put yourself in the position of risking such a tragedy.

The danger of a combination of strong winds, heavy rain, and inadequate clothing was tragically underlined at the Eighth Annual Four Inns Walking Competition (45 miles over high ground) in England in 1964. Only 22 of 240 healthy young competitors finished the race. Many competitors collapsed from exposure, three died, and four nearly died; yet the air temperature never fell below 3°C. In the final analysis, the competitors who finished were those who were fit enough to compensate for excessive body cooling by sustained high heat production — i.e., a hill-walking pace of 12 to 13 minutes per mile. The vast majority of those who got into trouble wore cotton garments which had poor air-trapping characteristics to start with and became even worse as they became soaked with the driving rain.

Putting all of this together, we can lay down the following guidelines for cold weather jogging:

1. Wear layers of clothing which are suitably woven to regulate heat loss.
2. Always consult the wind chill chart on windy days and use the effective temperature rather than the air temperature as a guideline. If the effective temperature is below −10°C (15°F.) post-coronary joggers should question the wisdom of exercising out of doors. To be honest, over 90 per cent of my patients exercise at below this temperature during the wintertime, but only after they have been adequately instructed in all of the safety measures mentioned above. In their case, it is particularly important that they allow for wind, wet conditions, presence or absence of sunshine, and so on. But probably the most important factor is whether or not they enjoy cold weather. I know it is hard to believe in this day and age of science, but the only way to predict whether or not an individual functions better in the cold or in the heat is to ask him! There are some people who can happily work out of doors in temperatures down as low as 0°F; there are others who shiver misera-

bly at one degree below freezing. Your body metabolism is your affair, and only you know the type of climatic conditions most suitable to your own machinery.

3. Because the wind and sun conditions can change rapidly, a short out-and-back course should be chosen, the furthest point of which should be no more than a quarter of a mile from the starting point. This is particularly important for the less fit.

4. In wet and cold conditions, the clothing layers should include a light cotton/nylon mixture outer garment that will provide up to two to three hours of protection against moisture.

5. Head winds must be taken into consideration and the pace adjusted downward to maintain the prescribed level of energy expenditure. If one does not reduce pace in the teeth of a head wind, then premature fatigue will inevitably ensue, a slower pace will lead to inadequate heat production, and symptoms from chilling will occur.

By how much should the pace be slowed? Pulse rate during normal workout conditions should be used as a guideline. Alternatively, back off the pace until you are experiencing the same level of breathing rate and leg muscle exertion you usually associate with your customary jogging pace. This concept of "perceived exertion level" was introduced by the Swedish psychologist, Dr. Gunnar Borg, and has created some interest in exercise physiology circles in recent years. It presupposes that the average individual can relate these body signals to a given intensity of exertion and heart rate, and by re-creating them at any time can reproduce that same level of exertion under widely varying circumstances. For example, let us assume that the walking or jogging prescription, done under ideal conditions, calls for the intensity of effort which is perceived by the patient as being "somewhat hard" or "13" on the Borg scale. This will correlate with a specific heart rate, breathing rate, blood pressure, oxygen consumption, blood lactate level, etc. Reproducing an RPE of "13" under difficult or adverse conditions (e.g., head wind or hilly terrain) will supposedly give the same physical measurements, even though the speed of the jog is necessarily slower. I find this true for many of my patients, but it does cause problems in those "deniers" who consistently overestimate their prowess. It can also be a dangerous rule of thumb for patients who develop increased skipped beats with exercise, and who can only detect them by pulse taking.

6. Frostbite is unusual in the jogger, but can occur in poorly protected hands, ears, and faces exposed to temperatures below −1°C (30°F). Failure to take wind chill into account is usually the cause.

For more than sixteen winters, a high percentage of some five thousand patients on the Toronto program have trained outdoors on all but the severest day without ill effects. They are the finest testimonial to our approach. The trouble is, by the time winter has come to an end, they have to start acclimatizing to the heat again. Such is life!

THE OTHER SIDE OF THE COIN

Jogging has become one of the most popular participation sports in North America. I am delighted. I enjoy jogging for its own sake, and I am happy to see so many others, young and old, male and female, share my delight. One of the many spinoffs, because of the increased feeling of well-being which accompanies a regular jogging program, is the development of a greater interest in other physical pastimes. At last count, my post-coronary patients were actively engaged in and enjoying any one of a total of sixteen different sports and physical recreations. In addition to jogging and walking, they included cycling, golf, swimming, tennis, squash, curling, bowling, ice skating and roller skating, cross-country and Alpine skiing, ice hockey, ballroom dancing, square dancing, various types of calisthenics, horse riding, sailing, and canoeing. There is no doubt that North America is on the greatest exercise kick in history. Are there any disadvantages to this? Maybe. Whether you call them side effects, drawbacks, or just the inevitable consequences of the latest vogue depends on your point of view. In any event, a few comments on these various aspects are probably timely at this particular stage in the development of what I hope is now our mutual hobby.

The Cult of Jogging

Any mass movement tends to attract the cultist, the individual who by nature is impelled to add a ritualistic and mystic aura to the most mundane of pursuits. I am the last to gainsay the psychological advantages of jogging, but to listen to the cultist, every workout should be akin to a religious experience. This supercharged attitude makes me feel a trifle uncomfortable, and I feel that it should be put into perspective.

A recent book on jogging stated that 78 per cent of all the subjects questioned by the author admitted to experiencing a "high" at least once while jogging. They described the experience in various terms, but in essence it seemed to mean a feeling of increased self-awareness, often associated with a pleasurable heightening of sensory input. The colours of sunsets or sunrises seem more intense. Familiar objects such as buildings, bushes, trees, billboards, assume unfamiliar but intriguing shapes. The very air itself develops a texture, an odour and a dimension which it never had before. Some even describe a state bordering on self-hallucination, in which "the true meaning of life is revealed." All well and good, except that in questioning thousands of joggers on my program and talking to as many or more fun runners in the British Isles, Europe and Australia, I have never been able to find more than a handful of individuals in whom running induced such bizarre sensations. For most of us, there are days when every step is a drag and the nicest thing about the whole session is the hot shower and the glass of beer that follow it. Running too hard or too fast doesn't "grey out our peripheral vision" as one eloquent cultist put it, it merely makes our heart rate go up, puts us into oxygen debt, gives us a headache, and from time to time causes us to throw up at the end of the race.

Believe it or not, but I have even heard one "high priest jogger" describe how, at a certain stage in a marathon race, his ecstasy of superlative fitness reached such heights that he experienced an orgasm! The reaction of my post-coronary marathoners (admittedly more cynical and hard-bitten than most) to this announcement was something to behold! Some wanted to know the exact mile at which it happened (so that they could prepare for the great and eagerly anticipated event should it happen to them); others, with more practical turns of mind, were inclined to implicate an excessively tight jock strap rather than the "ecstasy of fitness." Our erstwhile captain, Harry B., put forward the theory that the 67-year-old marathoner in question was probably confusing ejaculation with micturition.

But surely, I hear you say, the jogging enthusiast who is experiencing the pleasures of exercise and fitness for the first time is bound to see things in a new light and with a different perspective, and cannot this induce a totally new philosophy and outlook on life? I agree entirely. My only point is that one must be constantly on one's guard against exaggerated claims. I have no quarrel with those of poetic bent and eloquent turn of phrase who express the pleasures of jogging in an appealing and attractive manner. My concern is with the zealot, the visionary, who promises Nirvana after a six-mile plod. When the newcomer to the sport fails to experience such spiritual bliss, he naturally blames himself. At which point, he drops the whole thing, and goes back to watching television.

The other problem with cultists, of course, is that they are notoriously fickle. One year it's jogging, the next, dynamic breath-holding. Since they don't stay long enough with anything to obtain all the benefits, and since they often have to rationalize their reason for forsaking the last craze, they tend to bad-mouth it. These are people who are constantly looking for the unattainable; they are rarely, if ever, satisfied. Jogging can do without them. Not only do they add complex, unnecessary and exaggerated dimensions to what is essentially a very simple activity, but they inevitably entice other undesirables. If I may paraphrase Wordsworth, "The huckster is too much with us; late and soon, getting and spending, he lays waste our powers." Hucksters are attracted to cults like flies to a jampot. What better market for their wares? Jogging magazines are full of ads for "jogging aids," which are of questionable value. Self-styled experts lacking any formal training and short on experience, to say the least, promise to advise you by book, correspondence course, seminar, or "running camp" how to achieve your jogging heart's desire — at a substantial price, of course! Pseudo-scientific mumbo-jumbo is used to impress the unwary and confuse the intelligent enquirer in search of genuine help.

The answer to all this? Merely be aware that it's happening. Try to get your advice, whether verbal or written, from individuals who have been running or jogging long before the present craze started. When reading a column or a book on jogging, make it your business to find out the author's qualifications. That's not to say that you need a piece of paper or a string of letters after your name to make you an authority. Some of the greatest track and field coaches in the world never had a formal lecture on the subject. But the true expert will never try to mislead you, either directly or by inference. If he speaks of scientific matters, he will invariably give you the source of his basic data, and when he expresses his own interpretation of that data, he will make it equally plain what he is doing. The bottom line for the huckster, naturally enough, is dollars and cents. Bear that in mind, and you shouldn't be too easy a mark!

The Fanatical Jogger

A few weeks ago, I had a phone call from an orthopedic surgeon friend of mine. He was treating a jogger patient who had developed a stress fracture but, against advice, had continued to jog and had now developed a second fracture. My friend, in a desperate attempt to enforce a period of rest, had decided to apply a below-knee plaster cast. To his astonishment, the patient was still reluctant to accept the inevitable six-week layoff and was demanding that "something else" be tried that would allow him to get back to jogging within a few days. "What in God's name," said my friend, "makes a guy like this tick? Are all joggers this crazy?" I assured him that not all of us were this crazy, but I admitted that from time to time there are some who go a trifle overboard.

I have referred earlier in this book to the "beneficial addiction." By that, I mean the development of a reliance on your jogging workout, so that when you miss a few days, you begin to feel the worse for it. You get a little irritable, you feel a little down, you don't sleep quite as well, and you certainly miss the familiar rhythmic movement of your body along the roads and paths of your customary route. I believe there is a chemical reason for these mild, quite bearable, withdrawal symptoms. The trouble is, we have not as yet identified the chemical. This makes me wonder if the fanatical jogger, the individual who cannot bear to stop running for even a day, becomes a great deal more dependent upon that chemical than the rest of us. Could it be that he is deficient in it even before he starts jogging?

The jogger who cannot stop is often the one who attains the greatest degree of mental satisfaction and contentment from the workout. Our own studies have shown that the most depressed post-coronary patient is the one who obtains the greatest alleviation of that depression as a result of the jogging program. The individual with the normal psychological profile shows little change as a result of jogging. He feels better, he enjoys life more, and he uses jogging just as much as a relief from the tensions and anxieties of his everyday life as his depressed counterpart, but scientific analysis does not reflect this. In short, if you have a normal outlook on life, jogging is not going to do anything other than reinforce it. If, on the other hand, you have deep-seated psychological problems, then they may respond very gratifyingly to a regular jogging regime. Not only that, but the improvement may be readily measured by the clinical psychologist or psychiatrist. Drs. Glasser, Hackett, Greist and Kostrubala are all psychiatrists who confirm that jogging therapy can be effective in the treatment of chronic depression, phobias, anxiety neuroses, schizophrenia, and anorexia nervosa. In the hands of such experts, jogging is a welcome alternative to, for instance, the excessive use of various psychotropic medications.

But what if a runner, all unwittingly, is practising running self-medication — in other words, treating himself for any of the above conditions without realizing it? All he knows is that until he started running, life was miserable; since he began to jog, he is happy and functioning at a level of contentment that he has never experienced before. If he stops running, the old feelings of insecurity and despair begin to return. Under these circumstances, is he not likely to minimize any symptoms, be they musculoskeletal or cardiovascular, which might prevent him from running? Herein may lie the explanation for my orthopedic friend's patient who continues to work out with two broken bones in his foot. Or the marathoner described by cardiologist Dr. Tim Noakes of Cape Town who, against medical orders, ran five marathons in the 28-month period between his first heart attack and his second fatal one, and whose training log book recorded numerous episodes of pain in the chest, jaws or arms during training runs, for none of which he sought medical advice. Or the American congressman jogger who had two exercise stress tests which indicated severe disease of the coronary arteries but who, spurning all warnings, continued to run vigorously — until he dropped dead some months later at the end of a fifteen-mile training run! The examples are frequent enough, I think, to make my point. Certainly the theory could explain the unaccountable behaviour of some apparently intelligent joggers.

There is a fine line between enthusiasm and fanaticism, between dedication and a death wish. I have nothing but congratulations for the individual who so successfully organizes his work schedule and his spare time that he can fit in his jogging session as part of his life. I have the greatest admiration for those who overcome

the vagaries of weather and the inevitable daily unexpected cri-
ses of life and still maintain their regular exercise schedule. But
there is a difference between reorganizing your social life and totally demolishing it. What of the jogger who, because of his early
morning workout, must get to bed between 9 and 10 o'clock every
night, weekends included? As far as his wife, family and friends
are concerned, he is strictly a party pooper. Not only that, but
evening theatre, movies or late-night dinner engagements become
a thing of the past. If this is the way it is, then something has to be
wrong.

Like everything else, moderation is the key to success. While
not gainsaying the mental and physical benefits of jogging, these
benefits must be put in perspective. As goals, they must never be
lost sight of, but to become compulsive about the method of attaining them is, paradoxically, to destroy their value. The compulsive jogger is an uptight, strung-out individual who is worrying
about his work schedule when he is jogging and about his jogging when he is working. He is the antithesis of the relaxed,
loping, easy-breathing image that he is aiming for. The compulsive jogger is sick and a complete pain in the buttocks to all the
normal people who have to share his life.

If, on reading this, you begin to see the beginnings of a self-
portrait, then do me a favour — stop running for two weeks, and
then, at the end of the second week, make a list of the reasons
which started you jogging in the first place. Do you still consider
these reasons worthwhile? If so, how many of them have you
realized? Finally — and be honest here — has there been any deterioration in your mental equanimity, your home life, your relationships with the members of your family or your oldest and dearest
friends, your social and cultural life, or your job? If the answer to
this last question is yes, then is it due to your new lifestyle? In a
nutshell, have the gains outweighed the losses? If not, then the
chances are that you have become a compulsive jogger. The remedy lies in your own hands. The fact is that if you don't change,
you'll wind up without any of the health advantages, and maybe
even minus your wife and friends. The choice is yours.

The Media

The recent explosion of interest in jogging has intrigued those
whose job it is to report and comment on the opinions, habits
and daily activities of the rest of us. The result has been consider-

able media coverage of mass marathon runs, as well as features about the jogger, the jogger's wife, the jogger's shoes, and almost every conceivable aspect of jogging that you can mention. The high incidence of heart disease, and its association with the sedentary lifestyle, has given added impetus to this trend. I find that a goodly number of media workers are themselves joggers. They are often highly intelligent individuals who are quick to perceive the validity of the pro-exercise arguments. As a group, they have traditionally tended to smoke too much, eat irregularly and unwisely, take little if any exercise, drink too much, put on too much weight, and to add insult to injury, live notoriously hectic and stress-filled lives. They are, in short, prime candidates for heart attacks, and they know it. Small wonder that some of the most enthusiastic joggers are now to be found in their ranks.

This is all to the good. Not only have the media done a great job in fostering public interest in a more healthy lifestyle, but both the style and substance of the message has usually been both mature and well-informed. There is so much information available today on exercise, training, fitness, and the like that one is hard put to keep abreast of it all. It is no exaggeration to say that the intelligent layman who merely touches base from time to time with the larger circulation jogging magazines, newspaper fitness columns, and occasional radio and television programs knows more about the topic than most coaches of ten years back — and certainly than the vast majority of present-day physicians. The North American jogger is now thoroughly familiar with such terms as HDL cholesterol, fast-twitch fibres, carbohydrate loading, and similar jargon.

A word of caution. All honeymoons must come to an end. The business of the media is to present the news. The time is approaching when stories about joggers will have become about as interesting as the contents of the obituary column. Before leaving the topic of jogging, however, the media can still extract some interest by panning it. The time will come when a freelance writer is much more likely to get an article accepted if it decries jogging as a highly dangerous activity than if it merely repeats all of its advantages. Ten years ago, my post-coronary joggers had to endure the ridicule and warnings of their neighbours and friends as they plodded through the streets. They showed admirable singleness of purpose, faith in the program, and imperviousness to public opinion. Patients who join the program today find things a good deal easier. The streets are full of joggers, old and young, ridicule is stilled, and the media are with them every step of the way. I hope that when the brickbats come, they will not be intimidated back into their old way of life. I don't think they will, because I feel we have taught them to do all the right things for the right reasons. But I suspect that there are a group of latter-day joggers who enjoy swimming with the stream, but who, at the first appearance of the anti-jogging articles, will quickly put away their sweat suit and jogging shoes, and paddle about waiting for the next wave to ride.

JOGGING DEATHS

Sudden, unexpected death is not a recent phenomenon; it has been with us since antiquity. The commonest cause in recent times is a malfunction of the heart. Interestingly, while 50 to 60 per cent of heart attack victims die within a few hours, it should not be assumed that all cases of sudden death are caused by a heart attack. Actually, on autopsy only about one-third exhibit classical evidence of blocked coronary vessels and death of heart tissue. The other two-thirds, while frequently showing atherosclerosis of their coronary blood vessels, have no evidence of a myocardial infarction. Why is this?

The prevailing theory is that death has occurred too quickly (within a matter of minutes) for the classical, pathological changes to take place. But this doesn't explain why the coronary arteries should show no signs of a recent blood clot. Another explanation is that the heart has "fibrillated" or developed a defect in its rhythm-conducting system which interrupts its continuous pumping action and leaves it quivering ineffectually, thus starving the vital organs of oxygen. Sounds reasonable enough, but what caused the electrical failure in the first place? At present we don't know for certain; all we have are a good many clues.

We may be close to a breakthrough, however. In the first place, we have begun to accept that while cardiac atherosclerosis is probably at the root of 90 per cent of sudden deaths (the rest have non-cardiovascular causes), a frank myocardial infarction is not the only, or even the major mechanism responsible. It has been noted that in a number of cases of sudden death, tiny vital microscopic blood vessels supplying oxygen to the leashes of rhythm-conducting nerves of the heart are blocked by what are called platelet microemboli. Platelets are tiny round cells, about half the size of a red blood cell, which circulate in the blood in large quantities and prevent bleeding from cut or broken blood vessels by clumping together, plugging the break, and initiating the formation of a blood clot. The trouble is that they can be fooled into mistaking an atherosclerotic plaque inside the blood vessel for a break in its wall, or a slowing down of blood flow in a fat-narrowed vessel for a compensatory slowing due to excessive bleeding; in which case, with true sense of duty, they clump together and block off the blood flow through the blood vessel in question entirely. Deprivation of oxygen supply to the heart's rhythm pacemaker (the sino-atrial node — see p. 162), or any of its message-conduction systems, can be fatal in a matter of minutes.

But whether sudden death is due to a large clot in a major coronary artery which leads to destruction of heart tissue, or a microscopic clot in a microscopic artery which leads to fatal cardiac rhythm disturbances, what's the difference? Well, reduction in the incidence of sudden death depends upon our concept of its cause. If we assume that practically all cases are due to classical heart attacks, then prevention becomes strictly a matter of eliminating coronary atherosclerosis. But if disturbance in platelet cell function, superimposed upon coronary atherosclerosis, is the major risk factor, then actions and drugs which reduce platelet clumping may be critical in reducing the incidence of sudden death.

This theory of the cause of some sudden deaths does explain some hitherto paradoxical and puzzling scientific findings. For instance, a four-year follow-up in Seattle of 234 patients who were successfully resuscitated after "dying" suddenly showed that the subsequent "sudden death" rate was more than three times higher in those who, after their first episode, failed to go on to a full-blown heart attack. It would seem, then, from this study, that risk from sudden death can be a characteristic separate from myocardial infarction risk. There have also been a number of drug trials which has shown that certain medications have been woefully deficient in preventing heart attacks, both primary and recurrent but, apparently coincidentally, have been associated with the reduction in sudden deaths. Could it be that such therapeutic agents, while not affecting atherosclerosis per se, have been acting as anti-platelet aggregation substances? Or, looked at another way, since we know that smoking accelerates platelet clumping, would this explain why sudden death is apparently much higher in smokers than non-smokers?

The precise cause of sudden death in all cases is still a matter of conjecture, which makes it difficult to evaluate the effect of any one of a number of activities which the unfortunate victim is carrying out at the time of his demise. If a jogger drops dead, was jogging the cause? Unless an autopsy has been carried out, not even the immediate mechanism of death is certain, never mind the reason. And even if a post-mortem uncovers the immediate cause as being myocardial infarction or "electrical failure," can we incriminate exercise, or is it merely a coincidental association? In other words, would the episode have occurred anyway, irrespective of the activity? For instance, a study by Yater *et al* on young U.S. army men showed that while sudden death was twice as frequent during strenuous activity, autopsy demonstrated the presence of recent coronary thrombosis, i.e. silent heart attacks. In other words, the exercise had not caused the heart attack. The coronary artery clot had already developed prior to the strenuous event.

But what about the newspaper reports which confront you from time to time? "Congressman Drops Dead While Jogging." "American Medical Association Journal Reports 18 Cases of Sudden Death in Joggers." "Two South African Physicians Report Death from Heart Attacks in Four Marathon Runners." Well, you must realize that deaths occurring during exercise are news, especially if the victims are well known; they occur in full view of onlookers. How often do you read of surgical deaths? Yet if it made headlines in the press every time a patient failed to survive a coronary by-pass procedure or died while undergoing a coronary arteriogram (x-ray of coronary arteries using injection of radio opaque dye), it would give a totally false impression. Both coronary arteriography and coronary by-pass surgery are now extremely safe procedures. That's not to say that from time to time a death doesn't occur on the operating table, but when you consider the complex and intricate procedures being carried out, and the critically severe nature of the disease in those who are being treated, this is not surprising.

Medical science uses statistical methods to assess the odds for success. The bottom line is the same as in any other endeavour: the greatest good for the greatest number. In the long run, it all comes down to a mathematical assessment of benefit achieved balanced against harm done. Does that sound callous? If so, I don't mean it to. I, like many physicians and surgeons before me, have watched one of my patients die. It's something you never quite accept, never quite get used to. You analyze the circumstances for a cause. You ask yourself if you could have prevented it.

Jogging and exercise deaths are no exception. It's no good merely noting their presence. The cause of death must be identified wherever possible. Not only that, but because of the relative rarity of exercise deaths, they must be estimated mathematically in terms of their occurrence relative to other activities. For instance, do more sudden deaths occur during sleep, or sexual intercourse, or at work, or watching a football game, or in the sauna, or in the doctor's waiting room, etc.? In order to discover this, we must look at a large number of sudden death cases, and examine the circumstances under which they occurred. Not only that, but we must ascertain the time spent by the group under study in various activities. For instance, if one-third of their day was spent on work, one-third in sleep, and one-third in recreation, then, statistically at least, you would expect the same relationship to apply to the incidence of sudden death. A disturbance in this distribution might incriminate any one of these three activities. For instance, if you were to postulate that jogging or exercise was associated with a high incidence of sudden death, then you have to ascertain the amount of time spent by the group under study in exercising, and calculate the anticipated incidence of death accordingly.

Actually, it has already been estimated that in the United States, given the current incidence of death from heart and blood vessel disease, for every 250,000 joggers as many as 6.5 deaths could occur during or within two hours of the workout by chance alone — and that assumes an average jogging session of only 20 minutes, three times weekly. Given the most recent Gallup poll estimate that there are now some 20 million Americans jogging, as many as 520 of them can be expected to die by chance while jogging — just as some will die while eating, sleeping, watching television, or carrying out some other activity of daily living. I think this sheds some statistical perspective on the relationship between jogging and sudden death.

Jokl and McClellan reviewed sudden death and exercise in a monograph and noted that "Not one instance was encountered in which death could be regarded as due to the effects of extreme exertion in a previously healthy heart. It is significant that there is no case in our list." Dr. Ilkka M. Vuori, of the University of Turku, Finland, published one of the classical reports on sudden death in the *Journal of Cardiology*. He examined the circumstances surrounding 2,606 sudden deaths, with the specific purpose of ascertaining whether or not they were associated with physical activity. He concluded that sudden deaths connected with sporting activities were rare. Ten sudden deaths occurred in connection with day-long ski-hikes, and strenuous physical exercise seemed to have played an important role in these cases. However, most of the subjects had serious cardiovascular risk factors which were known in advance or which could have been identified by medical examination. Daily physical activities or sports could not be incriminated as an important contributory factor in sudden death in the general population. However, he suggested that there was a risk of cardiac complications in connection with strenuous physical exercise in subjects who had cardiac disease.

Our own studies and investigations in Toronto have corroborated these findings. The immediate factor triggering a heart attack in about one-third of the patients referred to us for post-coronary rehabilitation seemed to have been intense and unaccustomed exercise, sometimes associated with emotional excitement. This is hardly surprising. The majority of epidemiological studies support the conclusion that prolonged inactivity increases the overall risk of myocardial infarction. Unaccustomed exercise, then, when it acts as a precipitant for a heart attack, does no more than reveal a previously damaged coronary system which is highly susceptible to both physical and emotional stress.

Are we saying, then, that exercise can be dangerous in individuals who have severe coronary artery disease? Of course. Otherwise there would be no need for the medically supervised type of post-coronary exercise program offered at the Toronto Rehabilitation Centre. For those males over 35 in the general population who have latent heart disease but are not aware of it, there must surely be a danger in ill-advised, excessive, and non-medically prescribed competitive jogging. The cardiac contra-indications to exercise are dealt with fully in Chapter 7 and, in the interests of space, will only be dealt with briefly here. However, they are obviously of paramount importance in this particular context and will bear reading again.

There are a number of circumstances surrounding exercise which, either alone or in combination, may precipitate irregularities of cardiac rhythm or maybe sudden death. First and foremost is *exercising when one has a fever*. This has been stressed previously, but one cannot over-accentuate the dangers of forcing the heart to work when it may well be suffering from an infection. Flu-like illnesses may often be harmless, but from time to time they will give rise to a myocarditis, or inflammation of the heart muscle cells, in which case any additional strain placed on the heart may be fatal. In order to prevent the unnecessary risk of exercise-related sudden death in association with myocarditis, we apply the absolutely strict ruling that anyone suffering from a flu-like illness must not exercise until a full seven days have elapsed since his temperature has returned to normal. An unexplained persistent rapid or irregular heart rate following or accompanying a flu-like illness is strongly suggestive of active myocarditis.

The problems of *exercise in the heat* have been discussed in detail already, but one cannot over-emphasize the dangers. When one exercises in high temperature, there is a progressive fall in the ability of the heart to pump blood. In these circumstances, output of blood from the heart can only be maintained by an increase of the heart rate. All of this is due to the fact that a significant proportion of circulating blood volume has to be shunted to the skin in order to dissipate heat. The entire detrimental consequence of this major hemodynamic fluctuation is not as yet fully understood, but on first principles it seems advisable to pay particular attention to adequate fluid intake, and cold sponging during prolonged exercise in the heat. Deaths during long distance runs in high temperature have been ascribed to heart attacks, and yet on more than one occasion autopsies have failed to reveal any evidence of coronary atherosclerosis. It is not unreasonable to assume that such deaths have been due to dehydration and consequent alteration in blood electrolytes. No one is immune to all of the terrible consequences of dehydration, but middle-aged males with latent coronary artery disease are more susceptible.

A less tangible, but nonetheless important, factor in the equation balancing the benefits and hazards of exercise is that of *personality*. The driving, ambitious individual, who tends to take on too many projects and may have some concealed hostility, once introduced to an exercise program is usually over-eager to excel. Such individuals must be rigorously controlled from misapplying their natural aggression and competitiveness. Not infrequently they become compulsive, and when business pressures mount will try to complete their workout in less and less time. Even worse, they may deny cardiac symptoms so that they can continue both their exercise program and still keep up their heavy business and social commitments. In effect, they ignore symptoms, attributing them to non-cardiac ailments, or else they dismiss them as being of no consequence.

The inherent danger in this attitude is that it always causes a delay before these symptoms are brought to the attention of the doctor. For this reason I take warning signs such as excessive fatigue, tiredness and especially anginal-type pain on exercise extremely seriously. They are an indication that the training must be immediately reduced, pending a detailed re-examination of the exerciser's cardiovascular status.

We have evolved five exercise rules as applied particularly to these deadline fighters:

- train regularly without excessive peaks of activity;
- avoid intensive competitions;
- adhere to the prescribed limits;
- reduce the exercise load when either physical symptoms, mental tension or depression develops;
- report all "cardiac type" symptoms such as exercise-related chest pain, arm pain, excessive palpitations, dizziness, "black-outs", or undue breathlessness — even if they appear for the first time after years of steady symptom-free training.

The tragic death in the United States of an outstanding young female tennis star while warming-down after a competitive tennis match illustrates another potential presage to sudden death. Although the post-mortem failed to establish a cause of death, a detailed inquiry revealed that prior to her death, she had suffered episodic black-outs. It was, therefore, assumed that these black-outs and her death were both due to a cardiac arrhythmia which on this occasion failed to reverse spontaneously — so-called "electrical death."

The lesson here is that all episodes of *loss of consciousness*, however brief, occurring during or immediately after exercise, should be assumed to be cardiac in origin. The patient should be subjected to a thorough physical and cardiovascular examination including an exercise test, and his cardiac rhythm should be monitored for prolonged periods until either a treatable abnormality is found, or until it can safely be concluded that the likelihood of further dysrhythmic episodes is remote.

To sum up, exercise-induced deaths are rare, but inevitably they do occur. Despite suggestions to the contrary, those physicians who are involved on a day-to-day basis in training individuals with latent and overt coronary artery disease can often recognize and prevent potential hazards. Needless to say, it is impossible to prove that anticipatory action in the form of anti-dysrhythmic medications, or advice regarding reduction of exercise intensity has been successful in preventing an exercise death. However, results of successful post-coronary exercise programs are revealing. The Toronto program has been in operation since 1968, and has exercised over five and a half thousand heart attack patients. The incidence of exercise-related non-fatal heart attacks has been one for every 271,359 hours of exercise, and that of fatal heart attacks one for every 193,821 hours of exercise. This compares very favourably with the findings of William Haskell, who summarized the experience of 103 different post-coronary exercise programs, involving a total of 1,629,634 patient hours of supervised exercise. The average complication rate for all programs was one non-fatal and one fatal event for every 34,673, and 116,402 patient hours of participation respectively. There is no doubt that a medically pre-scribed exercise training program is extremely safe even when applied to patients with proven heart disease.

In the final analysis, surely the fact that the recent worldwide explosion in the number of joggers has not been accompanied by an immediate and proportionate increase in sudden jogging deaths attests in the most dramatic and eloquent way possible to jogging's inherent safety.

CHAPTER TWELVE

The Marathon

Since the Toronto heart patients ran the Boston Marathon in 1973, marathon running has become the North American national participation sport. By the end of the 1970s, there were over 300 official marathon races held in the United States; the most prestigious of all, the Boston Marathon, had well over 5,000 official entrants, as well as 2,000 unofficial starters! A far cry from the mere handful of runners who customarily started out from Hopkinton, Massachusetts in the 1930s and 1940s. The upstart New York Marathon, with a route which winds through all five boroughs of the "Big Apple," had to cope with some 14,000 entrants in 1979. The London Marathon has a cut-off point — 19,000 entrants! And so it goes, with larger and larger numbers of people wanting to finish the gruelling 26¼ miles.

Who are these masochists? Are they the new wave of hippies and weirdos? Anything but. Many of them are business executives and professionals. Yet the number of honest-to-God hardcore competitive marathon runners has not increased significantly. Undoubtedly, there are more sub-2½ hour marathoners than there were ten years ago, but one swallow doesn't make a summer. No, the bulk of this new wave of joggers is made up of people who enter for the same reason that my post-coronary joggers did when they took part in their first Boston Marathon back in 1973. It is a goal, a target to aim for. In a world where regretfully (but all too frequently), the winner is not just the smartest on the job but also the one who happens to know the right people (and in the right order), one cannot deny the appeal of making it on your own. One of my post-coronary marathoning patients put it to me like this, "When you train for a marathon, you know that no-one can do your homework for you."

Certainly anyone who takes up marathon jogging for his health can expect it to provide the physiological and psychological advantages of long distance running in general. But there is no magic in the marathon distance. Actually, in recent years, the original Bassler theory (that the completion of the marathon distance in 4½ hours or less confers an immunity from a fatal heart attack for two to three years) has become magnified out of all proportion.

The story of the "marathon controversy" is worth the telling if only to demonstrate how, from time to time, even the most clear-thinking scientists can get themselves sidetracked. The stage was set when Dr. Tom Bassler, a Californian pathologist, stated that he had never performed an autopsy on a non-smoking marathoner and found the cause of death to be coronary atherosclerosis. Neither, he said, did he expect to. He then propounded his contentious theory maintaining that the marathoner's lifestyle was incompatible with fatal coronary atherosclerosis. Further, he challenged physicians to produce autopsy evidence that would contradict his statement.

The outcome was predictable. Most physicians, as well as the lay media, accepted the claim for what it was worth. After all, our own Toronto post-coronary program had already demonstrated in the most dramatic way that individuals with indisputable evidence of coronary atherosclerosis, including angiography, can train for and complete marathons. A few responded more vigorously, producing case after case which purported to destroy the Bassler hypothesis. But that wasn't as easy as it looked. Electrocardiographic evidence of heart disease was not acceptable, nor were classical symptoms of a heart attack. Nothing more than an autopsy would suffice! Not only that, but the findings at autopsy had to show that death was due to a heart attack brought about by recent blockage of a coronary artery, and Bassler demanded proof that the deceased had *completed* a marathon within a specified period of time. When subjected to these criteria, the counter-arguments failed. Meanwhile, as the increasing hordes of joggers went quietly about their daily training programs, the hard-core protagonists on both sides continued the debate as if it were of apocalyptic magnitude. For myself, I always saw Bassler's theory as a novel and provocative philosophy, something to discuss over a friendly beer or even during a fun marathon jog. Besides, even if I cannot accept Bassler's argument in total, I share his belief in the healthy value of jogging.

Attacks on the Bassler bastion have come from Cape Town, South Africa, where Dr. Tim Noakes reports four cases of autopsy-proved coronary atherosclerosis in marathon runners. One runner with severe coronary atherosclerosis died during a 15-mile race; another had a heart attack and died in hospital while awaiting coronary bypass surgery. Two others killed in an automobile accident were found to have coronary atherosclerosis on post-mortem examination. (Interestingly, one of the two runners who actually died as the result of a heart attack was a smoker. The other had only been running long-distance events for 14 months; in this period, he entered and finished eight standard marathons, a 35-mile race and a 56-mile race.) Thus it would now seem, at least on the face of it, that the Bassler imperative can be laid to rest. If so (and we have to see Bassler's rebuttal yet), then we can all take pleasure in the fact that the coup was delivered by a likeable young physician who is a keen marathoner himself and who, gracious in victory, is quick to comment: ''We cannot prove that marathon running did not reduce the rate of progression of coronary atherosclerosis in these or other athletes. Nor can we prove that if these men had not been marathon runners, they would not have died sooner.''

This attitude is in sharp contrast to the Jeremiahs who, startled by Bassler's approach, have attacked the whole concept of long distance running on the basis that it is too dangerous. I am all for caution; recklessness can never be the hallmark of a successful exercise program. But I think we should be very careful that we don't frighten people away from healthy, strenuous endeavour. After all, what is left for the individual to challenge in today's world? Politics, business, interpersonal relationships are all so complex that effort is synonymous with stress. In the sixties, the young turned left from all this; they dropped out, refused to play, made failure a fetish. The eighties generation has, I believe, developed a much healthier approach. Like the Greeks (and even the much despised Victorians), they sense the harmony that must exist between a healthy mind and a healthy body. They seem to be discovering that discord in this interrelationship can have disastrous consequences. Oh, I admit that the symbolism is obvious. We are all running away from something. But in a way, that is a perfectly healthy reaction. Nature intended that we only stand and fight if we have a good chance of winning. If we can't win, then we were meant to run. Standing still in the face of imminent danger or, to put it another way, leading a sedentary life of constant anxiety, is an inappropriate action which ultimately leads to health breakdown. Movement placates the primitive brain, keeps it happy and ensures the efficient operation of all those intricate bodily mechanisms which are totally independent of the brain.

All of the foregoing may help you decide whether or not you want to prepare for a fun marathon. In the final analysis, you have to make your own decision. But maybe it will help if we look at the practical pros and cons.

PROS

Despite the introduction of such unofficial distances as 50 miles and 100 miles, the marathon 26 miles, 385 yards (or, in metric, 42 kilometres) still remains the longest official foot-race held under the auspices of the International Amateur Athletic Federation, the world's governing body of track and field. Thus, all official marathon races have to receive approval of that body or its local representative. This means that the course must be over a road surface, must be very accurately measured, must be kept clear of vehicular traffic during the competition and, while being challenging, should not be "impossible." The officials, including the timers, must be certified as competent, and the timekeeping apparatus must be checked for accuracy. The official nature of the contest endows it with a considerable air of status. Make no mistake about it, there is a great feeling of achievement in finishing. You walk ten feet tall for weeks afterwards.

Even the start of a marathon race is exciting. The atmosphere is almost carnival-like. Gathered together behind the starting line are thousands of individuals with similar interests, but from all walks of life. You are all there for the same purpose—to test your body's capacity to finish the same course under the same climatic conditions and in accordance with the same rules. Favouritism is impossible. In such circumstances, one can appreciate the deep sense of camaraderie which exists among fun marathoners. For them, it is a paramount ingredient of the whole proceedings. In this regard, you have to pity the serious competitor who can only allow himself the luxury of empathizing with his fellow runner after the race is over. The occasion, then, is a great motivator. Wherever it takes place, be it New York, Boston, Detroit, Toronto or Honolulu, its anticipation sustains you through those days when cheerless circumstances all combine to make those first few steps of your workout a supreme triumph of will over won't!

As a benchmark of your cardiovascular fitness, you probably couldn't choose better than a marathon, for more than fitness is required. You also require self-discipline not only in training, but also on the day of the race when you must keep a pace that is well within your capacity. There is nothing like a marathon to expose the foolhardy, those who consistently over-estimate their own capabilities.

Finally, when all the shouting has died down, most of us have to agree that marathoners seem to have the sort of metabolic and biochemical programming that scientists have consistently associated with a low incidence of coronary heart disease: slim, almost skinny, with minimal body fat, non-smokers, possessing a slowly beating, powerfully stroking heart and with high levels of so-called protective (or HDL) cholesterol. It would be surprising if such types didn't have noticeably less incidence of heart attacks.

CONS

If you don't like crowds, then you'd better pick your marathons carefully. Since becoming a national craze, the number of entrants in most of the major events can be counted in the thousands rather than the hundreds. So you are now faced with the hassle of finding suitable accommodation before the race. The last time I brought thirteen of my patients to take part in the New York Marathon, we had to book our rooms six months ahead of time! On the plus side, the New York Marathon is a model of efficiency. The same cannot be said for many other less well-organized races. What worked beautifully for 300 or 400 competitors becomes a disaster area when applied to 5,000 or 6,000 runners. On balance, the increased numbers tend to bring out more cheering onlookers and enhance the carnival atmosphere, and so can't be entirely condemned. Nevertheless, the mass marathons are not for the fastidious!

Another side effect of mass participation is the arrival of the pseudo-scientific gimmickry, the exhibitions which are now associated with the run and in which one must endure the spectacle of stall after stall displaying running shoes, sweat suits, stop watches, socks, pedometers, vitamins, food supplements, insoles, arch supports, shoe repair outfits, heart rate monitors, energy drinks, T-shirts, I.D. bracelets, treadmills, wrist radios, head band radios, reflective tape, anti-chafe cream, anti-sunburn cream, books on running, magazines on running, audio cassettes on running, etc., etc., etc. Some of the products currently on the market are of great help to runners. But for those who relish the simplicity of jogging, today's commercialism comes as a bit of a jolt.

The decision to enter a marathon requires, as you will see later in this chapter, a considerable commitment on your part. If you are to do yourself justice, avoid injury or accident, then you must be prepared to invest roughly the equivalent of a day a week in training time. If you are compulsive, competitive or careless of the signals given out by a tired or strained body, then you should think twice before you take up marathoning. Remember that all athletic injuries are self-inflicted wounds invariably caused by 1) exceeding your current level of competence either in terms of speed, duration or frequency of workout session; 2) not allowing for the effect of external conditions such as hills, head wind or rough ground; or 3) ignoring the signs of fatigue, lack of sleep, infections, etc. You can only draw on your body's reserve of energy for so long; sooner or later, the debt must be repaid. The marathon is the day of reckoning. It tests your personality as much as your physical endurance. If you suspect that either is likely to be found wanting, then better give it a miss — at least until you come to terms with yourself.

Having read all of the above, let's assume you decide to have a go. What's the next step? You must prepare yourself. That means a training program. It is not my intention to compete with the avalanche of running books which have appeared on the market over the past ten years or so. My advice will be strictly limited to the middle-aged jogger who is planning to enter his or her first marathon, whose sole aim is to finish — not necessarily in good time, but certainly in good shape. Furthermore, it is assumed that you are already at the stage of being able to jog six miles in one hour (10-minute mile pace) five times weekly; that is, you are jogging 30 miles a week. If you are not yet at this stage, then you have to work up to it before following the marathon training plan. I do have some patients who have successfully completed a marathon and cannot jog faster than a 12-minute mile pace, but they are exceptions, and I invariably like to train them on a personal basis, running with them myself.

PREPARATION

First, pick your initial marathon carefully. Avoid a very hilly course or one that has a reputation for strong head winds. Try to stay away from the hot part of the year; if the temperature is likely to be high, make sure the organizers of the race have a good track record for supplying plenty of ice and fluid along the route. Most important of all, make sure that the race is one which welcomes joggers. A serious, competitive marathon attracts top-class runners whose sole purpose in being there is to win or make a good time. In such company, joggers will invariably get under the feet of runners and officials alike. Not only that, but it is expected that no one will be out on the course longer than 3 hours, or 3½ at the most. So when you cross the finish line in 4½ or 5 hours, you may be shattered to find there is no line; it has been erased, the timekeepers have gone home, and the changing rooms are probably locked. A large marathon nowadays often caters to both top-flight runners and fun joggers (the overwhelming numbers of joggers providing a most welcome bonanza in entry fees). In this case, the rule at the start is runners in the front rank, joggers behind. These days it is not unusual for joggers like myself to discover it takes five or six minutes from the time the gun goes off to reach the starting line! Incidentally, your best source of information for all of the above points is a good journal such as *Runners World* or, better still, another jogger. You will be surprised to find how anxious other joggers are to help.

Well, you've picked your first marathon. How do you train for it? Before getting into that, I would like to make one point which I suppose should be self-evident. If there were such a thing as the perfect training method, then every coach and every athlete would be using it. In reality, there are as many training schedules as there are athletes using them. The more one studies the training methods of world-class athletes, the more variations you see. Why is that? Again, I think the answer is obvious. When one is striving for excellence, every strength must be exploited, every weakness must be minimized. The game plan, if it is to be successful, must be custom-designed, not an off-the-shelf item. Your needs are not so critical. Nevertheless, you should take a lesson from your

betters. The smart thing to do is to learn the accepted basic training principles for your chosen event, and then use them to modify the program you are following. Tables printed in a book, no
matter how good that book is (and that includes this one), should
never be adhered to slavishly. Look at it like this: the more successful the book is, the more copies it will sell and, therefore, the
more individuals will read it. Do you honestly think that a training schedule drawn up for a million aspiring athletes is going to
suit all of them? I would be surprised if it worked for 50 per cent.

Basic Principles of a Long Distance Training Program

In order to jog 26 miles, 385 yards non-stop, you have to cover a
considerable number of miles in training. Furthermore, the mileage must consist of both medium and long distance runs. In addition to increasing your ability to utilize oxygen, long runs teach
the body to become more efficient in utilizing fat as a working
fuel. The primary source of energy used by muscle is carbohydrate,
in the form of glycogen (see Chapter 3). When the muscle burns
up all its available supply of glycogen, it is no longer able to
function. This is what happens when your legs give out on a long
run — "hitting the wall," they call it. But the muscles can also
burn fat and don't hesitate to do so when their glycogen store
starts to run low. Fat-burning becomes a significant factor in muscle metabolism on any run in excess of 6 miles, which is why that
distance has been chosen as the basic training unit in the marathon training tables that follow on page 286. It is only by running
six miles and up that you accustom your system to using fat as a
fuel, thus eking out the precious supply of energy-rich glycogen.

   Given that mileage is a prerequisite, the next obvious question
to be answered is, how much? There is a theory that if you want
to be sure of finishing a certain distance in a race, your average
daily mileage (seven days a week) for eight weeks before the
race should be one-third of the race distance; that is, for the marathon you would have to jog 62 miles a week for eight weeks prior
to the day of the race. This rule of thumb works quite well and
has stood the test of time. However, I have found that for the
fun jogger who is maintaining a year-round average of about
30 miles a week and who is not concerned with finishing times,
this order of mileage may be a little on the high side and can be
reduced by about 10 per cent. Is there a total mileage which you
should have completed before entering your first marathon? Em-

pirically and based on experience with post-coronary middle-aged patients, I have established the "1,000-mile rule." Simply put, it states that the beginning marathoner must have jogged a minimum of 1,000 miles in training before being allowed to enter. In addition, for the reasons stated above, the mileage should be calculated in units of six miles, in other words, anything less than six miles doesn't count — only six miles and over. In the final three months before the marathon, the requirement is for 48 to 60 miles a week (eight to ten six-mile units), using a judicious blend of six (one unit), twelve (two units) and eighteen (three units) jogs.

Build-up versus Breakdown

You can define training as the repeated application of measured doses of stress to the body to stimulate the development of beneficial chemical and biological changes. The net result is greater resistance to the stress applied. Strength through adversity, as it were. However, it is not too difficult to imagine a situation in which the amount or duration of stress is so great that it overwhelms the body's defences completely before it has had time to become stronger. In some ways, excessive training is worse than no training at all. This may seem obvious, but this is probably the most difficult point to put across to any athlete. It seems we always get back to the old business of "if one pill is good for you, then two pills are twice as good for you, and four pills are four times as good for you!"

It may help to look at it like this. Training is a two-stage process. The first stage consists of the application of the stimulus or, in our terms, the workout. The second stage consists of the body's responses to that stimulus. This latter stage is just as important as the first and, as a matter of fact, requires a greater period of time. Thus, if you are to get benefit from your workout, you must allow time for the body to complete the job. If you apply the stimulus again and again, not allowing for any response, a training effect can never occur. Worse, the whole system begins to break down, the athlete's performances rapidly deteriorate, resistance to disease drops, and illness occurs.

How can we avoid this? Firstly, by adopting a training schedule which alternates periods of heavy work with periods of light work, long runs with middle-distance runs, faster runs with slower runs. We can also be constantly on the lookout for signs of overtraining. The main ones are:

- fall in body weight below the usual training level;
- irritability and insomnia;
- muscle ache in the legs at night in bed;
- running nose, often lasting only for a day or two and frequently attributed to a cold or allergy;
- tendency to minor gastro-intestinal upsets (e.g., nausea, diarrhea);
- vague aching pain in the joints, not accompanied by redness or swelling;
- sore throat; enlarged glands in the neck, under the arms, or in the groins; and
- tendency to uncoordination (e.g., tripping, becoming ''accident-prone'').

If you suspect over-training, then obviously the first thing to do is check your average mileage over the previous few months. Remember to take into account the speed of the jogs, the presence of adverse physical conditions such as high humidity, hills, poor running surface. And finally, make sure you're not burning the candle at both ends. You can't expect to keep up a heavy training schedule if you are working twice as hard at your job.

Natural Endowment

Never forget that all the training in the world is not going to turn a cart-horse into a Kentucky Derby contender. As a fun jogger, that shouldn't worry you. But if you start to become too ambitious, you might bear it in mind. There are such things as born marathoners just as there are born sprinters. These days, exercise physiologists are prone to carry out what they call muscle biopsies and talk knowingly about fast-twitch and slow-twitch fibres. The procedure consists of removing a minute piece of muscle tissue from deep within the muscle by means of a small needle-like instrument. Examined under a microscope, the muscle is seen to contain two types of fibres, slow and fast twitch. The higher the percentage of slow-twitch fibres present, the more the individual is suited to endurance type running. Conversely, the greater the percentage of fast-twitch fibres, the greater the propensity for speed. While training is thought to be able to improve the metabolic efficiency of both types of fibres, it seems unlikely that it can effect any marked change in their relative proportion. So don't expect training to achieve miracles. You are in it for your health, not just to beat that scraggy guy with the thin legs who always seems to run farther and faster than you, no matter how hard you try to catch him.

The training tables that follow are designed for the fun jogger, post-coronary or otherwise, who has achieved Level 6 of Phase 3 of the general training tables: i.e., six miles at the 10 or 12-minute mile pace, five times weekly, and who has been carrying this out easily and without symptoms or discomfort for a period of at least three months. The aim is to enable you to finish a marathon safely in a time of between 4½ and 6½ hours, depending on your initial level of fitness. They incorporate the following principles:

1) There are five stages, each of three weeks, between the basic 30 miles a week level and the start of a three-month preparation period for the marathon itself. When you are "coasting" between marathons, depending upon the weekly mileage you wish to maintain, you can choose any one of the five stages as a "holding pattern."

2) Since endurance, not speed, is our goal, no training jog is shorter than six miles.

3) Distances in excess of six miles are at proportionately slower pace (see Table 8). The purpose of training is to build up, not tear down. I am well aware that you are capable of running these longer distances quicker than the times specified, just as I am also aware that a 60-minute six-miler can run one single mile in 8 minutes or less. The fact is that many world-class marathoners do the bulk of their training at speeds 30 to 40 per cent slower than their best competition times. If it is good enough for them, why not us? Try, therefore, not to exceed the prescribed speeds.

4) Included in the workouts are a number of "speed-play" sessions where only the actual duration of the training session is given; the distance covered is ignored. For instance, a 4-hour speed-play session means that you walk and jog, comfortably and easily, for that period of time. I enjoy these sessions. They make a pleasant break, boost your morale, and help to prepare you mentally for being out on the marathon course for that period of time. The trick is to start slowly, and introduce the walk/jog sessions (say 5 minutes walk followed by 10 minutes jog) right from the outset. Don't jog until you are too tired to go any further, and then have to start walking.

5) Because the body needs rest as part of its building-up

Table 6   You are already jogging 30 miles a week, comfortably

	Stage 1			Stage 2			Stage 3			Stage 4			Stage 5		
Week	1	2	3	1	2	3	1	2	3	1	2	3	1	2	3
Day															
1	R	R	R	R	R	R	R	R	R	R	R	R	R	R	R
2	6	6	6	6	6	6	9	8	9	8	9	8	6	9	6
3	6	6	6	6	6	6	7	8	7	8	9	8	9	9	9
4	6	6	6	9	9	9	7	8	7	8	9	8	9	9	9
5	6	6	6	6	6	6	7	8	7	9	9	9	9	9	9
6	R	R	R	R	R	R	R	R	R	R	R	R	R	R	R
7	9	9	9	9	9	9	10	8	10	12	9	12	15	SP	15
Total														(4 hr)	
Mileage	33	33	33	36	36	36	40	40	40	45	45	45	48		48

Key: R = Rest   SP = Speed Play   M = Marathon

Table 7   Three-month preparation leading to marathon

	Month 1				Month 2				Month 3				Marathon
Week	1	2	3	4	1	2	3	4	1	2	3	4	Week
Day													
1	R	R	R	R	R	R	R	R	R	R	R	R	R
2	8	9	8	10	10	6	6	8	R	8	9	9	10
3	9	12	9	10	6	10	10	10	12	6	9	9	R
4	9	10	9	6	10	10	9	8	10	12	9	9	R
5	9	10	7	12	9	12	10	6	12	10	9	7	R
6	R	R	R	R	R	R	R	R	R	R	R	R	R
7	18	12	20	SP	18	SP	18	SP	12	12	10	10	M
Total				(4 hr)	(4 hr)		(5 hr)						26¹/₄
Mileage	53	53	53		53		53		46	48	46	44	36¹/₄

Table 8   Pacing table

		Time
Miles	Min. per mile	Total (hours)
6	10	1:00:00
7	10	1:10:00
8	10	1:20:00
9	10¹/₂	1:34:30
10	10¹/₂	1:45:00
12	11	2:12:00
15	11	2:45:00
18	12	3:36:00
20	12	4:00:00

program, long, hard workouts are alternated with shorter jogs or rest days, both on a daily and weekly basis.

6) Our customary five days a week training schedule has been retained, and the highest weekly mileage has been held to between 45 and 53 miles. Admittedly, running six or even seven times a week will "up" the mileage considerably and produce faster racing times. But we are not racing, and 30 minutes or even 60 minutes saved in a marathon is scant compensation for the fun jogger whose hitherto enjoyable workout has become a relentless, deadly grind. So, if you want to race, or feel that you are too good for the 60-minute six-mile class, then skip these tables, and look elsewhere for advice.

THE BIG DAY

Finally, the moment of truth has arrived. Your training has gone to plan, you have by luck as much as by good management avoided injury, and in a matter of hours you will be embarking on one of the most interesting if not most exciting experiences of your life. If you are smart, you will have checked out all your final preparations with an experienced marathoner. If you are lucky, you will be in the company of such an individual who will inevitably save you from the classic beginner's mistakes. Failing both, you will just have to read this section carefully. If you find it a little trite, then I assure you you are the very person who needs it. Admitted, these are the sort of obvious comments which you won't find in the high-powered training manuals — but I'll bet the majority of marathoners would have welcomed them in the early stages of their careers.

The Week Before

To deal with the question of carbohydrate loading, we have to go back to the week before the big event. Even if you don't follow this procedure, you should know something about it. Carbohydrates, sugars and starches are the body's major sources of energy. After digestion, they are broken down into glucose, a substance easily burned up by working muscle. Glucose, however, is an immediate source of energy and so when we eat more carbohydrate than we need for the time being, the body changes it into glycogen and stores it in both muscle and liver. This store can be called upon in times of need (e.g., running a marathon) and converted back into the easily utilized glucose. Obviously the greater the store of glycogen in your muscles, the more muscular work you will be able to do. Carrying the argument further, the way to increase the glycogen stores is to increase the intake of carbohydrate foods while at the same time limiting muscular action to a minimum.

This is the basic theory of carbohydrate loading. There are one or two refinements. If you drain the muscle of its glycogen content first, then you can stuff more glycogen in during the high carbohydrate ingestion. How do you drain the muscle of glycogen? Once glycogen is stored in muscle, the only way to get it out is for the muscle to burn it. This means going for a run which is long enough and fast enough to make your legs ache and become a little wobbly — and then plod on for about another mile! Obviously the distance will vary with individuals, but for the fun jogger it is probably around six to ten miles. On the three succeeding days following this workout the muscle glycogen level is kept at extremely low levels by adhering to a diet which contains only minimal amounts of carbohydrates (about 60 grams a day), and is very high in fat and protein. During this ''depletion'' stage, you may jog three miles or so daily but don't be surprised if your legs feel like lead and you find yourself becoming increasingly ill-tempered and depressed. The three days of high-fat, high-protein diet finishes with another leg-aching depletion run of about five miles (if you really restricted the carbohydrates you may be labouring as early as two miles). Finally, you reward yourself by switching to very high carbohydrate foods for the final three days before the marathon. Since you are trying to conserve every gram of the extra muscle glycogen you have managed to store, you do not do any exercising or running at all during this stage. Eat little and often, use natural carbohydrates such as fruits, cereals and whole-wheat bread, rather than cakes and candies, which are loaded with refined sugar. If all works to plan, then you can expect to have a good deal more spring in your legs over the last four to six miles of the marathon run.

Are there any provisos? The first thing to note is that for every gram of glycogen stored by the muscle, three grams of water are stored at the same time. It is for this reason that you should drink plentiful supplies of water during the three-day carbohydrate loading phase. But this additional stored water means an increase in body weight, and all that much more to carry over

the 26 miles, 385 yards; which is why some world-class marathoners who are strong on endurance but slow on speed do not
carbohydrate-load before an important race. The additional
weight slows them up in the initial stages of the race, the period
in which they are most vulnerable. This increase in weight, as a
matter of interest, provides a method of checking the effectiveness of your carbohydrate-loading program during the high carbohydrate stage. You should weigh yourself every morning; when
maximum glycogen storage has been achieved, your weight will
increase by two or three pounds. So you must balance the advantages of the extra glycogen against the disadvantages of the additional weight. There is one set of circumstances in which the stored
water, extra weight or no extra weight, can come to your help.
When you know that the run is going to be held in conditions of
high temperature or high humidity and that dehydration is an
ever-present threat, then maximal glycogen loading means that
you start the run with a water storage of about 2½ pints. This
represents a reserve within the muscle cells which can afford to
be lost in heavy sweating.

I have one other reservation to make on the subject of carbohydrate loading. A preliminary high-fat, high-protein diet is the least
important aspect of the process — in fact, some authorities feel
that it has no value at all. But, more important from the point of
view of the middle-aged male, it may result in a precipitate rise in
blood fat levels, with all its attendant dangers to the cardiovascular system. For those of us in that age group, then, I suggest you
miss out this stage.

The Day Before the Day

This can be a critical period. Your diet should be light, easily di-
gested. You will receive all sorts of advice from faddists, ranging
from fruit juices for 24 hours to steaks for breakfast, and I suppose there will be the odd individual who performs well on these
regimes. In general, you will do best to stay with small amounts of
what you fancy. I never cease to be amazed by the unerring accuracy by which the long distance jogger's appetite chooses that
which his body needs the most!

But diet isn't everything. You should try and get an early night;
even if excitement keeps you awake until the early hours, console yourself with the thought that insomnia will not take its toll
on your physical performance until the day *after* the race. Of course,

you will have checked all the practicalities. You will have packed your shoes (in which you have run at least 200 miles) and also packed a spare pair of laces. There is nothing more frustrating than breaking a lace just before the start and not having a spare. I hate to admit it, but I have arrived in Reno the night before the Silver City Marathon and been devastated to find that I had forgotten to pack my running shoes. If it were not for the incredible tolerance and kindness of the race organizer who persuaded the proprietor of the local Athlete's Foot Store (another jogger) to open his establishment and help get me fitted with a pair of Etonics, I would have had to pad the entire distance in bare feet! I have even been known to pack two left shoes. Fortunately, my jogging patients are now familiar with this weakness and invariably check my running gear before I leave Toronto.

Another invaluable item is a jar of vaseline. There is nothing worse than trying to run the last three of four miles of a marathon with agonizingly chafing thighs. Never mind that flies, road dirt and assorted airborne items stick to your person, you should be sure to apply vaseline liberally to your inner thighs, nipples, armpits and anal area.

The Morning of the Race

No matter how early the race starts, you are obliged to get out of bed about four hours beforehand. Otherwise, you won't have left enough time to digest your breakfast. Many competitors are happy to go to the starting line with just a slice of toast and a glass of orange juice. Others require something more substantial. Whatever you do, try not to eat within three hours of the starting time; that will leave enough time for digestion. Breakfast should be light enough to have passed the stomach within a three-hour period which means that protein (bacon, sausage, steak) and fatty foods are prohibited.

Immediate pre-race nutritional needs are minimal. I advise my joggers to pre-hydrate, and so 20 minutes before the start, they drink half a pint of water. Don't worry about having to urinate during the run; marathon joggers, both male and female, never suffer from false modesty and always manage to find convenient bushes or stone walls along the route. Some runners have the false impression that high sugar content drinks or glucose tablets taken within 30 to 60 minutes of the start will provide extra energy. Nothing could be further from the truth! The intake of sugar just before physical exercise results in a compensatory drop in blood glucose; this leads to a premature breakdown of the glycogen store in the muscle in order to bring the blood glucose back to normal levels. Thus, the muscle glycogen is used at an earlier stage in the race than normal and, consequently, is used up all the more quickly.

During the Race

Try to drink fluid, about 8 to 10 ounces, every 20 to 30 minutes. Water is probably best, althought slight fruit flavouring may be more appealing to the taste.

The more efficiently your muscles burn fat, the more sparing you are of your glycogen store. Recently there has been some evidence to suggest that the ingestion of caffeine about an hour before a long run will stimulate the breakdown of fat. So you might try a strong cup of coffee or tea 60 minutes before the start; but remember that caffeine also has a diuretic effect (i.e. it makes you pass urine more frequently). This may be a nuisance under normal conditions, but in the hot weather, it could aggravate the risk of dehydration.

You are now ready to make your way to the starting line. Unless it is very warm, you should keep your sweat suit on until a few minutes before the one-minute warning gun. You have applied your vaseline, adjusted your sweat headband, double-tied your shoelaces, pinned your number to the front of your running vest, made the last of what seems to have been innumerable visits to the toilet over the past few hours, put a quarter in your sock in order to make a telephone call in case you get stranded along the way, and handed your carefully wrapped belongings to your long-suffering wife or the appropriate race official. You are ready to go.

For those who merely want to finish, the die is cast in the first two miles. This is especially true for the novice marathoner. It's not until you enter your first race that you have any conception of the excitement at the start. You need a will of iron not to go charging off with the other thousands, elbow to elbow and shoulder to shoulder, caught up in a human cavalry charge that will take you to the five-mile point at a speed you never thought you were capable of. By then, it's too late. You've blown it. By the tenth mile, you are uncomfortable; by the fourteenth, you are praying you can finish; and by the twentieth, you have accepted the inevitability of having to drop out.

The answer is obvious. *Start slowly!* I can't emphasize that enough. Don't worry about letting people get ahead of you. I can assure you that if you have trained properly, and if your only aim is to finish, you will invariably experience the ecstasy of passing people one by one in the last two to three miles. If you feel embarrassed at being so far behind in the initial stages of the run, console yourself with the thought that the onlookers reserve their cheers for the first 50 and the last 200 finishers. If it's crowd adulation you want, then you can always double the cheering by putting on a teeth-gritting, true blue, stiff upper lip expression over the final 100 yards.

Two other points. If you fall into a conversation with a fellow jogger along the way, make sure you don't unintentionally fall into running at his pace — unless you know him well and are sure that he plans to finish in the same time as you. It's easy to get carried along and find you've run two or three miles at a minute or more faster per mile than you had planned. Secondly, don't experiment with new drinks along the way. If you trained using water, then don't try some other type of drink. I can recall one of Canada's marathon champions, Jerome Drayton, experimenting with a proprietary electrolyte drink in the Fukuoka Marathon in Japan and having to drop out with severe cramps. There was nothing wrong with the drink, it was just that he wasn't used to it. If a runner of Jerome's stature and experience can fall into that trap, how much easier for you as a novice.

From time to time in the first 20 miles, remind yourself that the marathon really only starts at 20 miles! That will keep you from squandering your energy too early in the game. Let's face it, many people can complete a 20-mile jog. It's the last six that separates the men from the boys. If your legs begin to feel very tired before the finish, there is no shame in walking for a few hundred yards and then picking up the jog again. In fact, I believe that it is better to slow to a walk from time to time when you still have some strength left, rather than grimly plodding along in a pathetic semblance of the jog only to slow to a walk out of complete necessity. When that happens, it is extremely unlikely that you will be able to get back into jogging tempo again.

Above all, don't race! Leave that to the talented young guys — or the dumb old ones. I realize it may require will power, but it really isn't going to make that much difference whether you finish in 4 hours, 30 minutes or 4 hours, 20 minutes. If you have a problem with your ego, don't let your nearest and dearest watch you. They won't be impressed by the sight of their hero, slack-jawed and blue in the face, trying to grunt his way past a sweet, smiling old lady or a rotund, middle-aged executive with a "Joggers Make Better Lovers" message on his T-shirt. Actually, it is probably better not to have your nearest and dearest anywhere near the finish at all. You probably look so haggard by then that you might be delivered an ultimatum to stop all this marathoning nonsense immediately — or else!

You've finished! I won't attempt to describe the feeling. Any words of mine would be superfluous. Now it's time for that beer (after a light sandwich), a shower, change, and start to put together the step-by-step, mile-by-mile narrative with which you are going to bore the office staff for the next few months — or until the next marathon!

Epilogue

This book started with the story of a rehabilitation success. Eight men ran along a road in Boston, and proved a point. There was nothing miraculous in what they did. In a way, the whole purpose of the exercise was to prove that very point; namely, it does not require a miracle for men or women who have had a heart attack to perform feats of physical endurance with safety. What it does require is motivation on their part and some informed medical guidance. Given these two ingredients, any post-coronary patient can learn to function maximally.

The results of the Toronto Rehabilitation Centre's post-coronary exercise program have been most encouraging. Acceptance of the program by the community, family physicians and cardiologists has been high. Currently the referral rate is running at 10 to 15 new patients a week. To facilitate this high patient load, a two-storey addition to the Centre was opened in 1980. The new building contains a 120-seat patients' lecture theatre, a Tartan-floored gymnasium, two exercise test laboratories, changing and shower areas, and office facilities. Attached to the new wing is an oval 200-metre artificial surface jogging track — a unique feature for a public hospital!

The exercise compliance rate has been excellent. A careful follow-up in 1976 of our first consecutively referred 610 patients showed that 82.8 per cent continued to exercise at least three times weekly, and only 2.8 per cent have ceased to exercise altogether.

Considering that the compliance rate in most programs is less than 50 per cent after two years, it is apparent that these results are exceptional and indicate that in virtually all patients the program effects a sustained alteration in their exercise pattern. These facts also give the lie to the repeated charge that jogging is boring and that few individuals will ever stick with a regular exercise regime that emphasizes only jogging.

To date, some 50 of our patients have taken part in a total of over 200 official marathon runs. These cardiac marathoners have not differed greatly in terms of their clinical history and running experience from the general post-coronary population. On admission to the program their cardiovascular fitness level was similar to that of the other patients, but in response to long and careful training they showed as much as a 55 per cent increase in their maximum oxygen consumption. These post-coronary marathoners have been generous in sharing their experiences with other patients and have continued to provide a constant source of encouragement for everyone else involved in the program.

How have our patients fared in terms of a second heart attack? In following the history of our first 610 patients for a period of twelve years, there has been an annual fatal recurrence rate of 1.7 per cent and a non-fatal recurrence rate of 1.0 per cent. Fatal and non-fatal recurrence rates were particularly low among patients who had exercised on the program for more than two years. In this group the recurrence rate was only 0.85 per cent per annum. These rates are considerably lower than the usual annual mortality of between 4 per cent and 6 per cent per year in the first five years after a heart attack; they are also consistent with the reports of others who have found that recurrence rates are lower in exercising than in non-exercising post heart attack patients.

However, while detailed statistical analysis is not appropriate for a book of this type, some interpretation of these results is necessary. It should be recognized that while they are highly suggestive of the efficacy of exercise in reducing recurrence, they cannot be accepted entirely as proof positive. Too many factors must be taken into account. For instance, like most other studies, we did not have an adequate control group of heart attack patients who were not exercised and who therefore could be compared with our patients. Then again, were the patients referred to the program the ones with the lowest recurrence risk? Were they, in other words, pre-selected or self-selected? My impression is that this is not so, but without assessing every other patient in Toronto who had a heart attack during the same period of time, one cannot be absolutely certain. Even if the referred patients are truly representative of all the other post-coronary patients, is it the exercise per se which is exerting this specific beneficial effect, or is it some other as yet unsuspected factor in the program's format? Again, one cannot be sure. All we can say is that the results indicate that our patients do well, and that the carefully prescribed vigorous exercise which they undertake does not increase their risk of dying suddenly or of suffering a further heart attack. In fact, our data and the data of William Haskell indicate that the risk of a heart attack occurring *during exercise* in a medically controlled rehabilitation program is no greater that that for the non-exercising post-coronary individual by chance alone.

At the same time, we must never lose sight of our goal: to successfully rehabilitate. Academic righteousness and statistical propriety should not be allowed to deny patients a method of therapy which cannot harm, and is to all intents and purposes most effective in improving the quality even if not the quantity of life. After all, in the final analysis, it is the quality of life which matters most.

I daresay 43-year-old Al V. would be happy to think he had another thirty years to live, but right now he is delighted to be able to work full-time, look after his young family, and go jogging five mornings a week — especially when you consider that just after his heart attack five years ago, he was referred to the Centre with the label "suitable for modified sedentary work only." At that time, he was well on his way to becoming a complete neurotic, imagined every ache and pain was the sign of another heart attack, and was reluctant to try anything but the lightest type of work. An immigrant from Europe, his comprehension of the English language was not as good as it might have been, and he responded poorly to the usual rehabilitation techniques involving psychotherapy and work assessment. After attending the Centre daily for almost a year, he was still no closer to going back to work. Finally, he was discharged to the evening exercise program where the only form of therapy was supervised jogging. Almost immediately his mood began to improve. With each increase in his prescription came renewed confidence until by the time he was able to jog three miles comfortably in 30 minutes, he had enthusiastically started to look for a job again. Right now, his greatest problem is low back trouble resulting from the heavy lifting required in his trade!

For some, the attraction of the program lies entirely in its ability to make life more enjoyable. This type of individual will usually continue to enjoy his cigarettes, his double martini before dinner, and his late-night weekend party, despite the possibility that all of these things, especially the smoking, may increase the risk of a recurrence. One advertising executive put it like this, "I'm not jogging to live longer. I'm jogging because it's made me fit, and I can now enjoy certain pleasures in life which have always been important to me. I no longer have angina when I stay up late at night, I can play longer and harder than ever before, and for me that's what living is all about." Obviously this man is interested in something more than marking off the days on a calendar, and mortality statistics mean nothing to him.

While we have talked much of the healthy, simple life associated with recreational running, we shouldn't become cult-like in our approach. I do have two patients who have given up their jobs to become mailmen. One had his own business, and the other was a salesman. In both their cases, the combination of heart attack and the running program made them realize that they preferred an active, open-air job. It's fair to say, however, that the vast majority of patients have returned to their previous employment, and a significant number have obtained better positions than they held before the heart attack. An analysis of their economic situations showed that less than 1 per cent had suffered a drop in living standards since their heart attack and as a result of the illness. This is a far cry from the state of affairs which existed before the era of rehabilitation, when many state and provincial authorities reported sadly that as much as 50 per cent and higher of heart attack survivors never returned to work.

That the fit post-coronary patient is also successful at his job is hardly surprising. The old dictum "a healthy mind in a healthy body" may have some justification after all, since numerous reports have verified that fitness is frequently associated with a superior self-image, better emotional control, increased self-confidence, and improved mental activity.

With increased self-confidence may come both welcome and sometimes unexpected bonuses. An example of the first is the heavy drinker or borderline alcoholic who now finds that he doesn't need liquor to bolster his self-esteem. An example of the second is the bachelor who had open-heart surgery, went on to complete two marathon runs and, if that weren't enough, proceeded at the age of 48 to get married and start a family.

Or, in a lighter vein, there is the patient who came to us with a cholesterol phobia so big that he wouldn't eat in a restaurant until he had inspected the kitchens and satisfied himself that the cook was using unsaturated cooking oil; he weakened once, ate a shrimp cocktail, and didn't sleep for weeks. He can now dare to contemplate eating an egg, and has almost ceased driving his wife and family physician crazy.

But, I can hear you say, what of the failures? Surely every case history is not a success story. You are right. Life isn't a fairy tale, and there is no medical treatment or rehabilitation program which promises immortality. I have already referred to the men who have suffered a fatal recurrence. A small group, admittedly, but none the less important for all that. That is why their histories are continuously reviewed in order to see if they contain a clue as to what went wrong. In most cases, one can only surmise the answer. Wherever there is a lesson to be learned, it is quickly introduced into the program format for the benefit of the other patients.

And then there are the dropouts. These are the individuals who couldn't accommodate to the new lifestyle required of them. Again, they are small in number, but there is less comfort in that, for these are often the very people who need the most help. It might have been easier to retain them by asking for an easier commitment, by making fewer demands, by bending the truth so as to make it more palatable; but that wouldn't be doing them any favours, and it would hardly be fair to the vast majority who have been prepared to go the whole course, both uphill and downhill.

On balance, I would say that the failures are so heavily outweighed by the successes that their main value is not to deter but rather to help formulate a better program. This is not meant to sound callous. It is the customary approach taken with any form of medical treatment, and is both rational and humane. The problem for those who use exercise in the treatment of heart disease is that they are allowed little, if any, margin for failure.

It is this which, in my opinion, has been largely responsible for the medical profession's reluctance to mobilize the post-coronary patient. Consider for a moment what happens if a heart patient undergoing rehabilitation drops dead in your local Y. Chances are that the incident will be fully reported in the morning paper, will probably receive mention on the town radio station, and might just make the tail-end of the late night T.V. news round-up. What if that patient were to die during heart surgery? It would likely receive no mention whatsoever in the media, unless he or she were someone of great importance. I realize that the exercise death may seem to be a more dramatic occurrence, taking place as it does in full view of the lay public. On the other hand, in some areas, post-coronary exercise rehabilitation is more common than by-pass surgery, has been around for a longer period of time, and has a far lower mortality rate. Which may put things a little more in perspective.

Yet every achievement has its failure, and every success story has its sad note. On February 15, 1975, "Big John," one of the original eight who ran the Boston Marathon in 1973, died in his sleep. An autopsy, while revealing the scars from his previous two heart attacks, failed to show any recent thrombosis of the coronary vessels or, indeed, any acute myocardial damage. It must be assumed that he died from a cardiac arrest, possibly due to some form of electrical failure. A regular distance jogger, he had been faithful to his program, although remaining a fairly heavy cigarette smoker, and there is some indication that his cigarette consumption increased in the months before his death. He had not run a marathon since 1973, largely because of business and social commitments, but was planning to take part again in 1975. Of the men who ran with him in 1973, some returned to Boston again in 1983, and their elation at doing so well was tinged by sorrow at the loss of a good friend. The mood was not entirely melancholy, however, for at the post-race dinner we all recalled again the letter from his wife which expresses better than I can, the sum and substance of these pages. I can think of no better way to end than with an appropriate excerpt:

"Knowing John's temperament, no one could have wished him a lingering end. I feel the program gave him seven vigorous and enjoyable years, living life the way he wanted to—to the hilt.

"He was a fine man—so have a brandy or a martini for him and we'll all be with you in spirit at the 'Boston'."

Nomograms

Nomogram C
Nomogram for Prediction of Maximum Oxygen Intake in Men Aged 25 and 35 Years

A line joining your heart rate and actual oxygen consumption will intersect the centre line at your maximum oxygen consumption.

Nomogram D
Nomogram for Prediction of Maximum Oxygen Intake
in Women Aged 25 and 35 Years

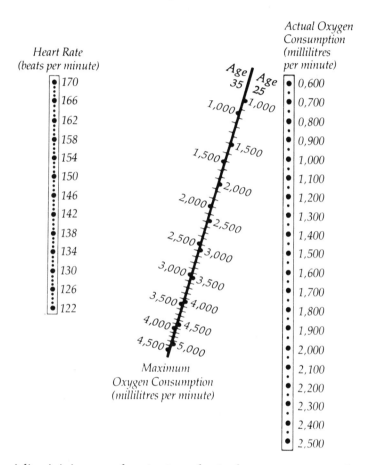

Heart Rate
(beats per minute)

Actual Oxygen Consumption (millilitres per minute)

A line joining your heart rate and actual oxygen consumption will intersect the centre line at your maximum oxygen consumption.

Nomogram E
Nomogram for Prediction of Maximum Oxygen Intake
in Men Aged 45 and 55 Years

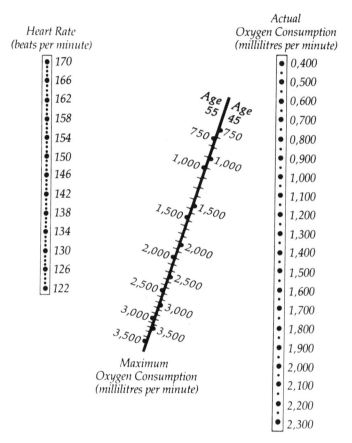

Heart Rate
(beats per minute)

Actual
Oxygen Consumption
(millilitres per minute)

Maximum
Oxygen Consumption
(millilitres per minute)

A line joining your heart rate and actual oxygen consumption will intersect the centre line at your maximum oxygen consumption.

Nomogram F
Nomogram for Prediction of Maximum Oxygen Intake
in Women Aged 45 and 55 Years

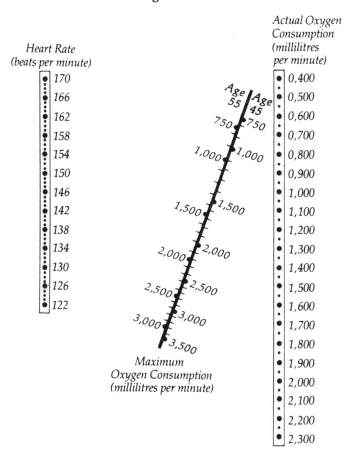

A line joining your heart rate and actual oxygen consumption will intersect the centre line at your maximum oxygen consumption.

Appendix

ˌ

TRAINING TABLES

To be used for determining your exercise prescription, *but* only after careful reading of the text.

If your predicted maximum oxygen consumption (VO_2 max.) is below 16 millilitres per kilogram per minute, or if you do not actually know what it is, begin at the Preliminary Phase, Level 1. If your maximum oxygen consumption is more than 16 millilitres per kilogram per minute, begin at the appropriate level in Phase 1 (see pages 132-33).

Ideally, in all Phases you should plan to exercise 5 times weekly.

Preliminary Phase

Levels to be taken in sequence.

Level 1   For 2 weeks walk 1 mile in 30 minutes
Level 2   For 2 weeks walk 1½ miles in 42 minutes
Level 3   For 2 weeks walk 2 miles in 50 minutes
Level 4   For 2 weeks walk 2½ miles in 57½ minutes

When you have completed the Preliminary Phase progress to Phase 1, Level 1.

Phase 1

For instructions on progressing through the levels of Phase 1, see page 129.

If you begin your exercise program at one of the levels in Phase 1 (see page 129), do not attempt at first the full prescription for your starting level. Instead, start with one third the starting prescription (e.g., at Level 1, walk 1 mile in 20 minutes if you are under age 45). After two weeks progress to two thirds the starting prescription (eg. 2 miles in 40 minutes, if under age 45 and at Level 1) for a further two weeks. Then, provided there are no adverse symptoms, proceed to the full three miles in the time prescribed for your starting level.

Phase 1

Level	Predicted maximum oxygen consumption (millilitres per kilogram per minute)	Distance (miles)	Time (minutes)	
			Under age 45	Over age 45
1	16.1 to 17.5 ml/kg/min	3	60	63
2	17.6 to 18.4 ml/kg/min	3	57	60
3	18.5 to 21.3 ml/kg/min	3	54	57
4	21.4 to 22.7 ml/kg/min	3	51	54
5	22.8 to 25.6 ml/kg/min	3	48	51
6	25.7 to 28.5 ml/kg/min	3	45	48
7	28.6 + ml/kg/min	3	42	45

Phase 2

For instructions on progressing through the levels of Phase 2, see pages 130-32.

Level	Under Age 45				Over Age 45			
	Distance (miles)	(metres)	Time (minutes)	Approx. Pace (mins./ mile)	Distance (miles)	(metres)	Time (minutes)	Approx. Pace (mins/ mile)
1	3	5,000	43½	14½	3		43½	14½
2	3	5,000	42	14	3		42	14
3	3	5,000	40½	13½(a)	3		40½	13½(a)
4	3	5,000	40½	13½(b)	3		40½	13½(b)
5	3	5,000	39	13	3		39	13
6	3	5,000	36	12	3		36	12
7	3¼	5,400	39	12	3¼		39	12
8	3½	5,800	42	12	3½		42	12
9	3¾	6,250	45	12	3¾		45	12
10	4	6,600	48	12	4		48	12
11	4	6,600	46	11½				
12	4	6,600	44	11				
13	4	6,600	42	10½	Metric equivalents are			
14	4	6,600	40	10	approximate			

If you have completed Phase 2, Level 11, and are now an enthusiastic jogger, you may progress to Phase 3.

Phase 3

For instructions on progressing through the levels of Phase 3, see page 132.

Level	Under age 45			Over Age 45	
	Distance (miles)	(metres)	Time (minutes)	Distance (miles)	Time (minutes)
1	4¼	6,800	42½	4½	51
2	4½	7,200	45	4½	54
3	4¾	7,600	47½	4¾	57
4	5	8,000	50	5	60
5	5½	8,800	55	5½	66
6	6	9,600	60	6	72

The predicted maximum oxygen consumption figures used in the Training Tables are based on values obtained from routine use of a sub-maximum, 9-minute, bicycle ergometer stress test.

Heat Safety Index

Wind Chill Factors

Wind Speed mph (km/h)*	Temperature °F (°C)*				
Calm	40(5)	35(2)	30(-1)	25(-3)	20(-1)
5(8)	35	30	25	20	15
10(16)	30	20	15	10	5
15(24)	25	15	10	0	-5
20(32)	20	10	5	0	-10
25(40)	15	10	0	-5	-15

Do not exercise out of doors when the wind chill factor is below the level indicated to the left of the heavy line.

*Metric equivalents are approximate

SOURCE: Adapted from a chart by Dr. Charles Egan

COLD WEATHER JOGGING MASK

The mask is made by attaching a simple plastic disposable oxygen mask to twelve inches of flexible plastic tubing. (Hudson No. 7 aerosol mask and Bennet No. 0848 flexible tube, ¾″ x 12″). A moleskin strip glued to the inner margin of the mask helps to prevent freezing around the edges. The mask fits over the nose and mouth and is held firmly in place by an elastic headband. The tubing extends beneath the subject's T-shirt to about the lower part of the chest. With this device angina patients can continue their outdoor exercise throughout the year.

CARDIOVASCULAR FITNESS LEVELS

The following is a rough guide to the level of cardiovascular fitness, expressed in walking or jogging pace, required for you to participate safely in various physical activities.

Sport	You should be able to comfortably walk/jog one mile or more, without stopping, at this pace:
Archery	20 min./mile
Badminton – social	17 min./mile
– competitive	12 min./mile
Basketball	12 min./mile
Bowling	20 min./mile
Canoeing – leisurely	20 min./mile
– 4 mph	15 min./mile
Cycling – 8 mph	20 min./mile
– 10 mph	15. min./mile
– 12 mph	12 min./mile
– 15 mph	10 min./mile
Gardening – raking	30 min./mile
– weeding	20 min./mile
– digging	12 min./mile
Golf – using power cart	25 min./mile
– pulling a club cart	20 min./mile
— carrying clubs	15 min./mile
Handball	11 min./mile
Field hockey	12 min./mile
Horseback riding – walking	25 min./mile
– trotting	14 min./mile
– galloping	12 min.mile

Judo	8 min./mile
Skating – leisurely	15 min./mile
– quickly	12 min./mile
Skiing – cross country (very leisurely)	14 min./mile
– cross country (4 mph)	12 min./mile
– cross country (5 mph)	10 min./mile
– cross country (8 mph)	7 min./mile
– downhill (easily)	14 min./mile
– downhill (vigorously)	12 min./mile
Snowshoeing	10 min./mile
Soccer	20 min./mile to 10 min./mile (depending) on position and level of play)
Squash	12 min./mile to 7 min./mile
Swimming (50 yds./min.) all strokes except:	10 min./mile
– butterfly	9 min./mile
– sidestroke	11 min./mile)
Tennis – doubles	16 min./mile
— singles	12 min./mile

	Height (no shoes)	MALE Weight (indoor clothing)		FEMALE Weight (indoor clothing)	
(in.)	(cm)	(lbs.)	(kg.)	(lbs.)	(kg.)
60	(152)	—	—	110	50
61	(155)	124	56.2	113	51.3
62	(157)	127	57.6	116	52.6
63	(160)	130	59.0	120	54.4
64	(163)	133	60.3	123	55.8
64.5	(164)	135	61.2	125.5	56.9
65.0	(165)	137	62.1	128	58.1
65.5	(166)	139	63.1	130	59.0
66.0	(168)	141	64.0	132	59.9
66.5	(169)	143	64.9	134	60.8
67.0	(170)	145	65.8	136	61.7
67.5	(171)	147	66.7	138	62.6
68.0	(173)	149	67.6	140	63.5
68.5	(174)	151	68.5	142	64.4
69.0	(175)	153	69.4	144	65.3
69.5	(177)	155	70.3	146	66.2
70.0	(178)	157	71.2	148	67.1
70.5	(179)	159.6	72.4	150	68.0
71.0	(180)	162	73.5	152	68.9
71.5	(182)	164.7	74.7	—	—
72.0	(183)	167	75.8	—	—
72.5	(184)	169	76.7	—	—
73.0	(185)	171	77.6	—	—
73.5	(187)	173.5	78.7	—	—
74	(188)	176	79.8	—	—
75	(191)	181	82.1	—	—
76	(193)	186	84.5	—	—

**Average "Ideal" Weights in Relation to Height and Sex for Persons
of Medium Build**

(Based on Data of Society of Actuaries, 1959, as modified by Shephard, 1972)

LOW ANIMAL FAT, CHOLESTEROL DIET

Allowed	Avoid
Skim or 2% milk (evaporated milk and yogurt) Cottage cheese, processed skim milk cheese Three egg yolks per week including those used in cooking; egg whites as desired; commercial egg substitutes without egg yolk	Whole milk, ice cream All cheeses except cottage cheese and processed skim milk cheese Egg yolks in excess of two per week Desserts made with cream or whole milk; frozen cream pies; commercially prepared pies, cakes, cookies Candies made with butter chocolate, cream, egg yolk or coconut; butter icings Dairy cream substitutes made with coconut oil or palm oil
Lean meat (trim all visible fat); chicken, turkey (with skin removed); wild game; fish; shellfish (except shrimp)	Heavily marbled and fatty meats; mutton; side bacon; spareribs; sausages, wieners; luncheon meats such as salami, bologna, etc.; duck, goose; shrimp; organ meats, e.g. liver, kidneys, brain, sweetbreads, tongue, etc.
Bread — whole wheat, rye, white, French, Italian, pumpernickel, and bran; muffins, quick breads, and pancakes using vegetable oil (without eggs); hot and cold cereals; rice; pasta (without eggs)	Egg and cheese bread; croissants; commercial cakes, doughnuts, quick breads, sweet rolls and other baked goods including mixes; party crackers; cereals containing coconut or coconut oil; egg noodles; premixed crumb coating for meat
All fruits and vegetables (may be cooked in vegetable oil)	Commercial vegetables packaged with sauces or butter
Clear broth, bouillon, consomme; commercial soups other than cream soups; homemade regular and cream soups (made with skim or 2% milk)	Commercial cream soups
Corn, safflower, and sunflower seed oil; specially labelled "soft" margarines (partially "hydrogenated" vegetable oil*); nuts such as almonds, Brazil nuts, peanuts, pecans, sesame seeds, sunflower seeds, and walnuts are allowed in moderation; peanut oil and olive oil may be used occasionally for flavouring	Butter, all "hard" margarines ("hydrogenated" vegetable oil), shortenings, lard; coconut and coconut oil; products containing coconut oil, palm oil and palm kernel oil; cashews and macadamia nuts; chocolate
Dairy cream substitutes made with soybean oil	

*N.B. Choose margarine with a polyunsaturated fat ratio of at least 2:1 (e.g. 35% PFA/18% SFA).

Roughage, e.g. wheat bran, ¼ to ½ cup daily

Reproduced with permission of the Ontario Hospital Association — Ontario Dietetic Association.

Category–Please check your group

Mon. ☐   Tues. ☐   Wed. ☐   Thurs.☐
Home☐   L.D.G.☐   Weight ____(lb. or Kg.)

EXERCISE DIARY
used at the Toronto
Rehabilitation Centre

NAME _____
Present Rx. _____
Resting pulse (average 3 a.m.'s ____

Day	Date (mo./day)	Type of exercise	Distance (miles)	Duration (min./sec.)	Just before exercise	After exercise within 10 sec	Observations of any symptoms during exercise	Remarks
Sun	FEB 8	walk/jog	3	42.15	11	19		
Mon	9	"	3	42.20	10	19		
Tues	10	"	3	42.0	11	18		
Wed	11	"	3	42.0	12	18		felt good
Thur	12	"	2	E	5	T		
Fri	13	"	3	44.10	11	19		
Sat	14	"	2	E	5	T		
Sun	15	"	3	42.0	12	21	Slight tightness in chest	
Mon	16	"	3	41.60	11	21	no problems	
Tues	17	"	3	42.15	11	20	"	
Wed	18	"	3	42.15	11	20	"	
Thur	19	"	3	42.15	11	19		
Fri	20	"	2	E	5	T		
Sat	21	"	2	E	5	T		

References

Abelmann, W.H. Virus and the heart. *Circulation*, 44:950-56, 1971.

Alcoholic Cardiomyopathy. *British Medical Journal*, 731-32, December 28, 1974.

Ammann L., W. Meesman, G. Schley *et al.* Der Einfluss gesteigerten laufband Trainings auf die Entwicklung von Koronarkollateralen und die Mortalitat nach akuter Koronarligatur bei Hunden. *Pfluegers Arch*, 332:R80, 1972.

Anderson, T.W. Serum electrolytes and skeletal mineralization in hard-and-soft-water areas. *Canadian Medical Association Journal*, 107:34-37, 1972.

———, G.H. Beaton, P.N. Corey *et al.* Winter illness and Vitamin C: the effect of relatively low doses. *Canadian Medical Association Journal*, 112:823-26, 1975.

———, W.H. LeRiche. Sudden death from ischemic heart disease in Ontario and its correlation with water hardness and other factors. *Canadian Medical Association Journal*, 105:155-60, 1971.

———, W.H. LeRiche and J.S. Mackay. Sudden death and ischemic heart disease: correlation with hardness of local water supply. *New England Journal of Medicine*, 280:805-807, 1969.

———, L.C. Neri, G.B. Schreiber *et al.* Ischemic heart disease, water hardness and myocardial magnesium. *Canadian Medical Association Journal*, 113:199-203, 1975.

Asmussen, E. Some physiological aspects of fitness for sport and work, in *Proceedings of the Royal Society of Medicine, Symposium No. 11:* "The Meaning of Physical Fitness," 62: November 1969.

Astrand, I, P.-O. Astrand and K. Rodahl. Maximal heart rate during work in older men, *Journal of Applied Physiology*, 14:562-66, 1959.

Astrand, P.-O. and K. Rodahl. Nutrition and Physical Performance, in *Textbook of Work Physiology*. New York: McGraw-Hill, 1970,455-88.

Auerback, O., E.C. Hammond and L. Garfinkel. Smoking in relation to atherosclerosis of the coronary arteries. *New England Journal of Medicine*, 273:775-79,1965.

Balke, B. Biodynamics, in Glasser, ed. *Medical Physics*. Chicago: Yearbook Publishers, 1960, 50-52.

Banister, E.W., and J. Griffiths. Blood levels of adrenergic amines during exercise. *Journal of Applied Physiology*, 33:674,1972.

Barnard, R.J., *et al*. Cardiovascular response to sudden strenuous exercise-heart rate, blood pressure and electrocardiogram. *Journal of Applied Physiology*, 34:833,1973.

Bartlett, R.G. Jr. Physiologic responses during coitus. *Journal of Applied Physiology*, 9:469-72,1956.

Biddulph, L.H. Athletic achievement and the personal and social adjustment of high school boys. *Research Quarterly*, 25(1):1,1954.

Birren, J.E., R.N. Butler, S.W. Greenhouse *et al*. *Human Ageing*. U.S. Dept. of Health, Education and Welfare. Public Health Services, Publication No. 986,1963.

Björntorp, P., K. DeJounge, L. Sjöström *et al*. The effect of physical training on insulin production in obesity. *Metabolism*, 19, 631-38, 1970.

Blackburn, H., H.L. Taylor, N. Okamoto *et al*. Standardization of the exercise electrocardiogram. A systematic comparison of chest lead configurations employed for monitoring during exercise, in *Physical Activity and the Heart*. M.J. Karvonen and A.J. Barry, eds. Springfield: Thomas, 1967,101-33.

Blankenhorn, D. Evidence for regression-progression of atherosclerosis. Presented at the Ontario Heart Foundation International Symposium on Atherosclerosis, September 1, 1975.

Blighton, P.H., and P.R. Richards. Cardiovascular disease in air travellers. *British Heart Journal*, 30:367-72,1968.

Booth, E.G. Personality traits of athletes as measured by the MMPI. *Research Quarterly*, 29(1):27,1958.

Borg, G. Subjective effort in relation to physical performance and working capacity, in *Psychology: From Research to Practice*. H.L. Pick, *et al.*, eds. New York: Plenum Publishing Corporation, 1978, 333-61.

Bortz, W.M.II, P. Angwin, J. Mefford *et al*. Catecholamines, dopamine, and endorphin levels during extreme exercise. *New England Journal of Medicine*, 305:466-67,1981.

Bowerman, W.J., and W.E. Harris. *Jogging*. New York: Grosset & Dunlap, 1967.

Boyer, J.L., and F.W. Kasch. Exercise Therapy in Hypertensive Men. *Journal of the American Medical Association (JAMA)*, 211:1668-71,1970.

Bruce, R.A. Prevention and control of cardiovascular complications, in *Exercise Testing and Exercise Training in Coronary Heart Disease.* J.P. Naughton and H.K. Hellerstein, eds. New York: Academic Press, 1973,355-63.

———, T.R. Hornsten, and J.R. Blackmon. Myocardial infarction after normal responses to maximal exercise. *Circulation,* 38:552-58,1968.

———, A.R. Lind, D. Franklin *et al.* The effects of digoxin on fatiguing static and dynamic exercise in man. *Clinical Science,* 34:29-42,1968.

Bruche, H. Energy expenditure of obese children. *American Journal of Disease of Children,* 60(5):1082,November 1940.

Brunner, D., and G. Manelis. Myocardial infarction among members of communal settlements in Israel. *Lancet,* 2:1049-51,1960.

———, G. Manelis, and S. Altman. Physical activity, lipoproteins and ischemic heart disease. *Pathologia Microbiologia,* 30:648-52,1967.

———, and N. Meshulam. Prevention of recurrent myocardial infarction by physical exercise. *Israel Journal of Medical Sciences,* 5(4):783-85,1969.

Bucher, C.A. Health, physical education, and academic achievements. *National Education Association Journal,* 54:38-40,1965.

Burkitt, D.P. Some diseases characteristic of modern western civilization. *British Medical Journal,* 1:274-78,1973.

Carlson, L.A., and F. Mossfeldt. Acute effects of prolonged, heavy exercise on the concentration of plasma lipids and lipoproteins in man. *Acta Physiologica Scandinavica,* 62:51-59,1964.

Carlsten, A., and G. Grimby. *The Circulatory Response to Muscular Exercise in Man.* Springfield:Thomas,1966.

Carr, D.B., B.A. Bullen, G.S. Skrinar *et al.* Physical conditioning facilitates the exercise-induced secretion of beta-endorphin and beta-lipo-tropin in women. *New England Journal of Medicine,* 305:560-63, 1981.

Carruthers, M., and P. Taggart. Paelocardiology and neocardiology. *American Heart Journal,* 48:1-6,1974.

Cash, J.D. A new approach to studies of the fibrinolytic system in man. *American Heart Journal,* 75:424,1968.

CASS Principal Investigators and their Associates: Coronary Artery Surgery Study (CASS). A randomized trial of coronary artery bypass surgery — Survival data. *Circulation,* 68(5):939-50,1983.

Cassel, J.C. Summary of major findings of the Evans County cardiovascular studies. *Archives of Internal Medicine,* 128:887-89,1971.

Chapman, J.M., L.S. Georke, W. Dixon *et al.* The clinical status of a population group in Los Angeles under observation for two to three years. *American Journal of Public Health,* 47:33-42,1957.

Choquette, G., and R.J. Ferguson. Blood pressure reduction in "borderline" hypertensives following physical training. *Canadian Medical Association Journal,* 108:699-703,1973.

Clausen, J.P. Circulatory adjustments to dynamic exercise and effect of physical training in normal subjects and in patients with coronary artery disease. *Progress in Cardiovascular Disease,* 18:459-95,1975.

————, Effect of physical training on cardiovascular adjustments to exercise in man. *Physiological Reviews,* 57:779-815,1977.

Clawson, B.J., and E.T. Bell. Incidence of fatal coronary disease in nondiabetic and in diabetic persons. *Archives of Pathology,* (Chicago), 48:105-106,1949.

Cobb, L.A., R.S. Baum, H. Alvarez *et al.* Resuscitation from out-of-hospital ventricular fibrillation: 4 years follow-up. *Circulation,* 52(Suppl.III):223-28,1975.

Cohen, M., and C. Goldberg. Effect of physical exercise on alimentary lipaemia. *British Medical Journal,* 2:509-11,1970.

Cooper, K.H. Effects of cigarette smoking on endurance performance. *JAMA,* 203:189,1968.

————, *The New Aerobics.* New York:Bantam Books,1970.

Coronary Drug Project Research Group. *JAMA,* 231:360,1975.

Corrigan, J.J., and F.I. Marcus. Coagulopathy associated with vitamin E ingestion. *JAMA,* 230(9):1300-3,1974.

Costill, D.L. Metabolic responses during distance running. *Journal of Applied Physiology,* 28(3):251-55,1970.

————. Physiology of Marathon Running. *JAMA,* 221(9):1024-29,1972.

————. R. Bowers and W.F. Kammer. Skinfold estimates of body fat among marathon runners. *Medicine and Science in Sports,* 2(2):93-95, Summer 1970.

————, and E. Fox. Energetics of marathon running. *Medicine and Science in Sports,* 1(2):81-86,1969.

————,W.F. Kammer, and A. Fisher. Fluid ingestion during distance running. *Archives of Environmental Health,,* 21:520-25,1970.

Council on Scientific Affairs, American Medical Association: Physician-Supervised Exercise Programs in Rehabilitation of Patients With Coronary Heart Disease. *JAMA,* 245:1463-66,1981.

Cowie, J., R.W. Sillett, and K.P. Ball. Carbon-monoxide absorption by cigarette smokers who change to smoking cigars. *Lancet,* 1:1033-35, 1973.

Daly, L.E., R. Mulcahy, I. Graham *et al.* Long term effect on mortality of stopping smoking after unstable angina and myocardial infarction. *British Medical Journal,* 287:324-26,1983.

Davis, R. Stress and hemostatic mechanism, in *Stress and the Heart,* R.S. Eliot, ed. New York: Futura Publishing, 1974,97-122.

Dawber, T.R., W.B. Kannel, N. Revotskie *et al.* The epidemiology of coronary heart disease — The Framingham Enquiry. *Proceedings of the Royal Society of Medicine,* 55:265-71,1962.

Dayton, S., M.L. Pearce, S. Hashimoto *et al*. A controlled clinical trial of a diet high in unsaturated fat in preventing complications of atherosclerosis. *Circulation*, 39-40(Suppl.2):1-63,1969.

DeMaria, A.N., A. Neumann, G. Lee *et al*. Alterations in ventricular mass and performance induced by exercise training in man evaluated by echocardiography. *Circulation*, 57:237-44,1978.

Detry, J.R., M. Rousseau, G. Vandenbroucke *et al*. Increased arteriovenous oxygen difference after physical training in coronary heart disease. *Circulation*, 64:109-18,1971.

Dill, D.B. Marathoner DeMar: Physiological studies. *Journal of the National Cancer Institute*, 35:185-91,1965.

——, Oxygen used in horizontal and grade walking and running on the treadmill. *Journal of Applied Physiology*, 20(1):19-22,1965.

Doan, A.E., D.R. Peterson, J.R. Blackmon *et al*. Myocardial ischemia after maximal exercise in healthy men: A method for detecting potential coronary heart disease? *American Heart Journal*, 69:11-21,1965.

Doll, R., and A.B. Hill. Mortality in relation to smoking: Ten years' observations of British doctors. *British Medical Journal*, 1:1399-410,1964.

Duguid, J.D. *The Dynamics of Atherosclerosis*. Aberdeen: Aberdeen University Press, 1976.

Eckstein, R.W. Effect of exercise and coronary artery narrowing on coronary collateral circulation. *Circulation Research*, 5:230-35,1957.

Eden, D., A. Shiron, J.J. Kellerman *et al*. Stress, anxiety, and coronary risk in a supportive society, in *Stress and Anxiety*, C.D. Spielberger and I.G. Sarason, eds. New York: Hemisphere Publishing, 1977, 251.

Ehsani, A.A., J.M. Hagberg, and R.C. Hickson. Rapid changes in left ventricular dimensions and mass in response to physical conditioning and deconditioning. *American Journal of Cardiology*, 42:52-56,1978.

——, W.H. Moslin, G.W. Heath, *et al*. Cardiac effects of prolonged and intense exercise training in patients with coronary artery disease. *American Journal of Cardiology*, 50:246-53,1982.

Elisberg, E.I. Heart rate response to the valsalva maneuver as a test of circulatory integrity. *JAMA*, 186(3):120-25,1963.

Ellestad, M.H., and M.K.C. Wan. Predictive implications of stress testing: Follow-up of 2,700 subjects after maximum treadmill stress testing. *Circulation*, 51:362-69,1975.

Engel, H.J., H.L. Page Jr., and W.B. Campbell. Coronary artery disease in young women. *JAMA*, 230:1531-34,1974.

Enos, W.F., J.C. Beyer, and R.H. Holmes. Pathogenesis of coronary disease in American soldiers killed in Korea. *JAMA*, 158(11):912-14,1955.

Fodor, J., G. Lamm *et al.* A co-operative trial in the primary prevention of ischaemic heart disease using clofibrate. *British Heart Journal,* 40:1069,1978.

Fox, S.M., and W.L. Haskell. Physical activity and health maintenance. *Journal of Rehabilitation,* 32:89,1966.

Frick, M.H. Coronary implications of hemodynamic changes caused by physical training. *American Journal of Cardiology,* 22:417-25,1968.

———. Significance of Bradycardia in relation to physical training, in *Physical Activity and the Heart.* M.J. Karvonen and A.J. Barry, eds. Springfield: Thomas, 1967,33-39

———, and M. Katila. Hemodynamic consequences of physical training after myocardial infarction. *Circulation,* 37:192-202,1968.

———, M. Katila, and A.-L. Sjögren. Cardiac function and physical training after myocardial infarction, in *Coronary Heart Disease and Physical Fitness,* O.A. Larsen and R.O. Malmborg, eds. Baltimore: University Park Press,1971,43-47.

Friedman, M., and R.H. Rosenman. *Type A Behavior and Your Heart.* Greenwich Ct: Fawcett Publications, 1974.

Gertler, M.M., and W.P. White. *Coronary Heart Disease in Young Adults. A Multidisciplinary Study.* Cambridge, Mass: Harvard University Press, 1954.

Gordon, T., W.P. Castelli, and M.C. Hjortland. High density lipoprotein as a protective factor against coronary heart disease — The Framingham Study. *American Journal of Medicine,* 62:707-14,1977.

Gottheiner, V. Long-range strenuous sports training for cardiac reconditioning and rehabilitation. *American Journal of Cardiology,* 22:426-35, 1968

Hall, V.E. The relation of heart rate to exercise fitness: an attempt at physiological interpretation of the bradycardia of training. *Pediatrics,* 32(PartII):723-29,1963.

Hames, C.G. Evans County cardiovascular and cerebrovascular epidemiologic study: Introduction. *Archives of Internal Medicine,* 128:883-86,1971.

Hammond E.C., and D. Horn. Smoking and Death Rates — Report on forty-four months of follow-up of 187,783 Men. *JAMA,* 251:2840-53,1984.

———. Smoking in relation to the death rates in one million men and women, in *Epidemiological approaches to the study of cancer and other diseases,* W. Haenszel, ed. Bethesda, Md: U.S. Public Health Service National Cancer Institute, Monograph No.19:127-204,1966.

Harger, B.S., J.B. Miller, and J.C. Thomas. The caloric cost of running. *JAMA,* 228(4):482-83,1974.

Haskell, W. Cardiovascular complications during exercise training of cardiac patients. *Circulation,* 57(5):920-24,1978.

Hattenhauer, M., and W.A. Neill. The effect of cold air inhalation on angina pectoris and myocardial oxygen supply. *Circulation,* 51:1053-58,1975.

Hellerstein, H.K. The effects of physical activity: Patients and normal coronary prone subjects. *Minnesota Medicine,* 52:1335-41,1969.

———, and E.H. Friedman. Sexual activity and the postcoronary patient. *Archives of Internal Medicine,* 125:987-99,1970.

———, T.R. Hornsten, A. Goldbarg *et al.* The influence of active conditioning upon subjects with coronary artery disease: Cardiorespiratory changes during training in 67 patients. *Canadian Medical Association Journal,* 96:758-60,1967.

Herbert, V.H., and E. Jacob. Destruction of Vitamin B_{12} by ascorbic acid. *JAMA,* 230:241-42,1974.

Hill, A.V. The air-resistance to a runner, in *Proceedings of the Royal Society,* London, Series B, 102:380-85,1928.

Hindman, M.C., and A.G. Wallace. Radionuclide exercise studies, in *Physical Conditioning and Cardiovascular Rehabilitation,* L.S. Cohen, M.B. Mock, and I. Ringqvist, eds. New York: John Wiley, 33-46,1981.

Hinkle, L.E.,Jr., S.T. Carver, and A. Plakun. Slow heart rates and increased risk of cardiac death in middle-aged men. *Archives of Internal Medicine,* 129:732-48,1972.

———, L.H. Whitney, E.W. Lehman, *et al.* Occupation, education, and coronary heart disease. *Science,* 161:238-46,1968.

Hirsh, P.D., L.D. Hillis, W.B. Campbell *et al.* Release of prostaglandins and thromboxane into the coronary circulation in patients with ischemic heart disease. *New England Journal of Medicine,* 304:684-91, 1981.

Hjermann, I., K.V. Byre, I. Holme *et al.* Effect of diet and smoking intervention of incidence of coronary heart disease: Report from the Oslo Study Group of a randomized trial in healthy men. *Lancet,* 2:1303-10,1981.

Holmgren, A., and T. Strandell. The relationship between heart volume, total hemoglobin and physical working capacity in former athletes. *Acta Medic Scandinavica,* 163:149-60,1959.

Horwitz, L.D. Alcohol and heart disease. *JAMA,* 232(9):1975.

Iatridis, S.G., and J.H. Ferguson. Effect of physical exercise on blood clotting and fibrinolysis. *Journal of Applied Physiology,* 18:337,1963.

Issekutz, B.,Jr., J.J. Blizzard, N.C. Birkhead *et al.* Effect of prolonged bed rest on urinary calcium output. *Journal of Applied Physiology,* 21: 1013-20,1966.

Jenkins, C.D., R.H. Rosenman, and M. Friedman. Development of an objective psychological test for the determination of the coronary-prone behaviour pattern in employed men. *Journal of Chronic Diseases*, 20:371-79,1967.

Jokl, E., and L. Melzer. Acute fatal non-traumatic collapse during work and sport, in *Exercise and Cardiac Death*, E. Jokl, and J.T. McLellan, eds. *Medicine and Sport*, Vol. 5. Switzerland:Karger,Basel, 1971,5-18.

Joslin, E.P., M. Root, P. White *et al*. *Treatment of Diabetes Mellitus*. Philadelphia: Lea and Febiger, 1959.

Kahn, H.A. The Relationship of reported coronary heart disease mortality to physical activity of work. *American Journal of Public Health*, 53: 1058-67,1963.

Kannel, W.B., T.R. Dawber, and P.M. McNamara. Detection of the coronary-prone adult: The Framingham Study. *Journal of the Iowa Medical Society*, 56(1):26-34,1966.

Karpannen, H., and P.J. Neuvonen. Ischaemic heart-disease and soil magnesium in Finland. *Lancet*, December 15,1973.

Karvonen, M.H., E. Kentala, and O. Mustala. The effects of training on heart rates: A "longitudinal" study. *Annales Medecine Experamentalis et biological fenniae*, 35:307-15,1957.

Katila M., and M.H. Frick. A two-year circulatory follow-up of physical training after myocardial infarction. *Acta Medica Scandinavica*, 187:95-100,1970.

Kavanagh, T. A cold-weather "jogging mask" for angina patients. *Canadian Medical Association Journal*, 103:1290-91,1970.

———. A conditioning programme for the elderly. *Canadian Family Physician*, July 1971.

———. Dehydration of athletics. *Canadian Physiotherapy Association Sports Medicine Newsletter*, 3:14-23,1978.

———. Distance running and cardiac rehabilitation: Physiologic and psychosocial considerations, in *Clinics in Sports Medicine*. Vol. 3. Philadelphia: W.B. Saunders Company, 1984,513-26.

———. Evidence to date for the beneficial effect of exercise following myocardial infarction, in *Controversies in Cardiac Rehabilitation*, P. Mathes and M.I. Halhuber, eds. Berlin: Springer-Verlag,1982,43-52.

———. Exercise and coronary artery disease, in *Therapeutic Exercise*, 4th Edition. J.V. Basmajian, ed. Baltimore, Ma: Williams & Wilkins, 1984,565-86.

———. General deconditioning, in *Medical Rehabilitation*. J.V. Basmajian, and R.L. Kirby, eds. Baltimore, Ma: Williams & Wilkins,1984,237-45.

———. Guidelines for cold weather exercise. *Journal of Cardiac Rehabilitation*, 3:70-73,1983.

———. Running away from heart disease. *Runner's World*, 18:50-53,74, 76,1983.

———. Exercise and the heart. *Annals, Academy of Medicine, Singapore, Rehabilitation Medicine*, 12:331-37,1983.

———. Exercise prescription. *Annals, Academy of Medicine, Singapore, Rehabilitation Medicine*, 12:434-37,1983.

———. The Toronto Rehabilitation Centre's cardiac exercise program. *Journal of Cardiac Rehabilitation*, 2:496-502,1982.

———. Intervention studies in Canada: primary and secondary prevention, in *Heart Disease and Rehabilitation*, M.L. Pollock and D.H. Schmidt, eds. Boston: Houghton Mifflin,1979,317-29.

———. Exercise training in post-coronary rehabilitation, in *Proceedings of the International Conference on Prevention of Heart Disease & Cardiac Rehabilitation*, sponsored by Society for Prevention of Heart Disease and Rehabilitation (SPHERE). C.V. Shah, and K.G. Nair, eds. Kemp's Corner, Bombay, India House No. 2, 1982,128-35.

———. and T. Noakes. Exercise prescription after MI: An approach and a philosophy, in *The South African Textbook of Sports Medicine*, I. Cohen, G. Beaton and D. Mitchell, eds. Sports Medicine Clinic, Johannesburg, 1979, 153-62.

———, and R.J. Shephard. Age and response to coronary rehabilitation. *Medicine in Science and Sports*, Vol. 3C,1971.

———, and R.J. Shephard. Testing the hypothesis that exercise is of benefit, in the rehabilitation of the post-coronary patient, in *Sport in the Modern World, Proceedings of Scientific Congress*, Munich,1972, 251.

———, and R.J. Shephard. The effects of continued training on the aging process, in *The Marathon: Physiological, Medical, Epidemiological and Psychological Studies — Annals of the New York Academy of Science*, 1977, 301:656-70.

———, and R.J. Shephard. Fluid and mineral needs of post-coronary distance runners, in *Sports Medicine (The International Congress of Physical Activity, Quebec City, 1976)*. F. Landry and W.A.R. Orban, eds. Miami, Fl: Symposia Specialists, 1978,143-52.

———, and R.J. Shephard. Conditioning of post-coronary patients: comparison of continuous and interval training. *Archives of Physical Medicine and Rehabilitation*, 57:72-76,1975.

———, and R.J. Shephard. Depression after myocardial infarction. *Canadian Medical Association Journal*, 113:23-27,1975.

———, and R.J. Shephard. On the choice of fluid for hydration of middle-aged marathon runners. *British Association of Sport and Medicine*, 2:26-35,1977.

———, and R.J. Shephard. Fluid and mineral needs of post-coronary distance runners, in *Sports Medicine*. Landry and Orban, eds. Miami, Fl: Symposia Specialists,1978, 143-51.

———, and R.J. Shephard. The immediate antecedents of myocardial infarction in active men. *Canadian Medical Association Journal*, 109: 19-22, 1973.

———, and R.J. Shephard. Importance of physical activity in post-coronary rehabilitation. *American Journal of Physical Medicine*, 52:304-13,1974.

———, and R.J. Shephard. Maintenance of hydration in post-coronary marathon runners. *British Journal of Sports Medicine*, 9:130-34,1975.

———, and R.J. Shephard. Maximum exercise tests on "postcoronary" patients. *Journal of Applied Physiology*, 40:611-18,1976.

———, and R.J. Shephard. Physical exercise and post-coronary rehabilitation. *Canadian Family Physician*, 121-128, September 1975.

———, and R.J. Shephard. Sexual activity after myocardial infarction. *Canadian Medical Association Journal*, 116:1250-53,1977.

———, and R.J. Shephard. Exercise for postcoronary patients: An assessment of infrequent supervision. *Archives of Physical Medicine & Rehabilitation*, 61:114-18,1980.

———, R.J. Shephard, A. Chisholm *et al.* Prognostic indexes for patients with ischemic heart disease enrolled in an exercise-centered rehabilitation program. *American Journal of Cardiology*, 44:1230-40,1979.

———, R.J. Shephard, H. Doney *et al.* Intensive exercise in coronary rehabilitation. *Medicine and Science in Sports*, 5:34-39,1973.

———, R.J. Shephard, and J. Kennedy. Characteristics of postcoronary marathon runners. *Annals of the New York Academy of Science, 301:* 455-65,1977.

———, R.J. Shephard, L.J. Lindley *et al.* Influence of exercise and lifestyle variables upon high density lipoprotein cholesterol after myocardial infarction. *Arteriosclerosis*, 3:249-59,1983.

———, R.J. Shephard, and V. Pandit. Marathon running after myocardial infarction. *JAMA*, 229(12):1602-1605,1974.

———,R.J. Shephard, J.A. Tuck *et al.* Depression following myocardial infarction: the effects of distance running. *Annals of the New York Academy of Sciences*, 301:1029-38,1977.

Kershbaum, A., S. Bellet, J. Jimenez *et al.* Differences in effects of cigar and cigarette smoking on free fatty acid mobilization and catecholamine excretion. *JAMA*, 195(13):117-20,1966.

Keys, A. Coronary heart disease in seven countries. *Circulation*, 1(Suppl): 41-42,1970.

———. Sucrose in the diet and coronary heart disease. *Atherosclerosis*, 14:193,1971.

Knochel, J.P. Environmental heat illness: An eclectic review. *Archives of Internal Medicine*, 133:841-64,1974.

Knox, E.G. Ischaemic-heart-disease mortality and dietary intake of calcium. *Lancet*, pp.1465-67,1973.

Kostrubala, T. Slow long-distance running as form of psychotherapy. Paper delivered at the Third Annual Honolulu Symposium on the Athletic Heart. *American Medical Joggers Association*, December 12, 1975.

Kozlowski, S., and B. Saltin. Effect of sweat loss on body fluids. *Journal of Applied Physiology*, 19:1119-24,1964.

Kramsch, D.M., A.J. Aspen, and B.M. Abramovitz. Reduction of coronary atherosclerosis by moderate conditioning exercise in monkeys on an atherogenic diet. *New England Journal of Medicine*, 305:1483-89,1981.

Larsson, Y.A.A., G.C.G. Sterky, Ekengren, *et al*. Physical fitness and the influence of training in diabetic adolescent girls. *Diabetes*, 11(2): 109-17,1962.

Leaf, A. "Every day is a gift when you are over 100." *National Geographic*, 143(1):93-118,1973.

Levy, R.I. Progress towards prevention of cardiovascular disease: A 30-year retrospective. *Circulation*, 60(1):1555-58,1979.

Lipid Research Clinics Program. The Lipid Research Clinic Coronary primary prevention trial results. I. Reduction in incidence of Coronary Heart Disease. *JAMA*, 251:351-64,1984.

Lopez, S.A., R. Vial, L. Balart *et al*. Effect of exercise and physical fitness on serum lipids and lipoproteins. *Atherosclerosis*, 20:1-9,1974.

Lord Moran. *Winston Churchill*, London:Constable,1966.

Mann, G.V., R.D. Shaffer, R.S. Anderson *et al*. Cardiovascular disease in the Masai. *Journal of Atherosclerosis Research*, 4:289-312,1964.

Mann, J.I., and W.H. Inman. Myocardial infarction in young women with special reference to oral contraceptive practice. *British Medical Journal*, 2(5965):241-45,1975.

——, M. Thorogood, W.E. Waters *et al*. Oral contraceptives and myocardial infarction in young women: a further report. *British Medical Journal*, 3(5984):605-60,1975.

Marble, A. Coronary artery disease in the diabetic. *Diabetes*, 4:290-97,1955.

Marcus, A.J. Aspirin as an antithrombotic medication. *New England Journal of Medicine*, 309:1515-16,1983.

Markoff, R.A., P. Ryan, and T. Young. Endorphins and mood changes in long-distance running. *Medicine and Science in Sports and Exercise*, 14:11-15,1982.

Mason, J.K. Asymptomatic disease of coronary arteries in young men. *British Medical Journal*, 2:1234-37,1963.

Mayer, J. *Overweight: Causes, cost, and control.* Englewood Cliffs, N.J.: Prentice-Hall,1968.

Mayou. R., A. Foster and B. Williamson. The Psychological and social effects of myocardial infarction on wives. *British Medical Journal,* 1:699-701,1978.

McDonough, J.R., C.G. Hames, S.C. Stulb *et al.* Coronary heart disease among negroes and whites in Evans county, Georgia. *Journal of Chronic Diseases,* 18:443-68,1965.

———, J.R. Kusumi and R.A. Bruce. Variations in maximal oxygen intake with physical activity in middle-aged men. *Circulation,* 41:743-51,1970.

McNamara, J., M. Molot, J. Stremple *et al.* Coronary artery disease in combat casualties in Vietnam. *JAMA,* 216:1185,1971.

Medical News. Inhaled cigar smoke can be particularly hazardous. *JAMA,* 232:1319-20,1975.

Mehta, J. Platelets and prostaglandins in coronary artery disease. *JAMA,* 249:2818-23,1983.

Mellerowicz, H. The effects of training on the heart and circulation, in *The Scientific View of Sport,* D. Grupe, D. Kurz, and J.M. Teipel, eds. Berlin:Springer-Verlag,1972,250-261.

Menon, I.S., F. Burke, and H.A. Dewar. Effect of strenuous and graded exercise on fibrinolytic activity. *Lancet,* 1:700,1967.

Mitrani, Y., H. Karplus and D. Brunner. Coronary atherosclerosis in cases of sudden death; the influence of physical occupational activity on the development of coronary narrowing. *Medicine and Sport,* 4: Physical Activity and Ageing, 241-48. New York:Basel-Kargel,1970.

Morganroth, J., B.J. Maron, W.L. Henry *et al.* Comparative left ventricular dimensions in trained athletes. *Annals of Internal Medicine,* 82(4):521-24,1975.

Morris, J.N. Towards prevention—and health. *Acta Medica Scandinavica,* Suppl.576:13-17,1974.

———, S.P.W. Chave, C. Adam *et al.* Vigorous exercise in leisure-time and the incidence of coronary heart-disease. *Lancet,* 333-37,Feb.17, 1973.

———, J.A. Heady, and P.A.B. Raffle. Physique of London busmen: Epidemiology of uniforms. *Lancet,* 2:569-70,1956.

———, J.A. Heady, P.A.B. Raffle *et al.* Coronary heart-disease and physical activity of work. *Lancet,* 2:1053-57,1953.

Nies, A.S., and D.G. Shand. Clinical pharmacology of Propranolol. *Circulation,* 52(1):6-15,1975.

Nikkilä, E.A., and A. Konttinen. Effects of physical activity on postprandial levels of fats in serum. *Lancet,* 1:1151-54,1962.

Noakes, T.D., L. Higginson, and L.H. Opie. Physical training increases ventricular fibrillation thresholds of isolated rat hearts during normoxia, hypoxia, and regional ischaemia. *Circulation,* 67:24-29,1983.

——, L.H. Opie, A.G. Rose *et al.* Autopsy-proved coronary atherosclerosis in marathon runners. *New England Journal of Medicine,* 301(2): 86-89,1979.

O'Leary, A.N. An assessment of patients' activity, knowledge and anxiety, after aortic-valve replacement. Paper presented at the *Annual Meeting of the Canadian Cardiovascular Association,* Winnipeg, October, 1974.

Paffenbarger, R.S.,Jr., and W.E. Hale. Work activity and coronary heart mortality. *New England Journal of Medicine.* 292(11):545-50,1975.

——, W.E. Hale, R.J. Brand *et al.* Work-energy level, personal characteristics, and fatal heart attack: A birth-cohort effect. *American Journal of Epidemiology,* 105:200-13,1977.

——, M.E. Laughlin, A.S. Gima *et al.* Work activity of longshoremen as related to death from coronary heart disease and stroke. *New England Journal of Medicine,* 282:1109-14,1970.

——, A.L. Wing, and R.T. Hyde. Physical activity as an index of heart attack risk in college alumni. *American Journal of Epidemiology,* 106:161,1978.

Parson, C.J., and W.P. Bobechko. Aeromedical transport: its hidden problems. *Canadian Medical Association Journal,* 126:237-43,1982.

Paterson, D.H., R.J. Shephard, D. Cunningham *et al.* Effects of physical training on cardiovascular function following myocardial infarction. *Journal of Applied Physiology,* 47:482-89,1979.

Pauling, L. *Vitamin C and the common cold.* San Francisco: W.H. Freeman, 1970.

Peffers, A.S.R. Carriage of invalids by air. *J.R. Call Physicians,* London, 12:136-42,1978.

Physical Fitness Research Digest. Series 4, No.3, July 1974. *Circulatory-Respiratory Endurance Improvement.* Published by President's Council on Physical Fitness and Sports.

Pollock, M.L. The quantification of endurance training programmes. *Exercise and Sports Sciences Reviews,* J.H. Wilmore, ed. New York: Academic Press,1973.

——, J. Broida, Z. Kendrick *et al.* Effects of training two days per week at different intensities on middle-aged men. *Medicine and Science in Sports,* 4:192-97,1972.

Pugh, L.G.C.E. Oxygen intake in track and treadmill running with observations on the effect of air resistance. *Journal of Physiology,* 207:823-35,1970.

——, J.L. Corbett, and R.H. Johnson. Rectal temperatures, weight losses, and sweat rates in marathon running. *Journal of Applied Physiology,* 23(3):347-52,1967.

Puranen, J., L. Ala-Ketola, P. Peltokallio *et al.* Running and primary osteo-arthritis of the hip. *British Medical Journal,* 424-25,May 24, 1975.

Raab, W. Training, physical inactivity and the cardiac dynamic cycle. *Journal of Sports Medicine and Physical Fitness*, 6:38,1966.

Rapaport, E. Exercise responses in patients with heart failure or valvular or congenital heart disease. *Journal of the South Carolina Medical Association*, Supplement, 61-64,1969.

Rechnitzer, P.A., H.A. Pickard, A.U. Paivio *et al.* Long-term follow-up study of survival and recurrence rates following myocardial infarction in exercising and control subjects. *Circulation*, 45:853-57,1972.

Redwood, D.R., D.R. Rosing, and S.E. Epstein. Circulatory and symptomatic effects of physical training in patients with coronary-artery disease and angina pectoris. *New England Journal of Medicine*, 286: 959-65,1972.

Report of the Joint Working Party of the Royal College of Physicians of London and the British Cardiac Society on Rehabilitation After Cardiac Illness. *Journal of the Royal College of Physicians of London*, 9:281,1975.

Rhoods, G.G., C.L. Gulbrandsen, and A. Kagan. Serum lipoproteins and coronary heart disease in a population study of Hawaii Japanese men. *New England Journal of Medicine*, 294:293-98,1976.

Richards, P.R. The effects of air travel on passengers with cardiovascular and respiratory disease. *Practitioner*, 210:232-41,1973.

Robb, G.P., and H.H. Marks. Latent coronary artery disease: Determination of its presence and severity by the exercise electrocardiogram. *American Journal of Cardiology*, 603-18, May 1964.

Rose, G. Cardiovascular mortality among American Negroes. *Archives of Environmental Health*, 5:412-14,1962.

Rosenberg, L., D.R. Miller, D.W. Kaufman *et al.* Myocardial infarction in women under 50 years of age. *JAMA*, 250:2801-2806,1983.

Russek, H.I. Emotional stress in the etiology of coronary heart disease. *Geriatrics*, 22:84,1967.

Saltin, B. Circulatory response to submaximal and maximal exercise after thermal dehydration. *Journal of Applied Physiology*, 19:1125-32, 1964.

———, and P.-O. Astrand. Maximal oxygen uptake in athletes. *Journal of Applied Physiology*, 23:353-58,1967.

Sarnoff, S.J., E. Braunwald, G.H. Welch *et al.* Hemodynamic determinants of oxygen consumption of the heart with special reference to the tension-time index. *American Journal of Physiology*, 192:148-56,1958.

Scheur, J., and C.M. Tipton. Cardiovascular adaptations to physical training. *Annual Review of Physiology*, 39:221-51,1977.

Selvester, R.H. Exercise and/or coronary by-pass surgery. Presented at the *International Symposium on Exercise and Coronary Artery Disease*, Toronto, October 1975.

Selye, H. *The Stress of Life*. New York:McGraw-Hill,1956.

Shaper, A.G. Soft water, heart attacks, and stroke. *JAMA*, 230:130-31,1974.

Shephard, R.J. Exercise test methodology, in *Coronary Disease*. Denver. Col:Dept. of Professional Education International Medical Corporation.

———. Intensity, duration, and frequency of exercise as determinants of the response to a training regime. *Internationale Zeitschrift für Angewandte Physiologic Einschliesslich Arbeitsphysiologie*, 32:1973.

———. Standard tests of aerobic power, in *Frontiers of Fitness*. Springfield: Thomas,1971,233-64.

———, P. Corey and T. Kavanagh. Exercise compliance and the prevention of a recurrence of myocardial infarction. *Medicine and Science in Sports and Exercise*, 13(1):1-5,1981.

Siegel, W., G. Blomqvist and J.H. Mitchell. Effects of a quantitated physical training program on middle-aged sedentary men. *Circulation*, 41: 19-29,1970.

Simonelli, G., and R.P. Eaton. Cardiovascular and metabolic effects of exercise. *Postgraduate Medicine*, 63:71,1978.

Slone, D., S. Shapiro, L. Rosenberg *et al*. Relation of cigarette smoking to myocardial infarction in young women. *New England Journal of Medicine*, 298:1273-76,1978.

Snow, C.C. Anthropologic and physiologic observation — Tarahumara endurance runners, in *Symposium on Sports Medicine*, American Academy of Orthopaedic Surgeons. St. Louis: C.V. Mosby Co., 1969,111-17.

Society of Actuaries. *Build and Blood Pressure Study*, Chicago, Ill.,1959.

Sonnenblick, E.H., J. Ross,Jr., and E. Braunwald. Oxygen consumption of the heart: Newer concepts of its multifactoral determination. *American Journal of Cardiology*, 22:328-36,1968.

———, J. Ross, J.W. Covell *et al*. Velocity of contraction as a determinant of myocardial oxygen consumption. *American Journal of Physiology*, 209:919-27,1965.

Stamler, J. Atherosclerotic coronary heart disease. *Connecticutt Medicine*, 28:675-92,1964.

Taggart, P., M. Carruthers, and W. Somerville. Electrocardiograph, plasma catecholamines and lipids and their modification by oxyprenolol when speaking before an audience. *Lancet*, 11,341-46,1973.

———, P. Parkinson, and M. Carruthers. Cardiac responses to thermal, physical, and emotional stress. *British Medical Journal*, 3:71-76,1972.

Taylor, H.L., A. Henschel, J. Brozek *et al*. Effects of Bed Rest on Cardiovascular Function and Work Performance. *Journal of Applied Physiology*, 2(5):223-39,1949.

Taylor, M.L. E. Kepetar A. Keys *et al.* Death rates among physically active and sedentary employees of the railroad industry. *American Journal of Public Health,* 53:1967,1962.

Theorell, T., and R.H. Rahe. Behavior and life satisfactions characteristics of Swedish subjects with myocardial infarction. *Journal of Chronic Diseases,* 25:139-47,1972.

Timmis, G.C., R.C. Ramos, S. Gordon *et al.* The basis for differences in ethanol-induced myocardial depression in normal subjects. *Circulation,* 51:1144-48,1975.

Tooshi, A. Effects of three different durations of endurance training on serum cholesterol, body composition, and other fitness measures. Doctoral Dissertation, University of Illinois, 1970.

Tuttle, W.W., and S.M. Horvath. Comparison of effects of static and dynamic work on blood pressure and heart rate. *Journal of Applied Physiology,* 10:294-95,1957.

Virchow, R.L.K. Die cellularpathologie in ihrer begrundung auf physiologische und pathologische Gewebelehre. Berlin: Hirschwald,1958.

Viruses and the Heart. *British Medical Journal,* No.5958:589,March 15,1975.

von Rokitansky, C. *A Manual of Pathological Anatomy.* London: New Sydenham Society,1852.

Vuori, I., M. Mäkäräinen and A. Jääskeläinen. Sudden death and physical activity. *Cardiology,* 63:287-304,1978.

Weinblatt, E., S. Shapiro, C.W. Frank *et al.* Prognosis of men after first myocardial infarction: mortality and first recurrence in relation to selected parameters. *American Journal of Public Health,* 58:1329-47,1968.

W.H.O., Committee of Principal Investigators: Clofibrate Trial: A cooperative trial in the primary prevention of ischaemic heart disease using clofibrate. *British Medical Journal,* 40:1069-118,1978.

Wright, V., D. Dowson, and A. Unsworth. The lubrication and stiffness of joints, in *Modern Trends in Rheumatology — 2,* A.G.S. Hill, ed. London: Butterworths,1971, 30-45.

Wyndham, C.H., and N.B. Strydom. The danger of an inadequate water intake during marathon running. *South African Medical Journal,* 893-96, July 1969.

Yater, W.M., A.H. Traum, W.G. Brown *et al.* Coronary artery disease in men 18-39 years of age. *American Heart Journal,* 36:334-72,1948.

Yudkin, J. *Sweet and Dangerous.* New York: Bantam Books,1973.

Zukel, W.J., R.H. Lewis, P.E. Enterline *et al.* A short-term community study of the epidemiology of coronary heart disease. *American Journal of Public Health,* 49:1630-39,1959.

Index